Breastfeeding and Media

Katherine A. Foss

Breastfeeding and Media

Exploring Conflicting Discourses That Threaten Public Health

palgrave
macmillan

Katherine A. Foss
School of Journalism
Middle Tennessee State University
Murfreesboro, TN
USA

ISBN 978-3-319-56441-8 ISBN 978-3-319-56442-5 (eBook)
DOI 10.1007/978-3-319-56442-5

Library of Congress Control Number: 2017936641

Printed on acid-free paper

This Palgrave Macmillan imprint is published by Springer Nature
The registered company is Springer International Publishing AG
The registered company address is: Gewerbestrasse 11, 6330 Cham, Switzerland

This book is dedicated to my sister.

Preface

Breastfeeding is intensely personal. It is a decision/commitment/struggle that a mother confronts daily, sometimes hourly, over weeks, months, or even years. Breastfeeding is intensely emotional. It impacts how you sleep, what you wear, how you feel—the nursing relationship is always on your mind. It is as much who you are as what you do. And because of how breastfeeding has been integrally connected to our conceptualizations of motherhood, it is also a touchy subject. Thus, to ask a mother, "Do/did you breastfeed?" is a loaded question, often more sensitive and intrusive than inquiring of one's political stance or religion.

With that in mind, I will state my intentions. My objective here is *not* to make readers of any infant feeding path feel inadequate, guilty, or emotionally troubled. This text is about identifying the cultural and institutional obstacles that impede women who want to breastfeed or do not get to nurse as long as they intended to do so, for the mother who was dissuaded by unhelpful mother-in-laws that deemed it "too hard," discouraging partners, or by well-meaning, ill-informed pediatricians that recommended weaning so that Mom could go on antibiotics. Or, the common situation of a breastfeeding mother who returns to work and discovers that the dedicated pumping space is actually just the women's restroom, her boss frowns upon missing work to pump, or that coworkers keep barging in, interrupting the pumping process. It is also for mothers who have painted their nipples purple with Genetian Violet in an attempt to curb thrush so painful that it brought tears to their eyes at each and every latch. This book is on behalf of any mother who has ever been stared at, ridiculed, or asked to "cover up" while nursing in public or asked "not to breastfeed around Grandpa because he's not used to such things." Or had friends and family exclaim in surprise that "You're *still* nursing?!" We can also celebrate the joy of hitting nursing milestones, milk dribbling down a grinning baby's chin, the first time a child purposely signs "milk," or a partner's amazement that you can feed the baby with your body.

Both struggles and positive experiences are usually ignored in public discourse, overlooked as if they do not matter. Instead the health benefits of the "liquid gold" are divorced from the women who produce it. Yes, breastfeeding is (and needs to be) considered a public health issue, but it is also deeply embedded in constructions of motherhood and womanhood. It is a Feminist issue. It is also an issue for populations beyond expectant and new parents, as culture profoundly influences success. Our understanding of breastfeeding is dervived from personal experience, as well as from mediated influences. At the center of this book is the assumption that media shapes our culture, and with that, our cultural perceptions of infant feeding.

I cannot write a book about breastfeeding without providing my own experience and intersectional position. I am an educated, Caucasian, heterosexual, married woman who had children relatively late (singleton term babies without complications at birth). I breastfed my oldest daughter until she was almost two, when I was well into my second trimester. I nursed my youngest daughter for much longer. On her third birthday, we mutually decided to be done. While I was privileged to have a supportive partner and enough flexibility to express and store milk at work, breastfeeding was not without struggles. I had some latching issues, mastitis with each child, and battled thrush for more than a year. I was fortunate to be set up for success. At the same time, I have witnessed friends whose breastfeeding goals were thwarted by a lack of support or health care providers. I have experienced living in a community in which breastfeeding is not the "norm," and resources are difficult to come by. Just as troublesome, I have observed the tactics of formula companies to derail and undermine breastfeeding rates through free samples, social media advertisements (ads), and complimentary dayplanners distributed at the first prenatal appointment. This book is about the constant negotiation between the various players in breastfeeding success. Through secondary and primary research on media's constructions, I argue that culturally, we have been swimming against a current of cultural resistance to adequately improve breastfeeding experiences and overall rates. How we, as a culture, perceive breastfeeding not only impacts how we treat and support women now, but also influences future generations.

Murfreesboro, USA

Katherine A. Foss

Acknowledgements

I would like to thank Shaun Vigil, Glenn Ramirez, and others at Palgrave Macmillan for publishing this book. It has been a pleasure working with you and a smooth process.

So many people have assisted me in this journey.

My academic study of breastfeeding in media began long before I had a personal interest in this area. As a new Ph.D. student, I took Dr. Brian Southwell's Media and Social Change seminar in 2004 at the University of Minnesota. For the final paper, I searched for a topic that explored shifts in women's roles in society and, ultimately, chose media discourse of infant feeding. It was admittedly not a great paper, but it got me started. The following semester, Dr. Southwell and I did a project that correlated breastfeeding rates with the number of infant feeding ads that appeared over 30 years in *Parents* magazine, which we published in the *International Breastfeeding Journal* in 2006. From there, I analyzed the infant feeding articles in *Parents* magazine (see Chap. 3 for a discussion of this study) and my interest continued to expand to breastfeeding in reality and fictional television, online discourse, and other related topics. I am very grateful to Dr. Southwell for helping me to cultivate and shape this interest, as well as mentoring me through the publication process.

Thank you to Kathy Forde, who helped me develop as a scholar and a writer, and who continues to serve as a mentor and friend. I will also always be grateful to Hazel Dicken-Garcia for her wisdom, guidance, and support.

I also would like to acknowledge the wonderful community of scholars and practitioners that I have gotten to know through the annual Breastfeeding and Feminism International Conference. I am grateful to Paige Hall Smith, Miriam Labbok (who is greatly missed), and Bernice Hausman for this conference and the *Beyond Choice* book. This group has truly been a gift for their amazing and diverse contributions to improving breastfeeding, along with their approachability and support for different kinds of work. I have enjoyed each panel, presentation, and poster and learned so much from discussions at the conferences and afterward.

I appreciate all of people who have answered my questions, provided articles, and helped me develop this manuscript. Thank you to Jackie Wolf for such thoughtful insights and direction. Additional thanks to Spring-Serenity Duvall, Erica Anstey, Deborah McCarter-Spaulding, Jennifer Lucas, Amanda Barnes Cook, Aunchalee Palmquist, Cecelia Tomori, Elizabeth Brooks, Jodine Chase, and Fiona Giles.

Thank you to those who have supported me in the writing process. Tanya Peres Lemons, you are still the best writing partner, even though you are far away. Reyna Gordon, I am glad you went to the La Leche meetings with me and I enjoyed our collaboration. Thank you to my other writing group members: Erin Anfinson, Melissa Lobegeier, and Suzanne Mangrum. I also appreciate Ken Blake's willingness to conduct two experiments with me on media's influence on breastfeeding perceptions.

This book also exists because of my resources and support from those at Middle Tennessee State University. Thank you to Dean Ken Paulson, Associate Dean Zeny Panol, former School of Journalism Director Dwight Brooks, current SoJ Director Greg Pitts, Sanjay Asthana, Jane Marcellus, Tricia Farwell, Jason Reineke, and other colleagues, Kimi Conro for our good "new mother" discussions, students, Denise Cathey, and the rest of the administrative staff.

As I will reiterate throughout this book, breastfeeding is personal and emotional. I am grateful to so many people for sharing their stories with me. Shortly after I began researching breastfeeding as a graduate student, I interviewed my grandmother about her experiences nursing children in the 1940s and 1950s. I will never forget that conversation (or how quickly my grandpa fled the room when he heard the topic). Even though this book is not an oral history project, such narratives influence how I think and write about breastfeeding.

Of course, I would like to thank family members and friends for sharing their experiences, listening to me, and passing along breastfeeding-related media examples. I received many texts from my dear sister, Kristi, about newly-discovered TV episodes that covered breastfeeding. I am grateful to her for so many reasons.

Finally, thank you to my husband, Eric, for supporting me as a breastfeeding mother and for giving me much-needed time to write. Finally, I am so fortunate to have two determined and curious daughters, Nora and Hazel, who gave me the experience to write this book and will help me celebrate when it is finished.

Contents

List of Figures

List of Tables

CHAPTER 1

Breastfeeding and Media

On January 17, 2015, the infant formula corporation Similac released a commercial entitled, "The Mother 'Hood Official Video."[1] This ad showcased the "Mommy Wars," demonstrating the tense polarization of contemporary parents based on parental philosophies and practices. With upbeat background music, the commercial features stereotypes of breast-feeding mothers, stay-at-home dads, bottle-feeders, and cloth diaper users, facing off on the playground until a child, briefly in peril, unites the parents. The video concludes with "No matter what our beliefs, we are parents first. Welcome to the Sisterhood of Motherhood," and fades into a dark screen with the Similac logo. Feedback was overwhelmingly positive, as over eight million people have voluntarily watched this video on *Youtube* and nearly 11 thousand people "liked" it on *Facebook*. The "Mother 'Hood" Similac video was even nominated for "Best Brand Content Campaign of the Year" for the Iris Awards, a ceremony that honors the year's best online parenting materials. News stories praised the video, with headlines such as "Similac Looks to End Mommy Wars Over Breastfeeding" (*Advertising Age*),[2] "This Ad Perfectly Parodies the 'Mommy Wars'" (*Time* magazine),[3] and "A Playful Reminder That Judging Other Parents is Wrong" (*The Huffington Post*).[4] Surprisingly, few people objected to its sneaky marketing tactic, dismissing or ignoring the fact that this video was obviously marketing commercial formula. With each "like" and "share," viewers willingly promoted formula, reinforcing bottle-feeding as a "normal" way to feed a baby. Media messages like this one obfuscate efforts to increase breastfeeding, suggesting that

K.A. Foss, *Breastfeeding and Media*,
DOI 10.1007/978-3-319-56442-5_1

to breastfeed (or especially to talk about breastfeeding) is to criticize other mothers, making it particularly difficult to celebrate success and to move toward the normalization of breastfeeding.

Contrary to the anti-breastfeeding discourse of the "Mommy Wars," it has been well-established that breastfeeding is best for babies, for mothers, and for the health of the American people. And yet, even with widespread recognition of breastfeeding's benefits and national efforts to improve duration rates, a disparity still exists between the number of women who initiate breastfeeding and the percentage of women who succeed overall. In other words, many women are not achieving their own breastfeeding goals and expectations. Gregory and colleagues noted that only 39.2% of the 1501 women surveyed had met their prenatal breastfeeding expectations at 2 months postpartum.[5] A study by Odom and colleagues found that as many as 60% of the women surveyed stopped breastfeeding sooner than planned.[6]

Why are mothers falling short of their goals? While the phrase "Breast is best" is accurate, it is also dripping with insinuation of a mother's inferiority and attributions of blame for not breastfeeding. Women who quit breastfeeding prematurely have reported feelings of shame and guilt for early weaning. As Dr. Miriam Labbok explained, responsibility, and the subsequent guilt for "failure," has been displaced onto individual women, who feel responsible for not breastfeeding, despite extensive research demonstrating that breastfeeding success rests on a complex intersection of factors, many of which are institutional and cultural.[7] This focus on individual responsibility for breastfeeding reflects the tradition of individualism as an American value. In the United States, we love to blame people, not organizations, businesses, fractured systems, or institutions. With breastfeeding, this spotlight on the individual means that we as a society ignore the social, economic, and political forces that impact breastfeeding success, and instead shape nursing as a choice, as individual action, as one woman's mothering assignment. Therefore, when these cultural forces fail the new mother, we hold her responsible.

News and entertainment media have been criticized for impeding breastfeeding success and contributing to this "breastfeeding as choice" myth. A statement released by the American Academy of Pediatrics (AAP) argued that media messages that depict bottle-feeding as "normal" have likely hindered breastfeeding rates.[8] Furthermore, the AAP recommended that media creators should "portray breastfeeding as positive and normative."[9] Historically, media—specifically corporations that marketed breastmilk substitutes—have been perceived as the primary detriment to rebounding breastfeeding rates in the 1970s, especially in developing countries. Concern over high levels of infant mortality for artificially-fed babies prompted international efforts to halt marketing of breastmilk substitutes. In 1981, a joint effort by the World Health Organization (WHO) and the United Nations Children's Fund (UNICEF) led to the creation of the "International Code of Marketing for Breast-milk Substitutes" (the Code) and its adoption by the World Health Assembly (with only the United States delegate opposing it).[10] The Codes contained a series of specific steps to reduce the marketing power of formula companies over consumers, especially those in developing countries.[11] This global objective of improving breastfeeding was reaffirmed with the 1990 WHO/UNICEF "Innocenti Declaration," stating a call to action to enforce the Code, emphasizing the importance of utilizing media in changing cultural norms about infant feeding.[12]

The Code's implementation has had mixed success. A 30 year follow-up found that only 19% of the 199 countries reporting have legislation that enforces all of the Code's recommendations.[13] Furthermore, 65% continue to allow the promotion of breastmilk substitutes.[14] The United States is among the few countries that have taken no action to restrict the marketing and distribution of commercial formula.[15] In "Breastfeeding for Public Health," Labbok articulated that media messages have undermined global efforts to improve breastfeeding by WHO, UNICEF, the U.S. Department for Health, and other organizations.[16] In 2011, the United States Department of Health and Human Services released "The Surgeon General's Call to Action to Support Breastfeeding," which identified media messages about breastfeeding as problematic and advocated for media to be better utilized as a tool to promote breastfeeding, cementing a long recognition that media influences public perception of breastfeeding.[17] So why hasn't the United States implemented legislation to uphold the Code? At the same time, with media's potential as a tool to positively promote breastfeeding, why haven't news and entertainment discourses promoted breastfeeding with the same intensity as pro-immunization or healthy eating campaigns?[18]

This book aims to answer these questions, exploring how breastfeeding has been constructed in American media and the influence of these messages on pregnant women, new mothers, and the general public. I confront the misperception that breastfeeding, and the failure to breastfeed, rests solely on the responsibility of an individual mother—attributions of blame that have also negatively impacted public health approaches to breastfeeding. Using research on media discourses of breastfeeding, I demonstrate that while media channels can and have been used to to help normalize breastfeeding, most mainstream products have provided and continue to provide a narrow definition of the breastfeeding woman, stigmatizing those who do not fit this ideal. Moreover, the marketing tactics of infant formula corporations have continued to undermine positive efforts at normalizing breastfeeding. Collectively, these media messages have contributed to cultural resistance of breastfeeding, at the same time perpetuating blame for women who wean prematurely (often because of institutional or cultural factors).

Establishing Breastfeeding as a Public Health Concern

To truly understand why rates matter, breastfeeding needs to be understood as a key component of public health, not just a mothering choice. International groups and federal agencies that include the Global Health Council, UNICEF, WHO, and the Centers for Disease Control & Prevention (CDC) recognize the importance of breastfeeding for optimal public health, and therefore advocate for its success. In a 2016 *Lancet* article, Rollins and colleagues estimated that worldwide, 823,000 deaths of children under five could be prevented if global breastfeeding goals were met, not to mention approximately 20,000 women's deaths from breast cancer (which is significantly less likely with extended breastfeeding).[19]

Extensive studies have demonstrated that breastmilk profoundly affects mental and physical health. Its immunological properties mean that breastfed babies have far fewer gastrointestinal and respiratory infections requiring hospitalization, fewer skin issues and ear infections.[20] Breastfed babies are significantly less likely to die from diarrhea, pneumonia or Sudden Infant Death Syndrome (SIDS), and have lower rates of mortality overall.[21] In other words, formula-fed children face higher risks of infectious morbidity, otitis media, and hospitalization for respiratory infections.[22] Formula-fed babies are also much more likely to die from Necrotizing Enterocolitis, especially if they are premature.[23] By 12 months, the body composition of formula-fed babies is higher in fat compared to breastfed babies.[24] Long-term, breastfed babies are healthier overall, experiencing fewer dental, vision, and respiratory issues, including asthma and allergies, and are less likely to develop eczema and childhood leukemia.[25] Children who were breastfed also have lower rates of obesity[26] and metabolic disorders.[27] For example, a study of 7798 children in Ireland found that formula-fed children were twice as likely to be obese at age nine than those who were exclusively breastfed for at least 26 weeks.[28] Those who had been breastfed for 13–25 weeks had a reduced risk of obesity of 38%.[29]

Cognitively, breastfed children also outperform their bottle-fed peers, scoring significantly higher on Intelligence Quotient (IQ) tests.[30] Moreover, Quigley and colleagues found that 5 year-olds who were breastfed score higher in pattern construction, vocabulary, and picture similarity.[31] Developmentally, they performed 1–6 months ahead of children who were not breastfed.[32] In another study, 10 year-olds who were breastfed for at least 6 months scored higher on achievement tests for mathematics, reading, spelling, and writing.[33] In this study, breastfeeding duration was especially influential for male children.[34] Breastfeeding can also positively impact long-term mental health. In a 14-year study of a birth cohort, Oddy and colleagues noted that shorter breastfeeding duration was association with higher mental health issues in childhood and adolescence.[35]

Women who breastfeed experience initial and long-term benefits. Breastfeeding reduces blood loss from childbirth and helps to shrink the uterus.[36] Within the first month after giving birth, breastfeeding mothers show higher brain responses (indicating greater maternal sensitivity) to infant cries compared to formula-feeding mothers.[37] Nursing mothers also lose their pregnancy weight faster on average than bottle-feeding women and have lower rates of weight retention between pregnancies, even when race, education, and other factors are considered.[38] Long after weaning, breastfeeding protects mothers, as those who breastfed their children are less likely to develop breast and epithelial cancer, osteoporosis, hip fractures, type 2 diabetes, and issues with high blood pressure later in life.[39] This protection increases with breastfeeding duration.[40]

Because benefits for mother and child increase with duration, the AAP and WHO recommend exclusively breastfeeding babies for at least 6 months and then continuing to nurse, with complementary foods, until at least a year or more.[41] And yet, breastfeeding rates in the United States do not reflect these guidelines. While approximately 81% of American women begin breastfeeding, only 44.4% exclusively nurse their infants to at least 3 months of age, according to the

CDC's 2016 "Breastfeeding Report Card."[42] Fewer mothers make it to at least 6 months or beyond, with only 22.3% exclusively breastfeeding at this point.[43] While the national averages for breastfeeding rates have increased over the past decade, they are still alarmingly low in certain states. For example, in Mississippi, only 52% of women attempt to breastfeed, with 9.3% exclusively nursing at 6 months—a decline from the 2014 Report Card.[44] Breastfeeding rates are also much lower in certain populations than others. Statistically, women who are younger, less educated, single, and of a lower socio-economic class are far less likely to breastfeed than those who are older, educated, and more affluent.[45] Tobacco use and a higher Body Mass Index (BMI) are also negatively correlated with breastfeeding.[46] Racial disparities also exist with breastfeeding rates, as African American women are less likely to breastfeed than those who are Hispanic or Caucasian.[47] It should be noted that these characteristics have been correlated with breastfeeding rates, but are not prescriptive for the group. Certainly African American women, teenage mothers, and other women do breastfeed, but recognizing disparities between groups can help with breastfeeding promotion and intervention efforts.

Low breastfeeding duration rates across groups of women have been recognized as a public health concern. A 2010 article in *Pediatrics* speculated that $13 billion in United States health care costs could be saved each year and more than 900 infant deaths could be prevented if 80–90% of women breastfed for at least 6 months.[48] Furthermore, a 2016 *Lancet* article estimated that $302 billion dollars in gross national income worldwide was lost because of the cognitive impact of short duration rates.[49] With its recognized role in lifelong health, major health initiatives have included increasing breastfeeding rates as a key objective to improving American health. "The Surgeon General's Call to Action to Support Breastfeeding" outlined 20 key components to improving national breastfeeding rates.[50] Furthermore, the U.S. Department of Health also outlined breastfeeding objectives as part of the *Healthy People 2020*, a strategic health promotion and prevention plan.[51]

Legislation to protect nursing women has accompanied the national objectives to raise breastfeeding rates. As of 2015, 49 states specifically protect mothers' rights to nurse in public or private, with 29 states exempting breastfeeding from public indecency laws.[52] In addition, 17 states excuse breastfeeding mothers from jury duty or allow them postpone it. Individual states have other laws to encourage breastfeeding.

Louisiana laws prohibit childcare workers from discriminating against breastfed babies.[53] They also do not tax breastfeeding items. Mississippi requires childcare facilities to provide space for breastfeeding mothers. And in Maryland, all child care centers must have policies and training to promote breastfeeding.[54]

National laws and policies have also been enacted to support breastfeeding for working mothers. In 2010, the Fair Labor Standards Act was amended to require employers to provide time and space to for mothers to pump or nurse.[55] Other components of the Affordable Care Act also support breastfeeding, including insurance coverage of lactation counseling and breast pumps.[56] Unfortunately, while legislation grants breaks and designated spaces for pumping in the first year, not all women work in breastfeeding-friendly environments.[57] Some groups of women have benefitted more than others from the legislation. Smith-Gagen and colleagues determined that laws protecting pumping time at work had a strong positive correlation with breastfeeding duration for Mexican-American women, much more than Caucasians.[58] However, legislation appeared to have less of an effect on African American mothers, suggesting that more research is needed to help carry out the laws to benefit specific groups of women.[59] In other words, a gap exists between legislation and its implementation—just one example of the inequity in breastfeeding access and support.

Predicting Breastfeeding Intention and Success

What creates a successful breastfeeding relationship is difficult, complex, and hard to pinpoint. Individual, institutional, and cultural factors impact if mothers breastfeed (initiation), for how long (duration), and whether or not only breastmilk is given (exclusivity). Breastfeeding knowledge has been shown to dramatically increase initiation and exclusivity.[60] Opinions of alternatives to breastmilk also impact exclusivity, as women who do not view breastfeeding as equal to formula are more likely to exclusively breastfeed.[61] Not surprisingly, intentions matter, as the expectant mother's plan to breastfeed can also help forecast whether or not she will try to breastfeed after birth.[62] Life experience also influences breastfeeding. Histories of violence and abuse can impact breastfeeding and maternal attachment. Abuse survivors are more likely to initiate breastfeeding, yet may face additional obstacles compared to those who have not experienced such trauma.[63] Furthermore, since most prisons do not allow women to breastfeed their babies or to maintain lactation through pumping, incarcerated women also have much lower breastfeeding rates.[64] Obviously, these are factors that correlate with higher breastfeeding rates, not the sole predictors of success.

Fertility, conception, pregnancy, and birth also influence rates. Cromi and colleagues determined that women who used Assistive Reproductive Techniques (ART) had similar initiation rates to those that conceived naturally, yet were more likely to wean by 6 weeks postpartum.[65] Overall, prenatal, birth, and postpartum experiences affect whether or not a woman intends to breastfeed, her success in doing so, and the length of her nursing relationship. When health professionals encourage and support breastfeeding, women are much more likely to succeed.[66] Birth experience also impacts breastfeeding success. Exclusive breastfeeding rates are lower for both elective and scheduled cesarean deliveries, likely due to the challenges in breastfeeding in the operating room after delivery.[67] Breastfeeding rates are lower for babies born prematurely and others who had to spend time in a neonatal intensive care unit.[68] Hospital practices that include policies against routine supplementation, rooming-in and skin-to-skin mother-infant contact immediately after birth also yield higher breastfeeding rates.[69] In addition, the routine distribution of discharge bags with commercial formula, and breastfeeding resistance within the health care system has also dramatically interfered with breastfeeding success rates.[70]

Just as important as the hospital staff, though, is the support team for the new mother at home. Attitudes toward breastfeeding can affect women's familiarity and comfort with breastfeeding. The opinions of expectant fathers, family, and friends significantly influence if and how long a woman breastfeeds.[71] Women are more likely to succeed if they have a strong support network.[72] Breastfeeding rates are higher for women whose partners are knowledgeable about breastfeeding. In fact, studies show that when expectant fathers participate in breastfeeding education classes, their partners are much more likely to initiate and sustain breastfeeding.[73] Women have reported feeling more confident and positive toward breastfeeding if they feel supported by their partners.[74]

For women who begin breastfeeding, a number of factors influence exclusivity and duration. Once mothers leave the hospital, common justifications for weaning prematurely include beliefs in insufficient milk (or disrupted lactation), sore nipples, and latching issues.[75] These physiological obstacles may result from misinformation about milk supply, nursing schedules, and nursing position, often due to poor advice from ill-informed health professionals.[76] Psychosocial factors also impact breastfeeding initiation and duration, as a key predictor in breastfeeding success is self-efficacy—the extent to which a mother believes she will succeed at breastfeeding.[77] And while some have used postpartum depression as justification for weaning, McCarter-Spaulding determined that the severity of postpartum depression did not significantly influence breastfeeding duration.[78] Routines at home can also impact success. Families who bed share with their babies are much more likely to breastfeed for at least 12 months.[79]

Breastfeeding interventions can profoundly help women overcome obstacles and increase breastfeeding success, particularly for low-income women.[80] The CDC's annual "Breastfeeding Report Card" highlights the importance of institutional and social support in breastfeeding success.[81] This report lists the State Maternity Practices in Infant Nutrition and Care (mPINC) score,[82] along with the number of Certified Lactation Consultants (CLCs), International Board Certified Lactation Consultants (IBCLCs), La Leche groups, and Baby Friendly hospitals by individual state.[83] Furthermore, peer counseling has been shown to improve the likelihood of exclusive breastfeeding in initiation and duration.[84]

Support of the general public can also influence breastfeeding rates.[85] Vari and colleagues found that breastfeeding rates varied regionally, with a clear relationship between positive breastfeeding attitudes and rates. In places in which breastfeeding was the cultural norm, men and women were more likely to support future breastfeeding or intend to breastfeed themselves.[86] On the contrary, when bottle-feeding is the cultural norm, women have more difficulty breastfeeding. Scott and Mostyn conducted focus groups with breastfeeding women from a community with low breastfeeding rates and found that these women were generally unprepared and surprised by nursing obstacles and felt unsupported by family and peers.[87]

A lack of cultural support can translate to resistance for breastfeeding in public. For example, in Scott and Mostyn's study, the breastfeeding women tried to avoid nursing in public for fear of scrutiny in a community of bottle-feeders.[88] Other research also suggests that the extent to which the public supports breastfeeding can impact a woman's willingness and comfort in nursing her child in public places, like the local restaurant or retail outlet.[89] Comfort with breastfeeding in public increases breastfeeding exclusivity and duration.[90] Even in childless populations, most people are aware of the health benefits of breastfeeding.[91] At the same time, breastfeeding attitude surveys reveal that the majority of participants are not comfortable with breastfeeding in public.[92] In a 2004 study of breastfeeding attitudes, Li and colleagues found that only 43% of people surveyed believed women should have the right to breastfeed in public.[93] Because of negative attitudes toward breastfeeding, nursing mothers have reported feeling "vulnerable" when nursing in public.[94] The public's discomfort with breastfeeding likely stems from the absence of breastfeeding images and positive stories in news and entertainment media. In fact, Scott and Mostyn cited the lack of positive breastfeeding representations as contributing to the "bottle-feeding culture," stating, "The way by which breastfeeding is currently represented by the media will do little to increase the social acceptability of breastfeeding and influence the choice and ability of mothers to breastfeed."[95] That said, multiple actions have been initiated in an attempt to change culture.

Programs and objectives to improve breastfeeding highlight the individual and institutional barriers to success. The 1981 Code addressed multiple sites of resistance for increasing breastfeeding rates: increasing the dissemination of accurate breastfeeding information to pregnant women and new mothers, changing health care to become breastfeeding-friendly, and radically curbing damaging, pervasive formula marketing practices.[96] In the early 1990s, the Innocenti Declaration and Baby-Friendly Hospital Initiative (BFHI) established specific strategies to transform health care facilities to become more conducive to breastfeeding.[97] To earn a "Baby-Friendly" designation, a facilty must prove that it adheres to the Ten Steps of Successful Breastfeeding, a plan that includes the creation of breastfeeding policies, training for health professionals, informing women about breastfeeding, and lactation support.[98] Hospitals seeking this designation must also adopt practices that increase breastfeeding success, including breastfeeding initation within 30 min of birth, when possible, newborns rooming-in with their mothers, nursing on-demand, no pacifiers, and no supplementing "unless medically indicated."[99] As of 2016, 18.48% of births in the United States occur in hospitals and birthing centers with a Baby-Friendly designation, a notable increase from the 2.9% of births in 2007.[100] State-by-state, this percentage ranges from under 1% of births (Arkansas,

Georgia, Kansas, Louisiana, Mississippi, Pennsylvania, Tennessee, Virginia, and West Virginia) to 35.98% (Connecticut).[101] Not surprisingly, some of the states with few or no Baby-Friendly facilities also yield the lowest breastfeeding rates.[102] Globally, 134 countries (including 12 developing countries) have Baby-Friendly designation on more than 15,000 facilities.[103] Still, the number of Baby-Friendly places varies substantially. Semenic and colleagues conducted an integrative review on obstacles to the BFHI, finding that socio-political factors, organization and implementation issues, knowledge and attitudes in individual health care settings, availability of breastfeeding resources, and the extent of formula marketing impacted the establishment of Baby-Friendly facilities.[104]

While the BFHI focuses on improving the quality of health care, the 2011 "Surgeon General's Call to Action" centers around social and institutional obstacles to breastfeeding success. This Call to Action identified seven types of barriers to improving breastfeeding rates: a lack of knowledge, family or social support, social norms that present "breastfeeding as an alternative rather than the routine way to feed infants," embarrassment about breastfeeding, short maternity leaves and employment policies that discourage breastfeeding, and problems with health professionals and the health care system.[105] The action steps address these barriers with individual, community, and societal actions to increase breastfeeding rates. Specifically, the actions include increasing support for new mothers, educating fathers and grandmothers, improving breastfeeding support in health care and employment practices, building community support through mother-to-mother and peer counseling, promoting breastfeeding through local organizations, launching a national breastfeeding campaign and, finally, minimizing the negative effect of formula marketing on exclusive breastfeeding.[106] This plan of action (and others) addresses multiple sites that can potentially impact breastfeeding, but has it been successful? Anstey, MacGowan, and Allen conducted a five-year follow-up on the success of the "Call to Action," finding some improvement in federal efforts to improve breastfeeding.[107] They noted the significant increase in hospitals with the Baby-Friendly designation, community-based campaigns that have been launched, targeting specific groups with lower-than-average breastfeeding rates, and the expansion of insurance coverage and employment protection for nursing mothers.[108] Furthermore, federal agencies have begun to use *Twitter* and other social media sites to disseminate breastfeeding information.[109] And yet, Anstey and colleagues pointed out that these action steps have been focused on federal improvements, and therefore, more campaigns and localized efforts are needed.[110]

As will be outlined in the next section, media play a significant role in creating a breastfeeding culture. In the Code, *Innocenti Declaration*, the "Call to Action," and other proclamations and strategies, challenging milk-substitute promotion and distribution, combined with better utilization of media in breastfeeding campaigns are central to shaping how health professionals, mothers, and the general public perceive breastfeeding.

Media and Breastfeeding

How do media fit into correlations and predictors of breastfeeding? News and entertainment messages help define what is considered "normal" about infant feeding. Indeed, past health campaigns on breastfeeding have demonstrated media's impact, improving awareness, increasing initiation rates, and producing positive attitudes toward breastfeeding.[111] For those without children, images of breastfeeding can help transform discomfort and spectacle into an everyday part of life. Breastfeeding promotion, education, and intervention can drastically counter many of the justifications for not nursing or for early cessation and increase support for the breastfeeding woman.[112] The source of information can also impact breastfeeding success.[113] On the negative side, media representations have been known to normalize bottle-feeding, destroy a new mother's confidence in breastfeeding through persuasive advertising and free samples, and convince health professionals to recommend formula, even when it may not be needed.[114]

Media play a significant role in shaping breastfeeding perceptions by disseminating information, defining what is considered "normal," and enacting changes in health behavior, particularly for those who lack breastfeeding education from other sources.[115] In an analysis of the Infant Feeding Practices Survey II, Chen, Johnson and Rosenthal noted that 64.1% of respondents received their infant feeding information from newspapers, television, books, newsletters, radio, and websites.[116] Moreover, 37.5% of those surveyed learned about breast pumps from media.[117] The quality of information can impact infant feeding choices. In one survey, bottle-feeding mothers indicated that they would have been more likely to breastfeed if they had gotten breastfeeding information from magazines, books, or television.[118]

Kornides and Kitsantas analyzed the correlation between the consumption of breastfeeding information from media sources and breastfeeding rates, noting a significant difference between women with low consumption and those who had medium to high rates.[119] Mothers who indicated low/no media sources of breastfeeding only had a 78.1% breastfeeding initiation rate, compared to 85.8% for high media consumption.[120] At 2 months, only 53% of these mothers were still doing any breastfeeding, as opposed to 62.8% for high media consumption.[121] Furthermore, only 32.8% of low media consumers were exclusively breastfeeding at 2 months, compared to 41.4% for medium consumers and 34.5% for high consumers.[122] These effects were less dramatic when other maternal characteristics were factored into the analysis, with the researchers concluding that breastfeeding knowledge, health professional encouragement, and family support significantly influenced initiation, duration, and exclusivity.[123]

Media messages can also impact perceptions of breastfeeding even if the audience is not consuming discourse specifically about breastfeeding. Ward, Merriwether, and Caruthers studied the relationship between consumption of men's magazines and television viewing, participants' belief in traditional masculine ideologies, and their attitudes toward childbirth and breastfeeding.[124] Higher media consumption correlated with more adherence to masculine ideologies and less support for public breastfeeding.[125] Furthermore, this group was more concerned that breastfeeding would interfere with sexual relations.[126] The researchers explained this relationship stating that by frequently reducing women to sexual objects, media content may make it difficult for men to see women any other way.[127] While it may seem tangential, men's opinions of breastfeeding matter significantly. Research shows that fathers' attitudes and support profoundly influence breastfeeding initiation and duration.[128] This study also highlights the fact that discusssions of infant feeding are heavily infused with connotations about women's bodies and status in society.

Obviously, formula marketing is tied into media's representations of breastfeeding. Formula is a multi-billion dollar industry, one that has grown significantly since the 1980s.[129] Since monetary value typically translates to cultural value, this commodification of breastmilk substitutes has placed them above breastmilk, which is especially problematic in developing countries.[130] Scholars and breastfeeding activists have questioned how breastfeeding (which is free) can or should compete with a commercial industry, turning to the sale of breastmilk online as an indication of its value.[131] Rollins and colleagues demonstrated the economic benefits of increasing global breastfeeding rates, with cost-savings in reducing infectious and chronic disease and chronic illness in children, as well as the environmental impact of formula production and consumption.[132] And yet, these economic benefits are generally hidden from consumers. Furthermore, as Rollins and colleagues argued, countries have not invested enough resources into improving breastfeeding rates.[133] This disparity in money spent on promotion of breastmilk substitutes, compared to breastfeeding promotion, helps to explain the pervasiveness of formula marketing. Even in countries that have adopted the Code, formula marketing has been abundant.[134] Such promotion has had dire effects on breastfeeding rates, presenting formula as the social norm, confusing consumers about health benefits and infant feeding, undermining a mother's confidence in breastfeeding, and interfering with policies to support breastfeeding.[135] While the effects are more damaging in developing countries, they are still problematic in the United States, particularly for groups with low breastfeeding rates. Formula advertising has a presence that is unparalleled in breastfeeding promotion. Mothers surveyed about infant feeding information can recall marketing materials far more than pro-breastfeeding information. Paula Bylaska-Davies interviewed women about their breastfeeding decisions, finding that most participants did not cite media sources as a reason to breastfeed, which was not surprising given that most participants had difficulty recalling specific pro-breastfeeding materials.[136] Comparatively, 90% of the women recalled receiving free formula samples and other forms of marketing and could provide much more vivid descriptions of formula advertising than they could breastfeeding material.[137]

Research on Infant Feeding in Media

Studies of infant feeding messages in media suggest its prevalence. Brown and Peuchaud reviewed studies on media coverage of breastfeeding, concluding that positive representations were lacking.[138] Research on media representations of breastfeeding has largely focused on quantitative studies of magazine content.[139] Formula advertising frequently appears in parenting magazines. Stang, Hoss, and Story studied 75 issues across 16 magazines, identifying 173 formula ads, with approximately 2.5 ads per issue.[140] Many of these ads used unsubstantiated health statements to sell their products.[141] The prevalence of these ads matter.

Foss and Southwell determined a negative correlation between breastfeeding rates and the number of commercial formula ads in a parenting magazine, from 1972 to 2000.[142] Breastfeeding trends in magazines and parenting manuals have suggested that contemporary media depict breastfeeding as positive, but difficult.[143] In a qualitative, historical study of infant feeding trends, Foss found a similar pattern, noting that experts have historically been used to support both bottle and breastfeeding.[144] This dependency on experts has been linked to short breastfeeding duration, given lack of breastfeeding training for health professionals.[145]

Even more disturbing, in *Mother's Milk: Breastfeeding Controversies in American Culture,* Bernice Hausman explained how media messages have framed breastfeeding as harmful, even dangerous, to infants, with stories of "dead babies" saturating media.[146] Bentley, Dee, and Jensen also argued that news stories exaggerate and sensationalize the few stories about breastfeeding tragedies, such as the case of Tabitha Walrond, whose breastfed baby died of starvation.[147] Likewise, Jacqueline Wolf outlined how media have ignored breastfeeding as preventative to childhood illness, but overstated and distorted the Walrond case, failing to mention the extenuating circumstances that contributed to that tragedy.[148] Media's hyperfocus on the Walrond case ignores the prevalence of tragedy from infant formula, like the six deaths and 300,000 sick babies from contaminated milk substitutes in China in 2008, or the significantly higher mortality rates for artificially-fed children overall.[149]

Even pro-breastfeeding media sites offer conflicting messages. Callahan and Lazard analyzed breastfeeding discourse in popular online parenting communities, concluding that the sites present breastfeeding as "natural."[150] At the same time, breastfeeding in public is construed as shameful, as the scholars noted sexualization of breasts.[151] The sexualization of breasts and other themes were also found in Bylaska-Davies' analysis of infant websites and noted by participants in her audience study.[152] Such disparate messages put tension on all types of infant feeding, demonizing both bottle-feeding and breastfeeding.

Media have also contributed to lower breastfeeding rates by normalizing bottle-feeding, perpetuating breastfeeding's difficulty, and placing restrictions on "acceptable" breastfeeding.[153] Breastfeeding mothers themselves have suggested that media present bottle-feeding as the "norm."[154] Scott and Mostyn noted a relationship between what they observed as a "bottle-feeding culture" to a lack of positive breastfeeding messages in media, stating:

> Television has the potential to serve as a proxy for real-life exposure to breastfeeding. However, the way by which breastfeeding is currently represented by the media will do little to increase the social acceptability of breastfeeding and influence the choice and ability of mothers to breastfeed.[155]

Bentley, Dee, and Jensen demonstrated the pervasiveness of a bottle-feeding culture in media, giving examples of news and entertainment media distorting breastfeeding tragedies, celebrities shown bottle-feeding, and abundant ads promoting commercial formula.[156] O'Brien, Zareai, and Fallon analyzed breastfeeding rates and cultural factors in a country with high breastfeeding rates (Iran) to a country with lower rates (Australia).[157] The scholars identified a vast difference in maternity leave policies, the number of BFHI, and support for breastfeeding mothers.[158] Just as important, they noted that the country with high breastfeeding rates held positive cultural attitudes, positively influenced by the high visibility of breastfeeding in Iranian media, which strongly conveyed breastfeeding benefits and formula risks.[159]

Media have likely influenced breastfeeding in other ways, defining appropriate ages and places for breastfeeding (that contradict public health recommendations), promoting milk substitutes to health care providers, and commodifying infant feeding so that breastfeeding is perceived as "less valuable" in our monetary-driven capitalist society. Beyond new and expectant parents, it is important that the general public supports breastfeeding so that nursing mothers feel comfortable, not scrutinized feeding in public. Since not all policymakers or employers are currently lactating, it is imperative that as a culture, we view breastfeeding as vital to public helath so those in positions of power can help create more breastfeeding-friendly conditions for nursing mothers. This book addresses these issues, building on existing studies, through a holistic look at the messages about breastfeeding and their connections to public knowledge and perception.

Theoretical Framework

This book draws from theories in Cultural Studies and Health Communication to explore the influence of media on public knowledge, perception, and behavior. Berger and Luckmann (1966) explained that our meaningful reality is socially constructed, or shaped, by the dominant institutions in society, including mass media, a perception labeled the social construction of reality theory.[160] Media, then, help shape public perception by perpetuating ideologies. In 1979, sociologist Todd Gitlin articulated this process:

> Commercial culture does not *manufacture* ideology; it *relays* and *reproduces* and *processes* and *packages* and *focuses* ideology that is constantly arising both from social elites and from active social groups and movements throughout the society (as well as within media organizations and practices).[161]

In other words, media reflect, perpetuate, and sometimes challenge the dominant ideas in society. Here, it is assumed then, that news stories, television shows, mothering blogs, online communities, and other media outlets impact how we, as a society and as individuals, understand infant feeding, define what is "normal" for breastfeeding, and assign value to infant feeding, often through the comparable commodification of formula. These constructions of infant feeding are not fixed, but change with cultural context. Hence, an investigation into media discourse over time can give insight into how society generally perceived infant feeding at a particular moment and provide an observation into shifting breastfeeding rates.

Power dynamics play a key role in this constructed world. Media gatekeepers do not exist in a bubble, but create and produce content based on historical precedents, preconceived notions about race, class, gender, family structure, geographic origin and other factors. Through the repetition of representations, certain notions become "commonsense," or what Antonio Gramsci called "hegemony."[162] Cultural hegemony positions certain groups in power, while others are delegitimized, ostracized, and marginalized—labeled "the Other."[163] Breastfeeding disparities are profoundly linked to inequities of race and socio-economic class, as reinforced through media constructions of the female body. Hausman contended that media stories of infant death (because of inadequacy in breastfeeding) have varied greatly with a woman's ethnicity, and that women of color are much more likely to be blamed for an infant's failure to thrive.[164] Linda Blum also stressed the importance of race and class, discussing how many African American women choose not to breastfeed because of the history of hypersexualization and its connection to the "animality" of these women in public discourse.[165] As she argued, to persuade more women from this cultural group to breastfeed, advocates must do more than preach about its benefits, but also address African American women's history in American culture.[166] Thus, to talk about breastfeeding success, is not just about the physiology of lactation, but also refers to a cultural resonance or understanding of the histories of different groups in American history.

This research assumes that media impact our understanding of health, shape our perceptions, and affect our behavior. Such influence has been extensively demonstrated. Other than personal physicians, media outlets, especially websites, serve as most people's primary source of health information.[167] These messages impact the overall public perception of breastfeeding. According to cultivation theory, developed by Gerbner and colleagues in the 1970s, heavy television viewers tend to perceive the world as it is presented on television. For example, those that watch crime dramas are more likely to believe that crime is more prevalent than people who do not watch these programs.[168] Expanding on Gerbner's research, scholars have noted that media consumption correlates with differing perspectives on gender and race. Heavy media consumers tend to hold greater racial biases and stereotypes, compared to light consumers.[169] Correlations have also been noted between news and television consumption and gender-damaging assumptions, notably higher agreement with statements that blame female victims for sexual assault.[170] In "An Explication of Social Norms," Lapinski and Rimal draw from social cognitive theory and cultivation to explain that media help to define social norms by creating misperceptions about what is common and prevalent in a society, as mitigated by personal experience.[171] One can also gather an understanding of the collective social norms of a society from observing trends in media.[172] With infant feeding, cultivation theory suggests that consumption of shows that present formula-feeding as "normal" would lead viewers to believe that breastfeeding is uncommon or "abnormal." Members of the general public may be less supportive of a breastfeeding woman, especially in a public space, if they perceive it as "abnormal" or unnecessary.

Media messages have also been shown to enact changes in health behavior. For example, in the 1980s media messages about the dangers of giving Aspirin to children helped to dramatically reduce the incidence of Reye's syndrome.[173] Following publicity of former First Lady Nancy Reagan's mastectomy, the frequency of breast-cancer patients choosing mastectomies over breast-conserving surgery (BCS) increased.[174]

Campaigns promoting behavior change are most effective if consumers believe that the benefits far outweigh the risk of not changing the behavior and if the behavior is somewhat easy to change.[175] With breastfeeding, it is not enough for women to know of the health benefits, but they need to believe that not breastfeeding is risky enough to their infants to make the action worth doing. As described by Jacqueline Wolf, in the 2000s, the Ad Council created a series of Public Service Announcements (PSAs) utilizing this approach.[176] These PSAs featured pregnant women riding bulls and partaking in other dangerous activities as a voice-over stated the risks of not breastfeeding.[177] Fears about these messages being too effective prompted commercial formula companies to protest.[178] This example demonstrates the influence of corporate power on risk prevention and suggests one reason why health promotion campaigns have not succeeded in significantly increasing breastfeeding duration, a concept that will be explored throughout this book.

Constructions of infant feeding are very much connected to cultural perceptions of motherhood and parenting. Discourses about infant feeding have been both polarizing and conflicting. On the one hand, the emphasis on breastfeeding's health benefits helps establish breastfeeding as a public health issue—one that is bigger than individual choice. However, as Paige Hall Smith pointed out, this approach can minimize the importance of women's experiences and their control over their own bodies, ignoring the need for gender equity.[179] Furthermore, it was the medicalization of infant feeding that initially stripped agency from mothers and their intuition. At the turn of the twentieth century, women were increasingly expected to turn to experts for parenting advice—a concept Rima Apple deemed the "scientific motherhood."[180] According to Apple, the "scientific motherhood is the insistence that women require expert scientific and medical advice to raise their children healthfully."[181] Apple noted that mothers were especially encouraged to rely on doctors' advice for infant feeding advice, instead of relying on other women or their own intuition.[182] While the advice has changed over time, health professionals continue to significantly influence infant feeding decisions and breastfeeding success.

Aside from the medical frame, breastfeeding discourse is often tied into societal ideals of womanhood and "the good mother." Callaghan and Lazard's study of discursive formations of infant feeding in parenting communities found that constructions of motherhood permeated the discourse about breastfeeding.[183] The scholars argued that the "breastfeeding as natural" message establishes a construct of "the 'unnatural' bottle feeder," "constituted as antithethical to ideas of natural, nurturing motherhood."[184] Douglas and Michaels argued that media have cultivated additional pressures for women, creating an unattainable definition of the "perfect mother," in which women have autonomy and choices, but are ultimately supposed to choose and excel at mothering.[185] As Hausman explained, the ideology of "the good mother" has been a staple part of breastfeeding promotion, blaming individual women who do not or cannot breastfeed as "bad mothers"—a tension that fuels what has been called the "Mommy Wars." Such a framework displaces fault on individuals, thus distracting from the economic and social changes needed to improve breastfeeding rates.[186] Unfortunately, media messages like the Similac ad described at the beginning of this chapter, exaggerate and fuel the false dichotomy of the "good"/"bad" mother, using the "Wars" to promote formula purchases, thus obfuscating the issue. Breastfeeding should not be considered as an individual mother's quest, but as a Feminist mission and public health objective that can help with gender equity, not distract from it with the "Mommy Wars."

The Book's Approach and Chapter Overview

In this book, I use case studies of different media to explore how media reflect, perpetuate, and sometimes challenge prevailing ideologies about breastfeeding. The first chapters specifically focus on media products and marketing materials geared toward expectant parents and new mothers. In Chap. 2, I incorporate analysis of nineteenth century newspaper ads for wet nursing and a study of *Ladies' Home Journal (LHJ)* as a means of tracing social constructions of the early history of infant feeding through the emergence of commercial formula. Chapter 3 continues this history, from the 1920s through the 2000s, addressing the decline of breastfeeding to its all-time low in the 1970s and then its revival as reflected and perpetuated in *Parents* magazine. In Chap. 4, I shift to contemporary times, looking at the marketing and distribution of infant feeding as I examine the role of health care providers in infant feeding, the history of formula marketing, national and localized breastfeeding promotion and campaigns, and other breastfeeding advocacy efforts. For Chaps. 5–9, I move to popular media and its audience reception. Chapter 5 looks at infant feeding messages for new parents and siblings through an examination of pregnancy and new parenting books, along with an analysis of infant feeding in children's books. Chapter 6 includes a purposive study of fictional television, analyzing representations from 1974 to 2015. In Chap. 7, I use reality television programs about motherhood to discuss how such "reality" shows and their deliberate product integration reinforces a "bottle-feeding" culture for viewers, even when the reality subjects and target audience significantly diverge. Chapter 8 moves to online discourse, in which I analyze breastfeeding messages in social media to show how new technologies have both hindered and helped breastfeeding success. And in Chap. 9, the issue of breastfeeding as spectacle and stigma is discussed, examining how media portrayals of "extreme" extended, erotic, and public breastfeeding have discouraged regular women from nursing. Finally, Chap. 10 questions and proposes changes to news and entertainment media, designed to transform the American cultural climate into one conducive to breastfeeding success. My intention with this book is not to look at all media—to do so would be impossible. Instead, I aim to analyze and discuss dominant messages about infant feeding in popular sites over time in order to showcase the relationship between media, breastfeeding, and shifting cultural perceptions.

Notes

1. *The Mother 'Hood Official Video.*
2. Neff, "Similac Wants to End Mommy Wars Over Breastfeeding: Abbot Brand Stages Playground Battle to Help End the Shaming."
3. Waxman, "This Ad Perfectly Parodies the 'Mommy Wars.'"
4. Bologna, "A Playful Reminder That Judging Other Parents Is Wrong."
5. Gregory et al., "Are Unmet Breastfeeding Expectations Associated With Maternal Depressive Symptoms?"
6. Odom et al., "Association of Family and Health Care Provider Opinion on Infant Feeding with Mother's Breastfeeding Decision."
7. Labbok, "Exploration of Guilt Among Mothers Who Do Not Breastfeed"; Hausman, *Mother's Milk*; Blum, *At the Breast*; Koerber, "'You Just Don't See Enough Normal' Critical Perspectives on Infant-Feeding Discourse and Practice"; Koerber, "Rhetorical Agency, Resistance, and the Disciplinary Rhetorics of Breastfeeding"; Wolf, "What Feminists Can Do for Breastfeeding and What Breastfeeding Can Do for Feminists."
8. Gartner et al., "Breastfeeding and the Use of Human Milk."
9. Ibid.

10. "International Code of Marketing of Breast-Milk Substitutes"; Shubber, *The WHO International Code of Marketing of Breast-Milk Substitutes.*
11. "International Code of Marketing of Breast-Milk Substitutes."
12. {Citation}.
13. "Country Implementation of the International Code of Marketing of Breast-Milk Substitutes: Status Report 2011."
14. Ibid.
15. Ibid.
16. Labbok, "Breastfeeding in Public Health."
17. "The Surgeon General's Call to Action to Support Breastfeeding - Calltoactiontosupportbreastfeeding.pdf."
18. Glik et al., "Health Education Goes Hollywood"; Grantham, Ahern, and Connolly-Ahern, "Merck's One Less Campaign"; Maddock et al., "Statewide Implementation of the 1% or Less Campaign."
19. Rollins et al., "Why Invest, and What It Will Take to Improve Breastfeeding Practices?"
20. Verhasselt, "Neonatal Tolerance under Breastfeeding Influence"; Duijts et al., "Prolonged and Exclusive Breastfeeding Reduces the Risk of Infectious Diseases in Infancy"; Kramer, "Breastfeeding and Allergy"; Stuebe, "The Risks of Not Breastfeeding for Mothers and Infants."
21. Khan et al., "Timing of Breastfeeding Initiation and Exclusivity of Breastfeeding During the First Month of Life"; Lamberti et al., "Breastfeeding for Reducing the Risk of Pneumonia Morbidity and Mortality in Children under Two"; Hauck et al., "Breastfeeding and Reduced Risk of Sudden Infant Death Syndrome"; Lamberti et al., "Breastfeeding and the Risk for Diarrhea Morbidity and Mortality."
22. Stuebe, "The Risks of Not Breastfeeding for Mothers and Infants."
23. Ibid.
24. Gale et al., "Effect of Breastfeeding Compared with Formula Feeding on Infant Body Composition."
25. Sonnenschein-van der Voort et al., "Fetal and Infant Growth and Asthma Symptoms in Preschool Children"; van Odijk et al., "Breastfeeding and Allergic Disease"; Palmer, "The Influence of Breastfeeding on the Development of the Oral Cavity: A Commentary"; Wright et al., "Increasing Breastfeeding Rates to Reduce Infant Illness at the Community Level"; Pratt, "Breastfeeding and Eczema."
26. It should be noted that while most research supports this correlation, independent studies in birth cohorts in Hong Kong and Belarus did not find a significant correlation between breastfeeding and obesity, suggesting that this link may be more pronounced in westernized countries, which have higher rates of childhood obesity (see Kwok et al., "Does Breastfeeding Protect against Childhood Overweight?"; Martin R.M. et al., "Effects of

Promoting Longer-Term and Exclusive Breastfeeding on Adiposity and Insulin-like Growth Factor-I at Age 11.5 Years").

27. Metzger and McDade, "Breastfeeding as Obesity Prevention in the United States"; Owen et al., "Does Breastfeeding Influence Risk of Type 2 Diabetes in Later Life?"; Villegas et al., "Duration of Breast-Feeding and the Incidence of Type 2 Diabetes Mellitus in the Shanghai Women's Health Study"; Shu et al., "Breast-Feeding and Risk of Childhood Acute Leukemia"; Beyerlein and Kries, "Breastfeeding and Body Composition in Children."
28. McCrory and Layte, "Breastfeeding and Risk of Overweight and Obesity at Nine-Years of Age."
29. Ibid.
30. Jacobson, Chiodo, and Jacobson, "Breastfeeding Effects on Intelligence Quotient in 4- and 11-Year-Old Children."
31. Quigley et al., "Breastfeeding Is Associated with Improved Child Cognitive Development."
32. Ibid.
33. Oddy et al., "Breastfeeding Duration and Academic Achievement at 10 Years."
34. Ibid.
35. Oddy et al., "The Long-Term Effects of Breastfeeding on Child and Adolescent Mental Health."
36. Labbok, "Effects of Breastfeeding on the Mother."
37. Kim et al., "Breastfeeding, Brain Activation to Own Infant Cry, and Maternal Sensitivity."
38. Jarlenski et al., "Effects of Breastfeeding on Postpartum Weight Loss among U.S. Women"; Amanda Yeaton-Massey, "Exclusive Breastfeeding Promotes Postpartum Weight Loss;" Østbye et al., "Effect of Breastfeeding on Weight Retention from One Pregnancy to the next."
39. Jordan et al., "Breastfeeding and Risk of Epithelial Ovarian Cancer"; Liu, Jorm, and Banks, "Parity, Breastfeeding, and the Subsequent Risk of Maternal Type 2 Diabetes"; Lupton et al., "Association between Parity and Breastfeeding with Maternal High Blood Pressure"; Labbok, "Effects of Breastfeeding on the Mother"; Enger et al., "Breastfeeding History, Pregnancy Experience and Risk of Breast Cancer."; Cumming and Klineberg, "Breastfeeding and Other Reproductive Factors and the Risk of Hip Fractures in Elderly Women."
40. Jordan et al., "Breastfeeding and Risk of Epithelial Ovarian Cancer"; Lupton et al., "Association between Parity and Breastfeeding with Maternal High Blood Pressure."
41. Breastfeeding, "Breastfeeding and the Use of Human Milk"; "WHO| Breastfeeding."

42. "Breastfeeding Report Card: United States, 2016 - 2016breastfeedingreportcard.pdf."
43. Ibid.
44. Ibid.
45. Jones et al., "Factors Associated With Exclusive Breastfeeding in the United States"; Bolton et al., "Characteristics Associated With Longer Breastfeeding Duration"; Ryan, Wenjun, and Acosta, "Breastfeeding Continues to Increase Into the New Millennium."
46. Al-Sahab et al., "Prevalence and Predictors of 6-Month Exclusive Breastfeeding among Canadian Women"; Hauff, Leonard, and Rasmussen, "Associations of Maternal Obesity and Psychosocial Factors with Breastfeeding Intention, Initiation, and Duration"; Jones et al., "Factors Associated With Exclusive Breastfeeding in the United States"; Wojcicki, "Maternal Prepregnancy Body Mass Index and Initiation and Duration of Breastfeeding."
47. Jones et al., "Factors Associated With Exclusive Breastfeeding in the United States"; Forste, Weiss, and Lippincott, "The Decision to Breastfeed in the United States"; Ryan, Wenjun, and Acosta, "Breastfeeding Continues to Increase Into the New Millennium."
48. Bartick and Reinhold, "The Burden of Suboptimal Breastfeeding in the United States."
49. Rollins et al., "Why Invest, and What It Will Take to Improve Breastfeeding Practices?"
50. "The Surgeon General's Call to Action to Support Breastfeeding - Calltoactiontosupportbreastfeeding.pdf."
51. "Maternal, Infant, and Child Health| Healthy People 2020."
52. "Breastfeeding State Laws."
53. Ibid.
54. Ibid.
55. Ibid.
56. Ibid.
57. Bai and Wunderlich, "Lactation accommodation in the workplace and duration of exclusive breastfeeding."
58. Smith-Gagen et al., "Breastfeeding Laws and Breastfeeding Practices by Race and Ethnicity."
59. Ibid.
60. Stuebe and Bonuck, "What Predicts Intent to Breastfeed Exclusively?"; Kornides and Kitsantas, "Evaluation of Breastfeeding Promotion, Support, and Knowledge of Benefits on Breastfeeding Outcomes."
61. Stuebe and Bonuck, "What Predicts Intent to Breastfeed Exclusively?"
62. Ibid.

63. Kendall-Tackett, "Violence Against Women and the Perinatal Period The Impact of Lifetime Violence and Abuse on Pregnancy, Postpartum, and Breastfeeding."
Stuebe and Bonuck, "What Predicts Intent to Breastfeed Exclusively?".
64. Cook, "Breastfeeding, Feminism, and Political Theory."
65. Cromi et al., "Assisted Reproductive Technology and Breastfeeding Outcomes."
66. Taveras et al., "Opinions and Practices of Clinicians Associated With Continuation of Exclusive Breastfeeding"; Arora et al., "Major Factors Influencing Breastfeeding Rates"; Odom et al., "Association of Family and Health Care Provider Opinion on Infant Feeding with Mother's Breastfeeding Decision."
67. Zanardo et al., "Elective Cesarean Delivery."
68. Al-Sahab et al., "Prevalence and Predictors of 6-Month Exclusive Breastfeeding among Canadian Women."
69. "Breastfeeding Report Card: United States, 2014 - 2014 breastfeedingreportcard.pdf"; Bramson et al., "Effect of Early Skin-to-Skin Mother–Infant Contact During the First 3 Hours Following Birth on Exclusive Breastfeeding During the Maternity Hospital Stay."
70. "Breastfeeding Report Card: United States, 2014 - 2014 breastfeedingreportcard.pdf"; Huang et al., "Association of Health Profession and Direct-to-Consumer Marketing with Infant Formula Choice and Switching"; Koerber, "'You Just Don't See Enough Normal' Critical Perspectives on Infant-Feeding Discourse and Practice"; Howard et al., "Office Prenatal Formula Advertising and Its Effect on Breast-Feeding patterns1."
71. Freed, Fraley, and Schanler, "Attitudes of Expectant Fathers Regarding Breast-Feeding"; Littman, Medendorp, and Goldfarb, "The Decision to Breastfeed The Importance of Fathers' Approval."
72. Schmied et al., "Women's Perceptions and Experiences of Breastfeeding Support"; Meedya, Fahy, and Kable, "Factors That Positively Influence Breastfeeding Duration to 6 Months."
73. Maycock et al., "Education and Support for Fathers Improves Breastfeeding Rates A Randomized Controlled Trial"; Wolfberg et al., "Dads as Breastfeeding Advocates."
74. Mannion et al., "Maternal Perceptions of Partner Support during Breastfeeding."
75. Stuebe, "Enabling Women to Achieve Their Breastfeeding Goals"; McClellan et al., "Nipple Pain during Breastfeeding with or without Visible Trauma"; Lewallen et al., "Breastfeeding Support and Early Cessation."
76. Lewallen et al., "Breastfeeding Support and Early Cessation."

77. de Jager et al., "The Role of Psychosocial Factors in Exclusive Breastfeeding to Six Months Postpartum"; Meedya, Fahy, and Kable, "Factors That Positively Influence Breastfeeding Duration to 6 Months"; Kools et al., "The Motivational Determinants of Breast-Feeding: Predictors for the Continuation of Breast-Feeding"; Khoury et al., "Breast-Feeding Initiation in Low-Income Women."
78. McCarter-Spaulding, "How Does Postpartum Depression Affect Breastfeeding?"
79. Blair, Heron, and Fleming, "Relationship Between Bed Sharing and Breastfeeding."
80. Khoury et al., "Breast-Feeding Initiation in Low-Income Women."
81. "Breastfeeding Report Card: United States, 2014–2014 breastfeedingreportcard.pdf."
82. This rating indicates the extent to which the maternity care practices support breastfeeding.
83. Ibid.
84. Chapman et al., "Effectiveness of Breastfeeding Peer Counseling in a Low-Income, Predominantly Latina Population."
85. Avery et al., "Factors Associated with Very Early Weaning Among Primiparas Intending to Breastfeed"; Sheeshka et al., "Women's Experiences Breastfeeding in Public Places."
86. Vari et al., "Community Breastfeeding Attitudes and Beliefs."
87. Scott and Mostyn, "Women's Experiences of Breastfeeding in a Bottle-Feeding Culture."
88. Ibid.
89. Sheeshka et al., "Women's Experiences Breastfeeding in Public Places."
90. Stuebe and Bonuck, "What Predicts Intent to Breastfeed Exclusively?".
91. Foss and Blake, "'It's Natural and Healthy, But I Don't Want To See It': The Impact of Entertainment Television on Breastfeeding Attitudes"; Kavanagh et al., "Breastfeeding Knowledge, Attitudes, Prior Exposure, and Intent among Undergraduate Students"; Li et al., "Public Beliefs about Breastfeeding Policies in Various Settings"; Marrone, Vogeltanz-Holm, and Holm, "Attitudes, Knowledge, and Intentions Related to Breastfeeding Among University Undergraduate Women and Men"; Spear, "College Students' Experiences and Attitudes Regarding Middle and High School–Based Breastfeeding Education."
92. Foss and Blake, "'It's Natural and Healthy, But I Don't Want To See It': The Impact of Entertainment Television on Breastfeeding Attitudes"; Kavanagh et al., "Breastfeeding Knowledge, Attitudes, Prior Exposure, and Intent among Undergraduate Students"; Marrone, Vogeltanz-Holm, and Holm, "Attitudes, Knowledge, and Intentions Related to Breastfeeding Among University Undergraduate Women and Men";

Spear, "College Students' Experiences and Attitudes Regarding Middle and High School–Based Breastfeeding Education."
93. Li et al., "Public Beliefs about Breastfeeding Policies in Various Settings."
94. Sheeshka et al., "Women's Experiences Breastfeeding in Public Places."
95. Scott and Mostyn, "Women's Experiences of Breastfeeding in a Bottle-Feeding Culture," p. 276.
96. "International Code of Marketing of Breast-Milk Substitutes."
97. "Baby-Friendly Hospital Initiative."
98. "The Ten Steps to Successful Breastfeeding."
99. Ibid.
101. "Find Facilities."
102. "Breastfeeding Report Card: United States, 2014 - 2014 breastfeedingreportcard.pdf."
103. Ibid.
104. "The Baby-Friendly Hospital Initiative."
105. Semenic et al., "Barriers, Facilitators, and Recommendations Related to Implementing the Baby-Friendly Initiative (BFI)."
106. ASH/OPHS, "The Surgeon General's Call to Action to Support Breastfeeding."
107. Ibid.
108. Anstey, MacGowan, and Allen, "Five-Year Progress Update on the Surgeon General's Call to Action to Support Breastfeeding, 2011."
109. Ibid.
110. Ibid.
111. Ibid.
112. McDivitt et al., "The Impact of the Healthcom Mass Media Campaign on Timely Initiation of Breastfeeding in Jordan on JSTOR"; Kim, "The Effects of a Breastfeeding Campaign on Adolescent Korean Women."
113. Martin RM et al., "Effects of Promoting Longer-Term and Exclusive Breastfeeding on Adiposity and Insulin-like Growth Factor-I at Age 11.5 Years"; Wolfberg et al., "Dads as Breastfeeding Advocates"; Chen, Johnson, and Rosenthal, "Sources of Education about Breastfeeding and Breast Pump Use"; Haroon et al., "Breastfeeding Promotion Interventions and Breastfeeding Practices"; Imdad, Yakoob, and Bhutta, "Effect of Breastfeeding Promotion Interventions on Breastfeeding Rates, with Special Focus on Developing Countries."
114. Chen, Johnson, and Rosenthal, "Sources of Education about Breastfeeding and Breast Pump Use."
115. Parry et al., "Understanding Women's Interpretations of Infant Formula Advertising"; "GAO-06-282 Breastfeeding: Some Strategies Used to Market Infant Formula May Discourage Breastfeeding; State Contracts

Should Better Protect Against Misuse of WIC Name - d06282. pdf"; Howard, Howard, and Weitzman, "THE PHYSICIAN AS ADVERTISER."

116. Conrad, *The Medicalization of Society*; Soumerai, Stephen, Ross-Degnan, and Kahn, "The Effects of Professional and Media Warnings about the Association between Asprin Use in Children and Reye's Syndrome."
117. Chen, Johnson, and Rosenthal, "Sources of Education about Breastfeeding and Breast Pump Use."
118. Ibid.
116. Arora et al., "Major Factors Influencing Breastfeeding Rates."
119. Kornides and Kitsantas, "Evaluation of Breastfeeding Promotion, Support, and Knowledge of Benefits on Breastfeeding Outcomes."
120. Ibid.
121. Ibid.
122. Ibid.
123. Ibid.
124. Ward, Merriwether, and Caruthers, "Breasts Are for Men."
125. Ibid.
126. Ibid.
127. Ibid., p. 712.
128. Wolfberg et al., "Dads as Breastfeeding Advocates"; Maycock et al., "Education and Support for Fathers Improves Breastfeeding Rates A Randomized Controlled Trial"; Nickerson, Sykes, and Fung, "Mothers' Experience of Fathers' Support for Breast-Feeding."
129. McFadden et al., "Spotlight on Infant Formula"; Piwoz and Huffman, "The Impact of Marketing of Breast-Milk Substitutes on WHO-Recommended Breastfeeding Practices."
130. Fentiman, "Marketing Mothers' Milk."
131. Ibid.
132. Rollins et al., "Why Invest, and What It Will Take to Improve Breastfeeding Practices?"
133. Ibid.
134. Piwoz and Huffman, "The Impact of Marketing of Breast-Milk Substitutes on WHO-Recommended Breastfeeding Practices."
135. Ibid.
136. Bylaska-Davies, "Exploring the Effect of Mass Media on Perceptions of Infant Feeding."
137. Ibid.
138. Brown and Peuchaud, "Media and Breastfeeding: Friend or Foe?"
139. Foss and Southwell, "Infant Feeding and the Media: The Relationship between Parents' Magazine Content and Breastfeeding, 1972–2000"; Frerichs et al., "Framing Breastfeeding and Formula-Feeding Messages

in Popular US Magazines"; Potter, Sheeshka, and Valaitis, "Content Analysis of Infant Feeding Messages in a Canadian Women's Magazine, 1945 to 1995"; Young, "American Conceptions of Infant Development from 1955 to 1984."

140. Stang, Hoss, and Story, "Health Statements Made in Infant Formula Advertisements in Pregnancy and Early Parenting Magazines A Content Analysis."
141. Ibid.
142. Foss and Southwell, "Infant Feeding and the Media: The Relationship between Parents' Magazine Content and Breastfeeding, 1972–2000."
143. Frerichs et al., "Framing Breastfeeding and Formula-Feeding Messages in Popular US Magazines"; Potter, Sheeshka, and Valaitis, "Content Analysis of Infant Feeding Messages in a Canadian Women's Magazine, 1945 to 1995"; Young, "American Conceptions of Infant Development from 1955 to 1984."
144. Foss, "Perpetuating 'Scientific Motherhood.'"
145. Schanler, O'Connor, and Lawrence, "Pediatricians' Practices and Attitudes Regarding Breastfeeding Promotion"; Freed, Fraley, and Schanler, "Attitudes of Expectant Fathers Regarding Breast-Feeding."
146. Hausman, *Mother's Milk.*
147. Bentley, Dee, and Jensen, "Breastfeeding among Low Income, African-American Women."
148. Wolf, *Don't Kill Your Baby: Public Health and the Decline of Breastfeeding in the 19th and 20th Centuries.*
149. Huang, "The 2008 Milk Scandal Revisited"; Rollins et al., "Why Invest, and What It Will Take to Improve Breastfeeding Practices?"
150. Callaghan and Lazard, "'Please Don't Put the Whole Dang Thing out There!'."
151. Ibid.
152. Bylaska-Davies, "Exploring the Effect of Mass Media on Perceptions of Infant Feeding."
153. Brown and Peuchaud, "Media and Breastfeeding: Friend or Foe?"
154. Bylaska-Davies, "Exploring the Effect of Mass Media on Perceptions of Infant Feeding."
155. Scott and Mostyn, "Women's Experiences of Breastfeeding in a Bottle-Feeding Culture."
156. Bentley, Dee, and Jensen, "Breastfeeding among Low Income, African-American Women."
157. O'Brien, Zareai, and Fallon, "Creating a Breastfeeding Culture."
158. Ibid.
159. Ibid.

Conrad, *The Medicalization of Society*, p. 276.

See note 115.
See note 113.
Foss and Blake, "'It's Natural and Healthy, But I Don't Want To See It': The Impact of Entertainment Television on Breastfeeding Attitudes"; Kavanagh et al., "Breastfeeding Knowledge, Attitudes, Prior Exposure, and Intent among Undergraduate Students"; Li et al., "Public Beliefs about Breastfeeding Policies in Various Settings"; Marrone, Vogeltanz-Holm, and Holm, "Attitudes, Knowledge, and Intentions Related to Breastfeeding Among University Undergraduate Women and Men"; Spear, "College Students' Experiences and Attitudes Regarding Middle and High School–Based Breastfeeding Education."
Avery et al., "Factors Associated with Very Early Weaning Among Primiparas Intending to Breastfeed"; Sheeshka et al., "Women's Experiences Breastfeeding in Public Places."
Chapman et al., "Effectiveness of Breastfeeding Peer Counseling in a Low-Income, Predominantly Latina Population."
McCarter-Spaulding, "How Does Postpartum Depression Affect Breastfeeding?".
Stuebe, "Enabling Women to Achieve Their Breastfeeding Goals"; McClellan et al., "Nipple Pain during Breastfeeding with or without Visible Trauma"; Lewallen et al., "Breastfeeding Support and Early Cessation."
Schmied et al., "Women's Perceptions and Experiences of Breastfeeding Support"; Meedya, Fahy, and Kable, "Factors That Positively Influence Breastfeeding Duration to 6 Months."
160. Berger and Luckmann, *The Social Construction of Reality.*
161. Gitlin, "Prime Time Ideology," p. 518.
162. Hall, Evans, and Nixon, *Representation.*
163. Ibid.
164. Hausman, *Mother's Milk.*
165. Blum, *At the Breast*, p. 119.
166. Ibid.
167. Hesse et al., "Trust and Sources of Health Information."
168. Gerbner and Gross, "Living With Television."
169. Dixon, "Black Criminals and White Officers"; Lubbers, Schneepers, and Vergeer, "Exposure to Newspapers and Attitudes toward Ethnic Minorities"; Northup, "Is Everyone a Little Bit Racist?"; Givens and Monahan, "Priming Mammies, Jezebels, and Other Controlling Images"; Dong and Murrillo, "The Impact of Television Viewing on Young Adults' Stereotypes Towards Hispanic Americans."
170. Kahlor and Eastin, "Television's Role in the Culture of Violence Toward Women"; Kahlor and Morrison, "Television Viewing and Rape Myth

Acceptance among College Women"; Franiuk et al., "Prevalence and Effects of Rape Myths in Print Journalism The Kobe Bryant Case."
171. Lapinski and Rimal, "An Explication of Social Norms."
172. Ibid.
173. Soumerai, Stephen, Ross-Degnan, and Kahn, "The Effects of Professional and Media Warnings about the Association between Asprin Use in Children and Reye's Syndrome."
174. Nattinger et al., "Effect of Nancy Reagan's Mastectomy on Choice of Surgery for Breast Cancer by US Women."
175. Hornik, *Public Health Communication.*
176. Wolf, "What Feminists Can Do for Breastfeeding and What Breastfeeding Can Do for Feminists."
177. Ibid.
178. Ibid.
179. Smith, "Breastfeeding Promotion through Gender Equality."
180. Apple, "Constructing Mothers."
181. Ibid., p. 161.
182. Ibid.
183. Callaghan and Lazard, "'Please Don't Put the Whole Dang Thing out There!'."
184. Callaghan and Lazard, "'Please Don't Put the Whole Dang Thing out There!'," p. 945.
185. Douglas and Michaels, *The Mommy Myth: The Idealization of Motherhood and How It Has Undermined Women.*
186. {Citation}.

CHAPTER 2

"Where the Mother's Milk is Insufficient…": The Commodification of Infant Feeding and the Demise of Breastfeeding

In May of 1867, one of the first ads for manufactured infant food (what would later be called "formula") appeared in *The New York Times*.[1] This marketing ploy for Liebig's formula touted its product as "a perfect substitute" for breastmilk.[2] Within just a few years, a number of manufactured infant food companies emerged.[3] Heavy advertising ensued, with each brand trying to persuade consumers that their product was the best alternative to breastmilk. While this early marketing certainly was not the sole cause of the trend toward bottle-feeding in the mid- to late-1800s, its pervasive messages suggested to women that breastfeeding would likely fail and that a "safe" alternative would protect their children through the perils of infancy.

Before the lucrative marketing of milk substitutes, it was commonsense that babies needed breastmilk to survive. The extent to which a woman was successful at breastfeeding would determine whether her baby would live or die.[4] Infants needed to either suckle at their mothers' breasts or at the breasts of wet nurses.[5] Those who were not lucky enough to be breastfed, particularly abandoned babies, had very little chance of survival, even if adopted by well-meaning caregivers.[6] Yet, by the late 1800s, many women did not breastfeed, opting to give their babies artificial food, often with dire results. In *Don't Kill Your Baby: Public Health and the Decline of Breastfeeding in the 19th and 20th Centuries*, historian Jacqueline Wolf estimated that 10–15 bottle-fed babies died for every one breastfed child, primarily due to diarrhea from contaminated cow's milk and other substitutes.[7]

K.A. Foss, *Breastfeeding and Media*,
DOI 10.1007/978-3-319-56442-5_2

Considering that women had been taught for generations that breastmilk was the *only* suitable food for babies, how did the tide turn? How do you move from a breastfed population to an artificially-fed one, particularly when the consequences were often fatal? This chapter seeks to answer this question, using literature on this time period and a primary study of media discourse of *LHJ* to identify and help explain the ideological shift from "only the breast" to a cultural preference for bottles.

Changing Ideologies About Infant Feeding

Scholars have speculated about the timing and primary causes of the increasing preference for artificial food and bottles during this time. According to Janet Golden, the popularity of wet nursing in the 1700s and 1800s instigated changes in infant feeding norms by making it common practice for (wealthy) mothers not to breastfeed their babies, instead hiring lactating women (usually of a lower socio-economic status) to nourish their infants.[8] This practice became so popular that by the mid-nineteenth century, people began to associate class with milk supply, falsely assuming that high-society women simply did not produce enough milk.[9] By the mid- to late-1800s, more and more women began weaning early, supplementing with bottles, or choosing not to breastfeed altogether.[10] Recognizing the high mortality risks of cow's milk and artificial food, nineteenth-century physicians continued to strongly encourage breastfeeding.[11] Yet, the rise in women's inclination for bottle-feeding gradually changed the position of the medical profession.[12, 13] By the early 1900s, this societal shift to bottle-feeding had become solidified by the medical profession's endorsement of artificial foods.[14]

Other factors also contributed to the erosion of women's confidence in breastfeeding and the decision to bottle-feed. In conjunction with other cultural shifts of the 1800s, the commodification of infant feeding, first with human milk, and then artificial food, profoundly influenced infant feeding.[15] Long before physicians encouraged artificial feeding, mass media, through articles and ads, persuaded mothers to use alternatives to their breastmilk, reinforcing and perpetuating bottle-use as the modern norm. In this chapter, I argue that nineteenth century media discourse spearheaded the ideological shift in infant feeding perceptions and practice, establishing justifications for not breastfeeding that are still used 125 years later. Examining the marketing of wet nurses and milk substitutes in the 1700s and 1800s demonstrates how and when women stopped trusting their bodies to feed their babies against medical recommendations, while discourse of the 1900s highlights the growing acceptance of artificial food by the medical community, both with homemade doctor-recommended concoctions and manufactured infant food.

Wet Nursing: The First Alternative to Mother's Milk

As Golden laid out, the first commodification of infant feeding emerged long before manufactured breastmilk substitutes. Some upper-class women sought wet nurses because their husbands disapproved of them breastfeeding, particularly with beliefs in abstinence during lactation.[16] Others hired wet nurses out of convenience. When mothers could not breastfeed, wet nursing was vital to infant survival. In fact, churches and townships would pay for wet nurses to breastfed orphaned babies well into the 1800s.[17] For the wet nurses themselves, breastfeeding other people's children provided a stable income to women who would have otherwise had a hard time.[18] Unfortunately, this occupation often came at the expense of the wet nurses' own children, many of whom died after they weaned them early in preparation to feed their clients' children.[19]

Beginning in the late 1700s, wet nursing was heavily advertised in newspapers, regularly appearing in the classified sections. Rich families routinely posted ads in which they saught a "respectable woman" with a "good breast of milk." Such ads were common and often described breast size and nipple shape as connected to the perception of good milk. Women would also advertise their services. For example, a 1795 ad labeled "A Wet Nurse," published in the *Weekly Museum*, called for "A healthy woman, 26 years of age, of a respectable and unexceptionable character, (having a good breast of milk), wishes to take a healthy child of reputable parents, to suckle in her own house."[20] Similarly, a woman advertised her lactation services in the November 25, 1815 issue of *The Intellectual Regale*, describing herself as "a respectable young married woman, who has lost her infant, wishes to take a child of reputable parents to suckle in her own house."[21] In addition to these individual ads, some printers and later, intelligence offices and maternity houses, served as brokers for wet nurses.[22] A 1797 ad appearing in *The Time Piece and Literary Companion* declared, "Any person wanting a wet nurse may be supplied by applying at Charles Coleman's... She has a new breast of milk and can be satisfactorily recommended: She would, if required, take a child into the house to nurse."[23] Comparable ads for wet nurses appeared throughout the newspapers of this era, often specifying class, marital status, religion, and other demographics, along with moral characteristics.

The way in which wet nursing was advertised highlights the difficulty of commodifying a product that is so intimately connected to a person. In these relationships, authority of the wet nurse's body was unclear, which became even more complicated when growing medical interest in infant feeding prompted wealthy families to use physicians to screen wet nurses for disease.[24] Furthermore, the belief that diet and lifestyle influenced milk quality raised more questions about the extent to which families should be able to monitor and control their wet nurses' behavior.[25] Fear of disease transmission and the challenge of satisfactorily controlling wet nurses contributed to wet nursing losing popularity in the late 1800s.[26] Even when physicians were still recommending hiring wet nurses, mothers began choosing artificial feeding, except in the most severe cases.[27] A search for "wet nurse" ads in the ProQuest Historical database illustrates the decline in this practice—at the very least, in its marketing. In the 1860s, 433 classified ads call for wet nurses. The number dropped to 350 ads in the 1880s, down to 117 ads from 1900–1909. And, in the 1920s, only 17 ads for wet nurses appeared, which declined to no ads by the 1930s.

Wet nursing first presented mothers with an alternative to what had been considered the natural progression after pregnancy. The prevalence of ads for wet nurses helped to normalize the practice and present it as the "modern" trend for families who desired to flaunt their status. However, cultural shifts of the 1800s, paired with the extensive marketing of manufactured food, drove women to choose bottles, not wet nurses, when they believed that their milk supply was inadequate.

The Nineteenth-Century Media Landscape: Infant Food as a Product

Commercial media boomed in the 1800s. The onset of industrialization and urbanization drastically changed the American landscape. Before this era, people made most of their goods or purchased them locally. The industrial age brought factory-production and mass distribution. This process largely separated producers from consumers.[28] And for the first time, people had choices in their products, particularly in rapidly-expanding urban areas.[29] Thus, the practice of branding and trade-marking became important, often conveyed through ads, which introduced and familiarized consumers with particular brands and products.[30] This practice cultivated a consumer lifestyle, creating, as historian James Wood stated, "New desires in the minds of readers, desires that grew into needs and resulted in purchases."[31] As part of this consumer culture, advertising became a lucrative business, aided by the reduced cost of printing, the expansion of places to advertise, and a growing audience due to increased literacy rates, higher incomes, and urbanization.[32] Furthermore, lack of federal regulation and knowledge about disease causality meant that advertisers could make any claims about their products, including curative properties.[33]

The development of what were marketed as breastmilk substitutes fit perfectly into this expanding climate of consumerism. Wet nursing had introduced the misperception that some women (or "class of women") could not produce enough milk. Urbanization and immigration had cut off many women from their extended families—generations of women who traditionally would have guided the birth and lactation process.[34] And, enough women had begun feeding babies alternatives to human milk that the medical community had begun investigating "safe" ways to modify cow's milk.[35] All that was needed was a product to fill that gap. In the 1860s, Justus von Liebig developed a "substitute" for human milk containing cow's milk, malt flour, bicarbonate of potash, and wheat flour.[36] Almost immediately, people rushed to create their own versions of the "breastmilk substitutes," with Mellin's Food, Nestlé's Milk Food, Hawley's Food, Wagner's Infant Food, Carnrick's Soluble Food, and other brands appearing in the 1860s and 1870s.[37] By 1873, 27 brands of infant formula had been patented.[38] It should be noted that these "breastmilk substitutes" were far from safe alternatives to mother's milk. In fact, they held very little nutritive value, and since most of them required cow's milk, babies fed manufactured food still faced steep mortality rates like other bottle-fed babies.[39] Nonetheless, these products were heavily marketed in newspapers and magazines as revolutionary and even curative alternatives to breastmilk.

At the same time, chemists and physicians were responding to the increase in bottle-feeding by developing their own recipes for artificial food. Many doctors believed that since women were already bottle-feeding, there needed to be a safer alternative to human milk. Dr. Thomas Rotch, a professor of Diseases of Children at Harvard University, spearheaded scientific efforts to develop alternatives to human milk. His 1893 address to the Children of the Pan-American Medical Congress captured three points of the medical profession's prevailing view of infant feeding at the time—acknowledging the superiority of human milk, establishing that an "infant feeding problem" existed because of the increase in bottle-feeding, and lastly, explaining how it was the role of science and physicians to both create a "safe" substitute and oversee the feeding process.[40] Rotch declared that only by duplicating "the changes in the various elements of the breast-milk which satisfy the individual... can we finally arrive at the proper solution of this intricate feeding problem."[41] Building on Alfred Meigs' 1884 descriptive analysis of the composition of human milk, Rotch led the creation of milk laboratories that developed scientific recipes for artificial feeding.[42] Using Rotch's theories, in 1897, Emmet Holt published 10 formulas for infants for physicians to prescribe to their patients—a number that continued to expand.[43] Most physicians preferred this approach, called the American Method or percentage feeding, over manufactured food.[44] While manufactured infant food would eventually dominate, the percentage feeding guidelines by Rotch and other physicians of the time set the stage for the medical profession's acceptance of bottle-feeding in the early to mid-1900s.[45]

Media's Role in the Shift to Bottle-Feeding

As Wolf has demonstrated, breastfeeding rates did not initially decline due to pressure from ill-informed physicians.[46] Rather, women changed their feeding preferences and patterns in the mid- to late 1800s, against their doctors' recommendations.[47] To understand this cultural shift, extensive sources were examined. In addition to secondary scholarship on the early history of infant feeding in America, I used the Proquest Historical Database to locate articles and ads from this time period. Searches were conducted for "infant feeding," "infant food," "breast milk," and early milk substitute brand names. Articles related to human milk and infant feeding appearing in the late 1800s were also identified (spanning from 1887 to 1905). A search indicating the frequency of wet nursing ads was also conducted, producing ads from 1797 to 1971. Furthermore, medical journal issues from the 1800s were consulted for discussions on infant feeding, milk substitutes and breastfeeding to help contextualize the role of "experts" in this time period. Specifically, the *Journal of the American Medical Association* (*JAMA*) and the *New England Journal of Medicine* were explored.

This prelimary analysis established the media landscape for how infant feeding, breastfeeding, wet nursing, and increasingly, bottle-feeding, were talked about in various media sources from the late 1700s to the early 1900s. The frequency of articles about infant feeding and ads for wet nursing, then milk substitutes, also sets the stage for further media analysis. Analysis of secondary sources, background literature, and trends in women's media consumption in the late 1800s established the magazine *Ladies' Home Journal* (*LHJ*) as one of the earliest and key magazines appealing to women in this time period. In addition, this magazine was a prime outlet for advertising home and childcare products. Thus, a case study of the articles and ads in *LHJ*, 1883–1907, provides a look into changing ideology and the rise of milk substitute marketing in this time period.

Infant Feeding in *LHJ*

By the 1880s, more and more niche publications were emerging, appealing to both readers and advertisers, who took advantage of the clearly defined targeted audience. *Ladies' Home Journal* began in December 1883 as one of the first magazines for women (under the title Ladies' Home Journal and *Practical Housekeeper*). This publication quickly became popular. Within a year of its first issue, circulation reached 25,000 readers.[48] By 1886, the magazine had 400,000 subscribers.[49] Its audience spanned socio-economic class lines and clearly recognized women as consumers.[50] Compared to other women's magazines at the time, *LHJ* was affordable, relying heavily on advertising to subsidize the cost. Historian Helen Damon-Moore described how the publisher, Cyrus Curtis, aimed for "a wide lower-middle-class to middle-class audience for the magazine, one to whom his advertisers could sell their new products."[51] Indeed, this approach was effective. By 1900, *LHJ* had more readers than almost any other magazine in the United States, with a circulation of more than one million.[52] Clearly, the messages in this magazine were widely received, including those about infant feeding. Therefore, this magazine allows a look into the changing attitudes toward breast- and bottle-feeding, as well as an exploration into the early marketing of manufactured infant food in an era with no regulation. To better understand the messages about infant feeding, articles about infant feeding and ads for milk substitutes and artificial feeding products were analyzed for the period 1884–1907.[53] This period encompasses the beginning of the shift toward bottle-feeding, as well as the early 1900s, in which "feeding experts" started recommending artificial feeding. A textual analysis was conducted on both articles and ads. Frequency of both was also noted. The end date (1907) was selected because of *LHJ* availability in the *American Periodicals* online database.

Breastmilk or Death: 1884–1889

In the articles of the early years, breastfeeding[54] is promoted as the only safe way to feed a baby. From 1884 to 1889, 23 articles address breastfeeding. *LHJ* writers in this era were 95% women. Drawing from their own experiences, their advice assumed that women planned to nurse for an extended period of time.[55] Writers offered tips to make nursing more comfortable. Nurse and regular writer Elizabeth Robinson Scovil, who later published a manual on childrearing, provided lengthy advice in an 1890 column, instructing readers on how to help draw out inverted nipples by using hot water to create a vacuum in a bottle.[56] She addressed the common problem of nipple pain, suggesting a variety of solutions that included "bathing the nipples twice a day for six weeks before the confinement with powdered alum dissolved in alcohol; or salt dissolved in brandy" and suggested treating cracked nipples with "a mixture of tannin and glycerine," which must be wiped off before nursing.[57] Furthermore, rubber nipple shields are recommended as a means to help with pain.[58] In an advice column on home issues, "Mrs. M. McO" recommended a tea to help with diaper rash, adding, "This same wash is excellent for sore nipples."[59] She also commiserated with readers about clogged ducts (what she calls "caked breasts"), describing how she found "relief in pouring on melted lard as hot as can be borne, and laying on a warm flannel" and massaging the breasts "so that the milk will flow freely."[60] If those remedies fail, she advised using "a common clay pipe," also useful for weaning.[61] Here, solutions do not include supplementing with bottles or early weaning, but instead address practical remedies to make breastfeeding more comfortable.

New mothers were expected to follow a set of very specific "rules" to produce quality milk. According to articles of the 1880s and 1890s, nursing women should consume sugar for constipation and "a cup of cocoa, gruel made with milk, good beef tea, mutton broth, or any warm, nutritive drink" after meals and before bed, avoiding vinegar and strong tea after meals and before bed.[62] Maintaining an "even" temperament was apparently part of the breastfeeding discourse, as emotion was believed to influence milk quality and the baby's health. For example, in a series entitled "Talks with Mothers, with Eminent Physicians," Dr. E.W. Watson explained that "Calmness and an equable temper on the part of the mother are necessary if she would be a good nurse."[63] Similarly, in "Timely Hints About Baby," Ada E. Hazell warned women about the transfer of one's demeanor to her child, stating,

> Aside from the diet, many other causes affect breast milk, and that mother who values the health of her child will persistently endeavor to preserve a cheerful, even temperament, and to avoid becoming overheated from violent or too-prolonged exercise, manual labor, etc. Anything that unfavorably affects her milk will manifest itself in the fretting and disposition of the babe.[64]

Likewise, in 1890, Scovil reminded breastfeeding women of the importance of a "sound mind," emphasizing, "If a woman is nursing her child, a fit of passion, or an imprudence in diet will affect the baby more disastrously than it will the mother."[65] She goes on to warn mothers against becoming overly tired or "excited," for "Self-control is as necessary on physical as on moral grounds."[66] Such advice is reminiscent of the beliefs about milk quality and emotion for wet nurses from earlier in the century. It also likely prompted mothers to question whether they were negatively impacting their milk if they became tired or upset—difficult to avoid with a new baby.

Writers offered strict, but sometimes conflicting, rules for breastfeeding. Hazell advised women to nurse every 2 h so that milk would not "spoil" in the breast.[67] Watson urged women to avoid nursing at night and if necessary, "Very small babies can be accustomed to drinking cool water out of a glass, and will be glad to get it, instead of an extra meal which they do not need."[68] This practice, he believed, would improve the "quality of [mother's] milk."[69] Very little justification was given for needing to switch to milk substitutes. In fact, even a "lack of milk" could be corrected with "persistency" and diet.[70] Regardless of the issue, women were encouraged to breastfeed through it.

Not breastfeeding posed great risk for babies, according to the discourse of this time. For example, in 1884, a cautionary tale written in the third person describes a baby that died after physician-recommended weaning at age 2 months. One character says: "Doctor to fiddlesticks! What do I care for a doctor? What do ye s'pose we did fifty year ago when half the time we couldn't get a doctor? We raised our children then; we didn't kill'em; but we didn't have anything to do with weak-kneed doctors, nervous gals, and milk-bottles."[71] An angry reader responded to this story, lamenting, "Let the women of fifty years ago step into *our* places and have twelve children and do their own work. Ah! I think they too would resort to some milk-bottles."[72] This reader's letter indicates that the cautionary tales conflicted with contemporary women's practice. And yet, a satirical piece entitled "Now to Kill the Baby" humorously emphasizes bottle-feeding's danger, stating that to harm one's children, one can give the baby castor oil, anise, or "Get some prepared food; try three or four kinds—you want the best. Alternate between them and nature's supply."[73] In serious pieces, writers outlined the dangers, with statements like "Babies who are fed from the bottle, either wholly or partially, are naturally more liable to bowel disorders."[74]

Writers cautioned women of early weaning, which they defined as ceasing breastfeeding before 12–18 months of age, or before "the Second Summer," a period of high mortality for babies and young children due to "Cholera Infantum" (severe diarrhea caused by contaminated milk). Indeed, they had reason to do so, given the prevalence of diarrhea-related deaths for bottle-fed babies at this time.[75] Stories were used to emphasize the risk of weaning early or not breastfeeding, connecting artificial food with infant diarrhea and death. The frequent columnist "John's Wife" described artificially-fed babies as "very large and fat, but their flesh is of a spongy texture, their teeth backward in cutting, and they are more apt to fall victims to cholera infantum and dysentery."[76] She pleaded with her readers to think of their babies' health, stating, "If it is possible, take care of yourself and your diet this summer and nurse baby till October."[77] In 1887, *LHJ* ran a three-month series on "The Summer Complaint," with Dr. Watson advising mothers on how to protect their babies. In "The Care of Babies in Summer-time," Dr. Watson declared, "The baby on the bottle however is the greatest problem of the summer."[78] The following month, Watson simply stated, "When a baby is nursed at the breast there is little to say" because the child is protected, followed by a lengthy description about the health complications of substitute feeding and the difficulties of keeping everything hygienic for the baby.[79] Watson went into detail in another article: "Summer Diarrhea is generally caused by the failure of an infant to properly digest its food; the food being generally not that designed for it by nature; hence; the great proportion of sickness of this sort in babies, is found in the bottle-fed, rather than in those at the breast."[80]

In the midst of these pro-breastfeeding articles, there is some acknowledgement of bottle-feeding. After outlining the importance of breastfeeding in the summer, Dr. Watson instructed women on how to help the bottle-fed baby and protecting him/her from Cholera Infantum.[81] Similarly, Anna E. Watson in "About the Baby," began her article with, "The heated term is approaching when so many babies die, and so many mothers, who are unable to nurse their infants are asking, 'What shall I feed my baby?'"[82] A lengthy discussion of mixing baby bottles answered this question. Yet, these articles on bottle-feeding are in the minority and overall position bottles as a far inferior second to breastmilk.

Writers even warned women against introducing any solid food. In a letter to the editor section, a woman urged mothers to delay complementary foods, declaring, "Above all don't give nursing babies 'tastes' of the food you eat. Let a mother feed herself with the most nourishing food she can get and the child will thrive without feeding until it is 10 months old."[83] "John's Wife," also spoke strongly against adding table food too early. She wrote of a woman who gave her 10 month-old a slice of cucumber because "he cried for it," and as a result, "the child was dead within twenty-four hours." "John's Wife" added that another child died after eating green corn.[84] This opposition to complementary foods would radically change within the next few decades, illustrating the wholehearted acceptance of alternatives to mother's milk.

False Promises of Early Milk Substitutes

Advertisements during this era tell a different story than the articles. Despite the pro-breastfeeding messages in the content of *LHJ*, ads for milk substitutes regularly appeared even early in the magazine. The five-year period of 1884–1889 included 74 milk substitute ads and two ads for bottles. During the early days of artificial feeding, companies pitched directly to consumers, targeting a wide audience. Milk substitutes were not solely marketed to babies, but to "invalids," "dyspeptics," "aged people," and occasionally even as beverages for breastfeeding women. While other groups were mentioned, however, the text and images of these ads focused on feeding babies, therefore, profoundly undermining the stern warnings of artificial feeding in the magazine's articles. With the lack of marketing regulation, milk substitute corporations positioned themselves as the optimal solution to when mothers "couldn't breastfeed." An 1886 ad for Lactated Food began with "It may be used with confidence when the mother is unable, wholly or in part, to nurse the child, as a safe substitute for mother's milk.... It cause no disturbance of digestion and will be relished by the child."[85] Lactated Food made a similar claim in an ad the following year, declaring, "Very many mothers cannot properly nourish their children, and the milk of many mothers produces bad effects in the child because of constitutional disease or weakness."[86] Likewise, Nestlé's Food declared, "Where the mother's milk is insufficient Nestlé's Milk Food is alone to be recommended."[87]

Other brands went so far as to claim their products were equal to breastmilk. A December 1884 Mellin's Food ad declared it as "The only perfect substitute for Mother's Milk."[88] Similarly, Carnrick's Soluble Food ad, from March 1888, stated, "Perfectly nourishes the child from birth, without the addition of cow's milk, and digests as easily as human milk."[89] Nestlé's Milk Food claimed to be "the best substitute known for mothers' milk.... Its chemical analysis is almost indentical (sic.) with that of human milk.... It is very nourishing and produces firm flesh, hard bone and tough muscle."[90] Another Carnrick's ad claimed that it was "The only food that removes from infancy all necessity, danger, and annoyance of a wet nurse."[91]

Another popular marketing strategy was to undermine the effectiveness of other products. For example, one ad stated that the recommendation of Nestlé's by a "prominent" physician "will be appreciated by mothers who are perplexed by the mass of boastful and extravagant advertising of infant foods, to know which is really THE BEST."[92] Similarly, an 1888 Nestlé's ad explained that "Each new compound put on the market in the past few years has either aimed at *imitating* Nestlé's food or *attacking* it, thereby testifying to its superiority."[93] Carnrick's Food also positioned itself as a finer product than its competitors. A long-running campaign for Lactated Foods touted its product as "the most nourishing, the most palatable, the most economical, of all prepared foods."[94] Attacks were paired with consumer testimonials that supported the superiority of the marketed product, such as "Our Baby thrives on Horlick's food."[95] Another tactic was to advertise these products through pseudo-articles, which appear to be magazine content but are clearly ads for manufactured food. For example, in August 1885, text in paragraph form read "The milk of a nursing mother becomes singularly venomous through the operation of certain powerful emotions." This statement is followed by the anecdote of a woman who received bad news and then nursed, causing her baby to die. Below this "article" is an ad for the milk substitute Ridge's Food.[96] This combination frequently and increasingly appeared in the magazine, undermining the pro-breastfeeding messages.

Despite evidence that babies were dying from contaminated milk, artificial food companies capitalized on concerns about hot weather mortality, claiming that their products offered protection against Summer Complaint. In fact, the ad campaigns for Nestlé's and others shifted to focus on hot weather with statements like, "Nestlé's Food is especially suitable for infants in hot weather. Requires no milk in its preparation, and is effective in the prevention of cholera-infantum."[97] Lactated Food took its claim a step further, declaring it as "The safest food in summer for young or delicate children: A sure prevention of cholera infantum. It has been the positive means of saving many lives where no other food would be retained."[98] The text of the ad then explicitly stated that the product "does not cause sour stomach, irritation, or irregular bowels."[99] Another Lactated Food ad from the same year described the product as "a predigested, non-irritating, easily assimilated food."[100] Later that year, Lactated Food promised to "surely prevent fatal results," while Mellin's Food positioned itself as "invaluable in cholera infantum and teething."[101]

Much like Dr. Watson and other medical experts in the magazine content, milk substitute companies often included a doctor's recommendation as part of the advertising text, with words like "Commended by Physicians," "Sold by Druggists Generally," "Hundreds of physicians testify to its great value," "England's *best known* medical authorities," "A prominent Boston physician," "The Physician's Favorite," and sales aided by "the influence of the medical profession."[102] Advertisers also use references to general "experts," as Nestlé illustrated with an 1888 ad reading "all the prominent writers on infant's feeding give this food the first place as a diet in hot weather as a preventative of summer complaints."[103] As with this Nestlé's ad, artificial food companies particularly used health "experts" during the summer months. An even bolder ad campaign that ran for years included the text "Ziemssen's Cyclopedia of the Practice of Medicine, Vol. VII., of the standard work, says; 'IN CASES OF CHOLERA-INFANTUM, NESTLÉ'S MILK FOOD IS ALONE TO BE RECOMMENDED."[104] This campaign illustrates the importance of science and medicine in this era, as these companies used the endorsement of a few physicians or scientists to make it seem as though the medical profession wholly approved of these products. To further emphasize their authoritative positions on infant feeding, most of the artificial food companies ended their ads with the offer of advice or samples. Readers could request free infant care books, or samples, or even "a pamphlet giving important medical opinions" from most of these companies, including Mellin's Food, Nestlé's Milk Food, and Lactated Food.

Ads were stacked together so that readers would see a string of milk-substitute brands, with Mellin's Food, Horlick's Food, and Anglo-Swiss Milk Food on one page.[105] And, unlike magazine articles, increasingly, artificial food companies used drawings to bolster their messages. Anglo-Swiss brand incorporated the image of a sophisticated woman next to its messages. Some of the Lactated Food for Infants and Invalids included a sketch of a woman holding her child as an old woman points at them. Carnrick's Soluble Food contained the most dynamic illustration. Its half-page ad featured two sophisticated women standing next to an elaborately decorated baby carriage.[106] The caption below the drawing details how the baby had been very ill until "we tried CARNRICK'S SOLUBLE FOOD, which agreed with him at once".[107] In an era with very few images and illustrations, these ads would have been particularly eye-catching and influential.

The juxtaposition of pro-breastfeeding articles with the pervasive artificial food ads offered mixed and confusing messages for readers at the time. Practical advice and sometimes difficult to decipher cautionary tales about bottle-feeding could hardly compete with Nestlé and other manufactured food companies declaring that their products could protect babies from intestinal distress, especially when the ads far outnumbered the articles. Furthermore, the use of science and "medical recommendations" in the ads, but not the articles, presented these products as part of the emerging scientific trend at the end of the nineteenth century.

When Mother's Milk Inevitably Fails… 1890s–1900s

In the *LHJ* articles of the 1890s, narratives began to shift, suggesting a growing population of women that "couldn't breastfeed" or who just did not produce "enough milk." In the transitional period, breastfeeding is briefly mentioned, followed by instructions on artificial feeding.

Writers who had previously focused on breastfeeding advice started to shift to a more neutral position on infant feeding. For example, in 1891, Nurse Scovil wrote, "If the mother cannot nurse her child, and it has to be fed, the best preparation to begin with is good cow's milk, diluted with the same quantity of *boiling* water; three tablespoonfuls of one and three of the other is enough at first, sweetened with sugar of milk, which is very inexpensive."[108] Likewise, in 1898, columnist Mrs. S.T. Rorer began her piece with "I have already strongly urged that the early food of a young infant should be the breastmilk of its own mother. Where this cannot be, a modified milk may be used," then launched into a detailed overview on pasteurizing milk and then mixing it with water, milk sugar, cream, egg whites.[109] Here, the lengthy instructions convey the necessity of the advice.

By the early 1900s, this magazine discourse suggested that bottle-feeding had displaced the breast as the means of feeding a baby, even though records show that even by 1911, approximately two-thirds of women still breastfed their babies.[110] Although *LHJ* writers acknowledged breastfeeding as the preferable food at birth, they focused on its difficulty and offered lengthy instructions for mixing and preparing artificial food. The prevalence of this shift suggests that nursing was no longer a given or the norm. Themes that emerged in the 1880s continued, with strict breastfeeding rules and concerns about "Summer Complaint" (death from diarrhea in warmer months). Increasingly, though, these issues became justifications for weaning, as recommended by the featured "expert"—now a staple part of the magazine. Earlier years (presumably) used mothers as advice columnists, with bylines that included "John's Wife" and "Mrs. McO," with the occasional M.D. By 1889, male participation in the creation of *LHJ* had increased to 15%, likely, in part, due to the rise of male "experts."[111] Both male and female "experts" tended to support bottle-feeding. In 1902, Dr. Emelyn Lincoln Coolidge began regularly writing infant feeding-related articles. Coolidge became well-known as a childrearing "expert" even outside of *LHJ*, with multiple books published on infant feeding, including *The Mothers' Manual: A Month by Month Guide for Young Mothers* (1909) and *First Aid in Nursery Ailments* (1911). From 1902–1907, Coolidge published at least 35 articles on infant feeding in *LHJ*. Unfortunately, Coolidge was also a staunch advocate of modified milk and other foods for babies, perceiving breastfeeding as often inadequate and difficult to control. She even offered readers the service of prescribing the modified milk formulas through the mail, closing her articles with, "If the mother or nurse will send me a stamped and addressed envelope I will be glad to send a set of formulas with explicit directions for preparing the food, taking care of the bottles and nipples, etc."[112] Coolidge's prominence and personal connection to the readers set the stage for messages about infant feeding during this time period.

Under the "right" circumstances, experts and others alike encouraged breastfeeding at birth, for, as "Mrs. S.T. Rorer" wrote in 1900, "a child nursed even for a few weeks at the beginning of his life will have a far better foundation than the child who is given the bottle as soon as he is born."[113] However, there was a persistent assumption that exclusive breastfeeding was unsustainable, likely due to the rigid advice about breastfeeding. Writers advised new mothers to wait 12 h to nurse their newborns and then once the milk came in, breastfeed at fixed intervals of every 2 h, following a prescribed suckling time and maximum number of feedings per night.[114] Coolidge proposed longer intervals, with women only breastfeeding every 6 h for the first 3 days, then every 2 h, except at night.[115] This rigid advice, of course, would likely lead to an underfed baby and a low milk supply, as contemporary breastfeeding experts recommend intervals of no longer than 2–3 h for new babies.[116]

This advice on how to keep babies healthy continued, extending to the mother's habits, diet, and emotional state. Mothers were cautioned against indulging their babies' suckling desires, as it was recommended to keep the nipple "out of sight until the baby forgets it," and providing "boiled water" between feeding intervals.[117] A nursing mother was expected to maintain a strict diet of cornmeal, cocoa, cooked cereal, eggs and soups, get regular exercise, and "never allow a day to pass by without a free movement of her bowels."[118] Furthermore, the misperception that a woman's disposition transfers to her nursling persists in the 1890s and 1900s. A nursing mother was expected to "exercise great self-control of her emotions," otherwise her excitement could result in indigestion or colic.[119] For example, in "What to do when the baby is sick?" (May 1903), the author proposed that the mother's lack of exercise and regular bowel movements has been causing her baby's illness.[120] This advice likely undermined new mothers' confidence in breastfeeding, particularly when paired with bottle-feeding instructions and encouragement to supplement. "Experts" did not advocate for exclusive breastfeeding, stating, "There is no harm whatever in partly nursing and partly bottle-feeding a baby" to give mother more sleep.[121] Introducing bottles by at least 4 months was strongly encouraged so that "should the mother's milk then suddenly fail or should she be obliged to leave the child for a short time there will be no struggle which would be especially hard for the baby in the coming hot weather."[122]

Breastfeeding was framed as regimented, controllable, and restrictive. Obviously, such "rules" contradict contemporary knowledge of the importance of establishing one's milk supply and the detrimental impact of supplementing on breastfeeding initiation. The assumption, then, was that breastfeeding would ultimately fail, and when it did, experts in this magazine, other media outlets, and real-life would carefully prescribe a "scientific" concoction of branded milk substitutes and/or cow's milk, gruel, broth, eggs, sugar, baking soda, lime water, and other ingredients believed to be nutritious for babies.

Writers presented milk substitutes as the immediate and obvious solution to breastfeeding "problems," particularly Dr. Coolidge, who used "case studies," to demonstrate the need for breastfeeding mothers to supplement or wean completely. Coolidge often recommended supplementing with barley water and modified milk or complete weaning for a variety of new mother "problems," including fatigue from babies waking at night, small plateaus in infant weight gain, or for babies who cried after eating, which she suggested signified that the mother "has not enough milk or the milk is not strong enough."[123] Coolidge also advised mothers to dilute their breastmilk with barley water to help with teething.[124]

In comparison to earlier years when writers strongly encouraged nursing until 18 months or so, by the 1900s, weaning was recommended between nine and 12 months. Scovil warned mothers, "A child should never be nursed more than a year."[125] She echoed this message throughout her columns, even recommending earlier weaning. As with older articles, weaning continued to be connected to concerns about Summer Complaint (Cholera Infantum or severe diarrhea). Scovil added to one of her weaning declarations of 9 months, "unless this time comes in very hot weather, or the infant is so delicate that a change of food would be injurious."[126] Yet, the importance of nursing during the summer came with the caveat, "If the mother is not strong her nursling will sometimes thrive better upon artificial food than on its natural nourishment."[127] In July 1902, Coolidge similarly stated, "Although, of course, it is safer for a mother to nurse her baby through the summer months it is much better to wean the child if he is losing steadily in weight or shows marked signs of indigestion."[128] In a later article, Coolidge suggested that extended breastfeeding could even be dangerous, declaring, "Very few mothers can nurse their babies after the twelfth month without either injuring the child or themselves."[129] She endorsed nursing after a year only during the second summer and then in conjunction with gruels and broths.

As with other articles at this time, writers focused on bottle-feeding. Coolidge briefly acknowledged some protection of mother's milk against Summer Complaint, telling readers, "The breast-fed babies are not so likely to have attacks of summer complaint, and if they do have them the attack will, in most cases, be a short one, recovered from quickly."[130] At the same time, Coolidge recommended supplementing the breast-fed baby in hot weather, stating "If the child is breast-fed give him one ounce of boiled water or barley-water before nursing, when the day is very warm, and this will reduce the strength of the mother's milk after it is in the baby's stomach."[131] Coolidge strongly discouraged breast-feeding babies who developed diarrhea, arguing, "The general rule in treating cases of summer complaint now is to stop all milk at once."[132] She instructed nursing mothers to withhold breastmilk and instead give "nothing but gruels for twenty-four hours and using a breast pump for the mother during this time."[133]

Increasingly, writers emphasize the "deficits" of breastfeeding, presenting it as the source of health problems. One author explained that "sometimes a nursing baby will be constipated because he does not get enough food to form a residue in the intestines. If this is the case he will not gain in weight."[134] The solution then is to switch to "modified milk made with oatmeal gruel as a substitute for the same number of meals from the breast."[135] And even though bottle-fed babies also experience constipation, they are, according to this article, "easier to treat."[136] Doctors of this time conveyed that breastfed babies are at risk of rickets, asthma, anemia, and rheumatism.[137] The suggestion of these risks, again, weakened claims about bottle-feeding mortality and provided further justification for not breastfeeding.

Even with brief recommendations of breastfeeding at birth, the assumption in this era was that breastmilk would inevitably fail. Considering that the nursing advice given would almost certainly have destroyed a milk supply, it was not surprising that women began weaning earlier or not breastfeeding. Furthermore, should a mother succeed at nursing, supplementing was still encouraged, "just in case" the milk fails later on, especially because most mothers did not perceive the hiring of a wet nurse as an option. According to discourse in *LHJ*, wet nursing was outdated, except for extreme cases in which mothers "couldn't" breastfeed and the babies would not suckle from bottles. In 1904, Coolidge stated her opinion on wet nurses, explaining, "As a rule I advise wet-nurses as a last resort only. In the first place it does not seem fair to the nurse's own baby to deprive him of his mother's milk; then wet-nurses are, as a rule, expensive and very uncertain as to temper, sometimes making a great deal of trouble in a house."[138] She described how an extremely premature baby survived because of a wet nurse. One other article mentioned wet nursing: a story describing how an Italian immigrant abandoned her baby. A doctor examined the child, declaring that he wouldn't survive "unless a wet nurse could be found, and even then it would be one chance in a hundred if he pulled through."[139] They hired a wet nurse and the baby lives. However, this tale was more about the generosity of caring for "foundlings," than focused on the practice of wet nursing. The scarcity of recommendations for hiring wet nurses emphasized the acceptance and normalization of artificial food as the alternative to mother's milk. This discourse fits with Golden's overall discussion of wet nursing at this time, as still occurring, but invisible, and only as a last resort for ill babies.[140]

As Coolidge and others touted the difficulty of breastfeeding and the ease of artificial feeding in the early 1900s, advertisers continued to bombard *LHJ* readers with milk substitute propaganda. Like previous decades, the ads often began by stating the importance of breastmilk and then presenting their products as the next best choice for *when* breastfeeding fails, as Nestlé's Food illustrated, stating, "The mother's milk is the best food for the baby, but when this fails, Nestlé's Food is the best substitute" with a large picture of a stork.[141] Another Nestlé's Food ad also exemplifies this tactic: "When a mother is unable to nurse her child, mature and medical skill demand a substitute that shall as closely as possible resemble the mother's milk—not only in composition, but in the entire absence of all drugs and stimulants, like opium, malt or alcohol."[142] Eskay's Albumenized Food declared, "It is the ONLY FOOD that perfectly corresponds to mother's milk."[143] Sanipure milk made a similar assertion with "the most perfect substitute for mother's milk ever prepared."[144] Lactated Food stated that "Dame Nature provides the best food for babies, but there are often cases where it is impossible to feed the child naturally or where such feeding, because of some unhealthy condition, is absolutely dangerous."[145] This text was paired with a drawing of a plump, smiling baby, demonstrating the "quality" of its product.

As in earlier times, companies used science and experts to vouch for the effectiveness of their products, quoting mothers and physicians. The text in a Ridge's Food ad from 1890 illustrates this emphasis, declaring, "Its superiority to other similar preparations rests not only on scientific analysis, but on the crucial test of thirty years' experience. It has successfully reared more children than all other foods combined."[146] This connection to science and the use of experts helped support the milk substitute company's claims, which became much more outrageous in this period. Lactated Food was marketed as "far better than medicine. It keeps babies healthy, and is the perfect substitute for mother's milk."[147] Three years later, the company went a step further with its claims, adding, that "by regulating the digestion and supplying the natural elements for proper growth, it prevents and overcomes colic, poor sleep and the other troubles that afflict infants."[148] Companies asserted that their products even protected against Summer Complaint, as Nestlé's Food proclaimed to be "recognized by physicians in all countries as the safest and most natural substitute for the mother's milk, particularly in hot weather" and that it is "fortified against the severe strain of summer heat."[149] Testimonies and anecdotes were used to bolster these claims. An 1889 Lactated Food ad stated in large letters, "Baby's Life Saved." The text describes a baby who was "at the point of death with Cholera Infantum" until "Lactated Food saved her life."[150] Likewise, an Eskay's Food ad includes a picture of a baby next to, presumably, its story. The doctor said he would die "for the baby could not retain mother's milk, or any of the substitutes that the doctor prescribed" until he was saved by Eskay's Food.[151] These testimonies, combined with drawings of babies and endorsement by physicians in the text, normalized bottle-feeding, suggesting to an audience that bottle-feeding babies could have a positive outcome (even if the mortality rates of the era conveyed a starkly different message).

The marketing of nipples, bottles, and other artificial feeding supplies dramatically increased in the 1890s. To put it in perspective, between 1884 and 1889, only two ads for bottles or nipples appeared in the 60 issues of *LHJ*. In the next 5 years, *LHJ* included 59 ads for feeding supplies—a number that held steady for the follow 10 years, with 183 ads for bottles and nipples from 1889 to 1907. These messages conveyed the ease, convenience, and "health" benefits of their products. Mizpah Valve Nipples claimed to "Make nursing easy, and prevent much colic."[152] The Best Nurser bottle announced that it "prevents sickness, wind, colic, indigestion."[153] A Davidson Health Nipple ad featured a picture of a baby sitting up, with "Here comes my bottle" underneath the image.[154] Like the substitute ads, the prevalence of these messages conveyed that bottle-feeding was the new way of life.

Feeding products often addressed fears of illness from hidden dangers. An 1899 ad for The King Silver Nipple began with "Don't Risk the Baby's Health by using rubber nipples. They are neither clean nor sanitary; therefore not healthful, and not fit to convey food to the infant. The King Silver Nipple made of Sterling Silver."[155] Similarly, the Security' Nipple described itself as "Secures cleanliness; no ribs or collars to collect milk or germs."[156] While it is certainly not clear how these specific products would thwart contamination, this language demonstrates the growing widespread adoption of the germ theory of disease causality.

Over the 1800s, a dramatic ideological shift occurred in how mothers and health professionals viewed infant feeding. Industrialization, urbanization, immigration, changes in family life, the birth process, and other factors certainly influenced perceptions of how babies should be fed. Yet, what validated these justifications together was the heavy unregulated marketing of milk substitutes in the late 1800s and early 1900s. The commodification of infant feeding, first with the marketing of wet nursing, and then the far more lucrative sale of various milk substitutes successfully undermined women's confidence in breastfeeding. Shifts in discourse in the articles of *LHJ* conveyed the effectiveness of this advertising. In the early years, writers desperately encouraged women to breastfeed, offered advice on overcoming obstacles, and emphasized the dire risks of not nursing, through warnings of Summer Complaint and cautionary anecdotes of infant death from artificial feeding. Yet, amid these pro-breastfeeding articles were pages of ads whose language countered every pro-breastfeeding claim. The prevalence of these ads started to normalize artificial feeding, bolstered by eye-catching text and images and scientific wording that touted this approach as the modern way.

The articles and ads of the 1890s onward gave no indication of the frequency at which bottle-fed babies died from the concoctions administered instead of breastmilk. While writers gave a brief nod to "breast is best," the immediate jump to artificial feeding, paired with rigid rules for breastfeeding that would have likely destroyed milk supply, firmly established bottle-feeding as the means of feeding babies—"safe" as long as the "right" recipe was determined.

What did this shift mean for babies and mothers? The increase of artificial feeding held dismal consequences for children. Bottle-fed babies were 10–15 times as likely to die, compared to breastfed babies, yet women still made this choice.[157] In addition to high mortality rates, babies faced malnutrition and other health problems. At this time, milk substitutes did not contain many vitamins needed for healthy development. The absence of vitamin C in commercial milk substitutes and home-made formulas caused many children to develop infantile scurvy—a term coined in this era, demonstrating its prevalence.[158] And, while writers in *LHJ* argued that breastmilk increased the risk of rickets (caused by a vitamin D deficiency), its condition was more common in artificially-fed babies.[159] Rather than returning to the breast as the solution, physicians advised adjusting the "formula" or switching milk substitute brands as the answer. By the 1910s, while most women still initially breastfed, supplementation and weaning occurred much earlier than decades before. Increasingly, bottle-feeding was becoming the normal long-term means of feeding a baby, while breastfeeding, especially after the newborn stage, had become passé. It would take 60 more years before breastfeeding rates would rebound. As media messages had played a significant role in shifting dominate ideologies about infant feeding in the nineteenth century, they continued to do so throughout the next century.

Notes

1. "Breast Milk for Infants."
2. Ibid.
3. Apple, *Mothers and Medicine: A Social History of Infant Feeding.*
4. Ibid.; Wolf, *Don't Kill Your Baby: Public Health and the Decline of Breastfeeding in the 19th and 20th Centuries.*
5. Golden, *A Social History of Wet Nursing in America.*
6. Ibid.
7. Wolf, *Don't Kill Your Baby: Public Health and the Decline of Breastfeeding in the 19th and 20th Centuries.*
8. Golden, *A Social History of Wet Nursing in America.*
9. Ibid.; Wolf, *Don't Kill Your Baby: Public Health and the Decline of Breastfeeding in the 19th and 20th Centuries.*
10. Wolf, *Don't Kill Your Baby: Public Health and the Decline of Breastfeeding in the 19th and 20th Centuries.*
11. Ibid.
12. Scholar Rima Apple (1987) argued that bottle-feeding became popular because of the emergence of "scientific motherhood"—a twentieth-century paradigm in which women relied on experts for childrearing

advice, including guidance on infant feeding (Ehrenreich and English 1978). However, other historians have placed this change earlier, arguing that the medical community's involvement with infant feeding was a response to existing infant feeding choices (Wolf 2001).

13. Wolf, *Don't Kill Your Baby: Public Health and the Decline of Breastfeeding in the 19th and 20th Centuries.*
14. Apple, *Mothers and Medicine: A Social History of Infant Feeding*; Wolf, *Don't Kill Your Baby: Public Health and the Decline of Breastfeeding in the 19th and 20th Centuries.*
15. Golden, *A Social History of Wet Nursing in America*; Wolf, *Don't Kill Your Baby: Public Health and the Decline of Breastfeeding in the 19th and 20th Centuries.*
16. Fildes, *Breasts, Bottles and Babies—a History of Infant Feeding.*
17. Golden, *A Social History of Wet Nursing in America.*
18. Ibid.
19. Ibid.; Wolf, *Don't Kill Your Baby: Public Health and the Decline of Breastfeeding in the 19th and 20th Centuries.*
20. "A Wet Nurse," March 21, 1795.
21. "A Wet Nurse," November 25, 1815.
22. Golden, *A Social History of Wet Nursing in America.*
23. "A Wet Nurse," August 25, 1797.
24. Golden, *A Social History of Wet Nursing in America.*
25. Ibid.
26. Ibid.
27. Wolf, *Don't Kill Your Baby: Public Health and the Decline of Breastfeeding in the 19th and 20th Centuries.*
28. Wood, *Magazines in the United States.*
29. Ibid.
30. Ibid.
31. Ibid., p. 276.
32. Ibid.
33. Ibid.
34. Wolf, *Don't Kill Your Baby: Public Health and the Decline of Breastfeeding in the 19th and 20th Centuries.*
35. Ibid.
36. Apple, *Mothers and Medicine: A Social History of Infant Feeding.*
37. Ibid.
38. Baumslag and Michels, *Milk, Money, and Madness: The Culture and Politics of Breastfeeding.*
39. Apple, *Mothers and Medicine: A Social History of Infant Feeding*; Wolf, *Don't Kill Your Baby: Public Health and the Decline of Breastfeeding in the 19th and 20th Centuries.*

40. Rotch, "The General Principles Underlying All Good Methods of Infant Feeding."
41. Ibid., pp. 505–506.
42. Apple, *Mothers and Medicine: A Social History of Infant Feeding.*
43. Ibid.
44. Fomon, "Infant Feeding in the 20th Century."
45. Apple, *Mothers and Medicine: A Social History of Infant Feeding*; Fomon, "Infant Feeding in the 20th Century."
46. Wolf, *Don't Kill Your Baby: Public Health and the Decline of Breastfeeding in the 19th and 20th Centuries.*
47. Ibid.
48. Damon-Moore, *Magazines for the Millions: Gender and Commerce in the Ladies' Home Journal and the Saturday Evening Post, 1880–1910.*
49. Ibid.
50. Ibid.; Zuckerman, *A History of Popular Women's Magazines in the United States, 1792–1995.*
51. Damon-Moore, *Magazines for the Millions: Gender and Commerce in the Ladies' Home Journal and the Saturday Evening Post, 1880–1910*, p. 26.
52. Wood, *Magazines in the United States.*
53. For the 1884–1889 database, a search was done using the keyword "milk." Relevant articles were then identified for further analysis. In the "1889–1907" database, "milk" yielded too many results. "Breast" AND "Milk," as well as "Bottle" were then searched, restricted to articles. Advertisements for milk substitutes and bottle-feeding and breastfeeding supplies were also collected, using the terms "milk substitute" for all dates, "Nipple OR Bottle" for the early years and "Nipple" OR "Nursing Bottle" for the latter years. Furthermore, ads for the specific milk substitute brands Nestlé, Carnrick, Ridge's Food, Lactated Food, Allenburys, Sanipure, Eskay's, and Anglo-Swiss were also searched.
54. Nursing, not breastfeeding, is the term used, with breastmilk and mother's milk as the substance. Writers use "bottle-feeding," "modified cow's milk," "artificial food," and "milk substitutes" for the non-breastmilk substances given to babies. The word "formula" to mean milk substitute does not appear in *LHJ* until 1906.
55. Damon-Moore, *Magazines for the Millions: Gender and Commerce in the Ladies' Home Journal and the Saturday Evening Post, 1880–1910.*
56. Scovil, "Words for Young Mothers," October 1890.
57. Ibid.
58. Ibid.
59. Mrs. M. McO.
60. Ibid.
61. Ibid.

62. Hazell, "Timely Hints About Baby"; Scovil, "Words for Young Mothers," October 1890.
63. Watson, "Talks with Mothers, By Eminent Physicians: The Care of Babies in Summer-Time."
64. Hazell, "Timely Hints About Baby."
65. Scovil, "Words for Young Mothers," October 1890.
66. Ibid.
67. Hazell, "Timely Hints About Baby."
68. Watson, "Talks with Mothers, By Eminent Physicians: The Care of Babies in Summer-Time."
69. Ibid.
70. John's Wife, "An Answer to 'Mrs. S.'"
71. "'Nater' vs. Milk-Bottles."
72. Morice, "'Nater' vs. the Milk-Bottle Again."
73. "Now to Kill the Baby."
74. Hazell, "Timely Hints About Baby."
75. Wolf, *Don't Kill Your Baby: Public Health and the Decline of Breastfeeding in the 19th and 20th Centuries*; Golden, *A Social History of Wet Nursing in America*; W.S., *Summer Complaint and Infant Feeding*.
76. John's Wife, "An Answer to 'Mrs. S.'"
77. Ibid.
78. Watson, "Talks with Mothers, By Eminent Physicians: The Care of Babies in Summer-Time."
79. Watson, "Talks with Mothers, By Eminent Physicians: Babies' Summer Hygiene."
80. Ibid.
81. Ibid.
82. Watson, "About the Baby."
83. The Mother of Five, "The Mother of Five."
84. John's Wife, "When Shall the Baby Be Weaned?"
85. "Lactated Food," 1886.
86. Lactated Food, "Crying Babies."
87. "Nestlé's Food."
88. "Mellin's Food," 1884.
89. "Carnrick's Soluble Food," 1888.
90. "Nestle's Milk Food," 1885.
91. "Carnrick's Soluble Food," 1887.
92. Nestlé's Milk Food, "Ringer's Ringing Recommendation."
93. Nestlé's Milk Food, "Winter Diet."
94. "Lactated Food," 1886.
95. Horlick's Food, "Our Baby."
96. "Article 2."

97. Nestlé's Milk Food, "Hot Weather."
98. "Lactated Food," 1886.
99. Ibid.
100. "Lactated Food," 1886.
101. "Lactated Food," 1886; "Mellin's Food," 1887.
102. "Mellin's Food," 1884; "Anglo-Swiss Milk Food"; "Lactated Food," 1886; Nestlé's Milk Food, "Ringer's Ringing Recommendation"; "Nestlé's Milk Food," 1887; "Lactated Food," 1887; Nestlé's Milk Food, "Secure Strong Hard Teeth for Baby."
103. Nestlé's Milk Food, "About Your Baby's Teeth."
104. Nestlé's Milk Food, "Hot Weather."
105. "Mellin's Food, Horlick's Food, Anglo-Swiss Milk Food."
106. "Carnrick's Soluble Food," 1887.
107. Ibid.
108. Scovil, "Feeding Very Young Babies."
109. Rorer, "Proper Cooking for the Nursery: New Cooking Lessons: Number Three."
110. Baumslag and Michels, *Milk, Money, and Madness: The Culture and Politics of Breastfeeding.*
111. Damon-Moore, *Magazines for the Millions: Gender and Commerce in the Ladies' Home Journal and the Saturday Evening Post, 1880–1910.*
112. Coolidge, "The Young Mothers' Home Club: An Ounce of Prevention Is Better Than a Pound of Cure."
113. Rorer, "The Proper Food for a Child in Summer."
114. Rorer, "Proper Cooking for the Nursery: New Cooking Lessons: Number Three"; Scovil, "Feeding Very Young Babies."
115. Coolidge, "The Young Mothers' Home Club: An Ounce of Prevention Is Better Than a Pound of Cure."
116. Sears and Sears, *The Breastfeeding Book.*
117. Coolidge, "The Young Mother and Her Child." Coolidge, "What to Do for a Baby Month By Month."
118. Coolidge, "The Young Mother and Her Child: The Proper Management of Breast-Fed Infants."
119. Ibid.
120. "What to Do When the Baby Is Sick."
121. Coolidge, "The Young Mother and Her Child: The Proper Management of Breast-Fed Infants."
122. "What to Do for a Baby Month by Month."
123. Coolidge, "Mother's Calendar: Four Breast-Fed Babies Who Did Not Thrive, and How"; Coolidge, "What to Do for a Baby Month By

Month"; Coolidge, "The Young Mother's Calendar: Why Four Babies Could Not Sleep."
124. Coolidge, "The Young Mother's Calendar: The Baby's Mouth and Teeth."
125. Scovil, "Feeding Very Young Babies."
126. Scovil, "Words for Young Mothers," 1890.
127. Ibid.
128. Coolidge, "The Care of the Baby in Summer."
129. Coolidge, "The Young Mother and Her Child: The Proper Management of Breast-Fed Infants."
130. Coolidge, "The Young Mothers' Summer Club," 1906.
131. Coolidge, "The Young Mothers' Summer Club," 1906.
132. Coolidge, "The Young Mothers' Summer Club," 1906.
133. Coolidge, "The Young Mother's Calendar: What to Do for Summer Complaint."
134. "What to Do When the Baby Is Sick."
135. Ibid.
136. Ibid.
137. Coolidge, "The Young Mothers' Home Club: The Prevention of Rheumatism in Children"; "The Eleventh and Twelfth Months"; "What to Do When the Baby Has the Rickets."
138. Coolidge, "Mother's Calendar: The Care of Premature and Backward Children."
139. Toby, "A Mother to Five Hundred Babies: A New York Woman's Beautiful Work."
140. Golden, *A Social History of Wet Nursing in America.*
141. Nestlé's Milk Food, "When the Stork Has Brought the Baby."
142. Nestlé's Milk Food, "Natural Law in the Baby World."
143. Eskay's Albumenized Food, "It's Worth Crying for."
144. Sanipure, "Have Your Baby Thrive."
145. Lactated Food, "Proper Food for Infants."
146. "Ridge's Food for Infants and Invalids."
147. Lactated Food, "Baby's Life Saved."
148. Lactated Food, "Proper Food for Infants."
149. Nestlé's Milk Food, "Natural Law in the Baby World"; Nestlé's Milk Food, "One Minute's Talk with Baby's Mother."
150. Lactated Food, "Baby's Life Saved."
151. Eskay's Albumenized Food, "It's Worth Crying for."
152. "Mizpah Valve Nipples."
153. "The Best Nurser."

154. "Davidson Health Nipple."
155. King Silver Nipple, "Don't Risk the Baby's Health."
156. "Security Nipple."
157. Wolf, *Don't Kill Your Baby: Public Health and the Decline of Breastfeeding in the 19th and 20th Centuries.*
158. Dobson, *Disease.*
159. Apple, *Mothers and Medicine: A Social History of Infant Feeding.*

CHAPTER 3

Infant Feeding in the Twentieth Century: Shifting Media Messages and the Role of the "Expert"

> Parents are often confused by the conflicting advice of relatives and well-meaning friends! Consult the doctor on all questions directly concerning baby's health… Always ask his advice before making feeding changes. ("Redhead," May 1945, p. 53)

This advice, given in a 1945 ad for Heinz Baby Foods in *Parents* magazine, captures the overarching belief of the twentieth century—that infant feeding decisions were best left to medical professionals and "scientific" evidence, not mother's intuition. This dependency on "experts" would dominate throughout this century, even as the specific mode of feeding changed. Examining two parenting manuals of the early 1900s, followed by a case study of infant feeding discourse in *Parents* magazine, demonstrates the changing ideologies and the role of "experts" in these shifts.

As stated in Chap. 2, at the beginning of the twentieth century, most women started out breastfeeding their babies. In 1911, approximately two-thirds of babies in the United States were breastfed.[1] Yet, times were shifting. By the 1920s, physicians largely supported and recommended artificial feeding. Thus, began the era in which Apple attributed

A portion of this chapter first appeared as Foss, K.A. (2010). Perpetuating "scientific motherhood": Infant feeding discourse in *Parents* magazine, 1930–2007. *Women & Health*, 50(3), 297–311. Reprinted with permission.

K.A. Foss, *Breastfeeding and Media*,
DOI 10.1007/978-3-319-56442-5_3

low breastfeeding rates to the "scientific motherhood," a time in which "educators, social commentators, physicians, health reformers and mothers themselves, promoted the idea that mothers needed to learn about science and medicine."[2] As part of this expectation, mothers were encouraged to learn about "scientific" approaches to childrearing, including infant feeding, from physicians, child care manuals, general interest journals, and women's magazines.[3]

Interestingly, "experts," like those that regularly contributed to *LHJ* did not generally promote, nor condemn breastfeeding. The influence was less direct. Instead, the "experts" would encourage mothers to adhere to strict rules and scheduling, which was often detrimental to milk production.[4] Childrearing and mothering handbooks were common. For example, both *LHJ* contributors Dr. Elizabeth Robinson Scovil and Dr. Emelyn Lincoln Coolidge published manuals in the early twentieth century. Scovil's *How to Bring Up a Baby: A Hand Book for Mothers* (1906), was a free manual, distributed "with the compliments of the manufacturers of Ivory Soap."[5] Scovil offered meticulous advice on various topics, such as "Children's hair should not be cut until they are at least 3 years old" and after bathing a child, you must "dry by 'patting'—not rubbing—with the towels."[6] Breastfeeding was mentioned once, in the midst of a lengthy discussion of feeding, "A mother need not stop nursing her baby because her milk does not seem to agree with it. By diet and exercise, by increasing or shortening the length of time between the nursing, the character of the milk can be changed until it suits the digestion."[7] This advice is followed by a long discussion of how to modify milk and prepare bottles.[8]

Coolidge published several manuals on childrearing. *The Mothers' Manual: A Month By Month Guide For Young Mothers* (1909) offered recommendations on salient issues for each of baby's first 12 months and then older children. The book's introduction established the credence of both Coolidge and the book itself (reinforcing the "scientific motherhood") as Margaret E. Sangster declared, "With the utmost confidence that not a line of this book is other than trustworthy and immediately helpful, as well as in-touch with the latest developments of medical science, *The Mothers' Manual* is sent forth to the mothers of America."[9] Like Scovil's book, Coolidge outlined very specific rules and schedules, along with prescribing ointments and other remedies for good health, including treating the umbilical stump with "bismuth," and dipping a baby's hand in quinine to cure thumb-sucking.

Feeding advice was abundant in this book, with rules in every chapter dictating scheduling and quantity. Scovil encouraged mothers to breastfeed at birth, stating, "Unless there is some very good reason to the contrary, a mother should nurse her own child."[10] For newborns, Scovil advised intervals of every 2 h, with two night feedings, and giving baby "boiled water" between feedings.[11] This paragraph was followed by over two pages on how to modify and administer milk-substitutes in bottles. After the newborn stage, Scovil offered additional feeding advice, including washing out baby's mouth and wiping the breasts with boric-acid. By 4 months, she suggested starting babies on bottles (if they have not done so already). Scovil asserted, "Should the mother's milk then suddenly fail, or should she be obliged to leave the child for a short time, there will be no struggle, which would be especially hard for the baby if it happened to be in hot weather."[12] This rationale was followed by lengthy advice on how to introduce bottles. Scovil firmly proclaimed:

> If a baby has always been fed from the breast he should be weaned completely by the end of his first year, unless there is some especial reason for continuing his mothers' milk. Children who are nursed too long are apt to have rickets or anaemia.[13]

Coolidge and Scovil's assumptions in their advice reinforced and showcased prevalent attitudes of the early 1900s. Yes, women were breastfeeding, but for shorter periods of time and supplementing earlier. It should be noted here that these parenting manuals, like *LHJ*, were very much geared toward white, upper-class, literate women who had the time and the means to implement the advice.

In the early 1900s, health professionals would encourage women to breastfeed, but only in "ideal" situations. At the first sign of "trouble" for babies (crying, poor sleeping, eating "too much," appearing to eat "too little," illness, etc.) or mothers, doctors were quick to recommend artificial feeding.[14] Physicians then advised women to prepare a complicated concoction based on the "percentage" system or use manufactured milk substitutes.[15] With the difficulty of the percentage system, increasingly, this manufactured food ("formula") became the dominant substitute.[16] Media discourse reinforced and perpetuated this bottle-feeding trend, which fueled the perception of commercial formula as a symbol of "modernity" and status, due to its cost and the scientific design of the product.[17] Infant feeding was very much tied to socio-economic class and poverty. While "high society" women were choosing to wean earlier, working-class mothers had little choice in using milk substitutes. As Wolf pointed out, without refrigeration to safely keep expressed milk, the babies of working-class women were fed artificial food, often with dire results.[18] Despite some health interventions to increase breastmilk for babies, especially in impoverished families, breastfeeding rates dramatically declined over the first half of the twentieth century.[19] By the late 1940s, approximately 25% of women breastfed and fewer than 5% were still nursing at 6 months. What bottle-fed babies were consuming had also shifted. By the 1960s, more than 90% of bottle-fed infants used commercial formula, instead of concocting their own modified-milk recipes themselves.[20] Breastfeeding rates continued to decline until their record low of 21% in 1971.[21]

Interestingly, during this era of steady decline, artificial food marketing, which had played a significant role in the initial switch to bottle-feeding, no longer directly targeted consumers.[22] By the early 1900s, medical professionals increasingly frowned upon the direct-to-consumer marketing of artificial food, perceiving the practice as dangerous to babies, as it bypassed the medical supervision that they believed necessary to ensure proper nutrition.[23] After the success of Dexi-Maltose and other milk substitute products that were sold "by prescription only," and endorsed by physicians, more artificial food companies began voluntarily advertising only to the medical community.[24] Formula companies began removing preparation instructions from their products' packaging, instead referring consumers to their doctors for feeding instructions.[25] The ban on direct-to-consumer marketing for formula became official in 1932, when the Committee on Foods (of the American Medical Association) restricted commercial formula advertising to health professionals only.[26] Companies that did not comply would not earn the AMA's "Seal of Acceptance."[27]

Despite this self-imposed ban, direct-to-consumer marketing did not cease entirely. Companies continued to advertise complementary foods and condensed milk products to the general public. Other media discourse reinforced and perpetuated the bottle-feeding preference that would dominate until the 1970s. The question is then, in this time of pro-bottle-feeding, what was media's role? How did narratives and advertising shift with the resurgence of breastfeeding in the 1970s? This chapter explores infant feeding messages in a popular women's magazine throughout the twentieth and early twenty-first centuries. An examination of *Parents* magazine (1930–2007) demonstrates the way in which media solidified artificial feeding as the modern way to feed a baby and then later changed with the cultural context to promote breastfeeding. Furthermore, this chapter will outline the rise of the "expert" in infant feeding decisions.

Context: Shifting from Trade to Profession

Dramatic changes occurred for medicine and journalism from the late 1800s to the early 1900s, as both shifted from trades to professions, impacting the role of "experts" in infant feeding and its media discourse. In the 1800s, physicians were generally not highly regarded, which was understandable given the little they could do to help their patients.[28] The discovery of anesthesia in the 1850s, acceptance of the "germ theory," and the subsequent adoption of antiseptic practices increased doctors' capabilities to successfully treat injuries and disease.[29] This growing understanding of disease causality, numerous scientific developments, and the standardization of medical schools in the 1910s helped bolster the credibility and trust in physicians as respected authorities on health.[30] Increasingly, this expertise included infant feeding.[31]

How information, including health information, was conveyed in both news and marketing was also shifting. The emergence of journalism schools standardized training for reporters and shifted journalism from a trade to a profession.[32] In newspapers, an objective model began to replace the nineteenth century literary preference for news writing.[33] Led by Adolph Ochs at *The New York Times*, this style emphasized "facts" and balance.[34] Advertising also changed in this era. The Food and Drug Act of 1906, combined with industry self-censorship by the newly-created American Advertising Association, forced advertisers to avoid making claims that could not be substantiated.[35] As a result of this censorship and a growing recognition of women as a target audience for goods, advertising messages with emotional appeals became dominant by the 1920s.[36]

These transformations resulted in changes in how products were marketed, including the promotion of milk substitutes. As Chap. 2 demonstrated, the artificial food (formula) ads in *LHJ* used powerful, exaggerated claims about the abilities of their milk substitutes to prevent and cure disease. Such ads were not published (at least not in reputable publications) in the twentieth century. Thus, advertising discourse had to shift dramatically in this later time. The question is then, how was artificial feeding talked about and advertised in this era of regulation, both as breastfeeding was declining (1910s–1960s) and then in its resurgence? Exploring media discourses over time can help identify the ideological shifts in infant feeding attitudes and trends over the next 60 years.

Shifting Discourses in *Parents* Magazine

An examination of *Parents* magazine from 1930 to 2007 illustrates how media may have shaped and impacted infant feeding decisions, even as breastfeeding rates plummeted (1930–1971) and then began to rise (1972–2007). *Parents* magazine replaced *LHJ* as the case study for this era for several reasons. In his thorough historical analysis of *Parents* magazine, Steven Schlossman explained the origins of this magazine in 1926, as part of a social movement on child development.[37] During the Great Depression, Schlossman stated that this magazine was the only periodical with steady growth in circulation numbers and advertising revenues and was "acclaimed as the most popular educational periodical in the world."[38] Furthermore, secondary literature on *LHJ* suggests its emphasis on creating a domestic identity in the 1900s, of which childrearing was important, but not the sole focus as in *Parents* magazine.[39]

Parents magazine provides a solid look at changing discourse over time in that it has been regularly published since 1926, has historically had a wide circulation and continues to be popular, consistently having a circulation of over two million.[40] This magazine is still one of the leading publications on parenting and regularly addresses infant feeding and other childrearing issues.[41] Much like the case study of *LHJ* in the late 1800s, following discussions of infant feeding in one popular magazine over 79 years allows a consistent examination of how infant feeding has been addressed longitudinally, even if the discourse itself has changed. 1930 marked one of the first years that *Parents* magazine was published, at a time in which breastfeeding rates were beginning to decline.[42] This year also fell in the middle of the AMA's creation of the formula marketing restrictions (1929–1932), which dramatically changed how infant foods would be advertised.[43] Finally, this time period allowed for an extensive study of how infant feeding discussions have shifted. To select a range of issues for the qualitative analysis, yet maintain a manageable sample size, I used a constructed year to determine the sample. To allow for differences in the time of year, the January, May, and September issues from these years were examined. A total of 237 issues, spanning 79 years, were analyzed.

To conduct the analysis, the magazine issues were examined to identify which articles and photographs addressed infant feeding. All non-advertising content was considered for this study, including feature stories, letters to the editor, and readers' questions and answers. Articles were selected for further analysis if any part of the text addressed infant feeding, such as the words, "bottle," "feeding," "nurse," "breast milk," "breastfeed," and "formula." Photographs that addressed infant feeding were also selected for more in-depth analysis. Articles and photographs did not need to focus on infant feeding to be included for further analysis. For example, an article that described the experiences of a visually-impaired man raising a child was included because he mentioned bottle-feeding his baby.[44]

Infant feeding messages in relevant articles and photographs were then examined. The following questions further guided the analysis: Did the author mention both bottle and breastfeeding? Which feeding method was listed first? What was said about the method of feeding? Did the author discuss the difficulties of breastfeeding without providing solutions to these problems? Was infant feeding advice limited to experts or did readers contribute? Images accompanying the articles were noted, serving as visual cues to the "preferred" (or normative) means of feeding a baby. Since commercial electric breast pumps were not available until the 1990s, unless an article or photo caption mentioned expressed breastmilk, this research assumed that references to bottle-feeding referred to formula consumption.[45]

Of the 237 issues studied, 95 addressed breastfeeding, bottle-feeding, or both. Thirty-five articles solely mentioned bottle-feeding and 29 only addressed breastfeeding. Additionally, 31 articles referred to both breast- and bottle-feeding. Forty-six images of bottle- or breastfeeding appeared in the issues studied: 23 of breastfeeding and 23 of bottle-feeding. The time period from the 1990s to 2007 contained the most articles and images.

Promoting the Bottle: 1930s to 1960s

Articles of the 1930s and 1940s primarily focused on bottle-feeding. During this time period, nine articles exclusively mentioned bottle-feeding, while three articles of this time exclusively mentioned breastfeeding. In other words, when only one form of feeding was mentioned, it was typically bottle-feeding. For example, feature stories on infant's schedules described giving the bottle as part of one's day. In a 1934 article entitled, "Feeding the new baby," Regina J. Woody described the experience of bringing an infant home from the hospital. Woody wrote, "Once you are at home and the baby safely tucked into his little crib, you will be confronted, almost immediately, with the practical necessity of warming and giving some of the formula which the hospital has so kindly provided your baby."[46] The reference to the hospital providing the formula suggested that a new mother would have made this choice, especially because breastfeeding was not mentioned.

In these early years, when writers referred to both feeding methods, they generally placed bottle-feeding first in the article, giving it more attention. For example, in a 1943 article on equipment for feeding baby, the writer described the modern supplies available to aid in bottle-feeding, adding "Even if you are fortunate enough to be able to nurse your baby, it is necessary to have heatproof, shockproof glass bottles for water, orange juice, or supplementary feedings."[47] The focus on bottle-feeding, combined with the writer's word choices, indicated that breastfeeding was so difficult that even breastfed infants likely require supplements of formula or other liquids.

The assumption that most women did not breastfeed was supported in a 1944 article, which described formula feeding as the preferred choice. Hazel Corbin stated, "Although mother's milk is the natural food for babies, there are still more babies who are 'artificially' fed than there are babies who are nursed," presenting breastfeeding as less common.[48] Corbin advised readers on proper formula preparation, writing, "Mothers should realize at the outset that preparing the baby's milk according to formula means work, takes time, and requires precise attention to details."[49] Photos of a woman carefully mixing bottles and a woman bottle-feeding her baby accompanied this story. From 1930–1959, images of infant feeding almost exclusively depicted bottle-feeding. In fact, until 1955, no images of breastfeeding appeared in the issues studied.

In articles of the 1930s and 1940s, writers referred to "outdated" practices of the past, emphasizing that "modern" readers preferred bottle-feeding. A 1938 article on feeding described the importance of utilizing "modern medicine" to raise healthy babies. Dr. Ernest Caufield explained, "Today the modern mother reads scientific articles, discusses the latest medical discoveries at afternoon teas, and takes her baby for periodic examinations."[50] Caulfield's writing exemplified thinking of the scientific motherhood—not only should women depend on medical doctors for help with infant care, especially their infant's nutrition, but they should seek out additional expert advice on their own.[51] Writers of this time period also celebrated "modern" technology in advising parents on how to feed their infants, using X-rays of an infant's stomach, for example, to demonstrate the best position for feeding babies.[52] Photos of the X-rayed infant further emphasized the importance of trusting technology, more than a woman's intuition or experience.

Such beliefs fit with the general acclamation and confidence in science at the time. In *Deliver Me From Pain: Anesthesia & Birth in America*, Jacqueline Wolf described the popularity of the drug-induced birth experience in the mid-twentieth century.[53] Physicians freely administered anesthesia and narcotics to laboring mothers, rendering them unconscious for the actual birth, which often included the use of forceps and routine episiotomies.[54] New mothers scarcely got to see their newborns, much less feed them, as babies stayed in nurseries and were only delivered to their mothers at four to five hour intervals in the day, with no night visits.[55] Even if women wanted to breastfeed, hospital practices at the time almost guaranteed failure.[56] And yet, media at the time applauded the "pain-free" birth and the "advances" of science.

Advertising Without Directly Marketing Formula

By the 1930s, most artificial food companies had agreed to solely advertise to the medical profession, ceasing direct-to-consumer marketing (excluding condensed milk).[57] This trend continued until 1989, when Nestlé released television commercials for formula, targeting the general public.[58] *Parents* magazine exemplifies this pattern, with only 45 ads specifically for formula appearing in the magazine from 1930 until 1988. However, marketing for products that supported formula usage frequently appeared in the magazine, including ads for bottles, nipples, bottle sterilizers, baby cereal, and condensed milk, often using experts and scientific language to promote the product. For example, a 1930 Pyrex Nursing bottle ad illustrated this medical endorsement, with "For *your* baby, *doctors urge* Pyrex Nursing bottle. Hundreds of doctors—all over the country—urge the use of these boil-proof Nursing Bottles… Physicians say these bottles promote higher infant health standards because they make absolute feeding regularity so much more certain."[59] As opposed to the 1800s ads, these products did not claim to prevent severe illness and death, but still declared their safety and health benefits, and encouraged a reliance on experts. A May 1938 ad declared: "Carnation Milk is safe, uniform, nourishing, more easily digested than is ordinary milk. And it's *irradiated*, to provide your baby with 'sunshine' vitamin D the year round... Ask your doctor about a formula for *your* baby containing Irradiated Carnation Milk."[60] A seal of approval from the Council on Foods of the American Medical Association visibly endorsed the ad.

Advertising for formula-feeding products was steady from 1930 until the 1970s. A study of these ads by Foss and Southwell suggested a negative correlation between the number of pro-bottle-feeding advertising and breastfeeding rates the following year, even without the promotion of formula itself.[61] Combined with articles that solely endorsed bottle-feeding, *Parents* magazine clearly reinforced formula as the means of feeding a baby, ignoring mothers during this time that did breastfeed.

Returning to the Breast: Transitions in the 1960s and 1970s

In the 1960s, tone and language shifted in the magazine articles, apparently marking a transitional period in perceptions of infant feeding. In 1960, Maja Bernath wrote, "Breast milk is nutritious, safe and easily digested; so is properly prepared formula," and then argued that the feeding experience mattered more than the means of feeding.[62] This neutral statement suggested the beginning of a shift from formula as the prevailing food to breastfeeding. Increasingly, articles encouraged women to breastfeed, conveying its benefits to the mother and infant. In a 1964 story, Dr. Ashley Montagu stated, "Biologically, psychologically, and physiologically, what better reassurance and promise of good things to come can the baby be given than to be held in his mother's arms, and encouraged to nurse at her breast?"[63]

As in previous decades, stories of the 1960s conveyed that breastfeeding could be challenging. However, unlike past articles, writers addressed overcoming breastfeeding obstacles like sore nipples, low milk supply, feeding premature infants, and nursing after a Caesarean section. In a 1970 article, Gloria Goldreich explained: "Some people believe, also incorrectly, that mothers delivered by Caesarean section cannot nurse their babies. But the production of breast milk is not affected by the means of delivery. Women who have Caesareans are free to nurse if they choose."[64] Acknowledging a shift from formula to breastmilk as the dominant infant food, another story encouraged mothers who did not nurse their older children to breastfeed their subsequent babies.[65]

In 1971, breastfeeding had reached an all-time low, with only 21% of mothers choosing to nurse.[66] By this point, the Second Wave Feminist Movement had encouraged women to take back their bodies from the medical profession, encouraging natural childbirth and birth reform.[67] Hospital practices and perceptions of infant feeding started to shift away from medicalized births, nurseries, and rigid schedules to more natural experiences, with prenatal childbirth classes, newborns rooming in and feeding on demand.[68] In addition, support for breastfeeding specifically also became more prevalent with the growing popularity of La Leche League (LLL) and other forms of support.[69]

By this time, most infant feeding articles promoted breastfeeding. Stories that described a new baby's schedule or a woman's labor and delivery included breastfeeding. For example, an article entitled "Hospital hints," told readers, "You'll be encouraged to breastfeed soon after you deliver. Nursing doesn't always come naturally, so ask ahead of time to see a lactation consultant."[70] During this time, articles about infant feeding generally referred to specific issues a breastfeeding mother might face, including breastfeeding rights, a nursing mother's nutrition, medication to avoid, exercising and nursing, and safely expressing and storing breastmilk. Unlike stories of the transitional period, however, stories seldom addressed specific health challenges, like mastitis and thrush.

"Breast is Best"—1980s, 1990s and Beyond

Over the next 30 years, breastfeeding rates fluctuated, yet still remained much higher than the 1970s. In 1982, 61.9% of mothers initiated breastfeeding.[71] This number decreased between 1983 and 1989, down to 51% (still much higher than the 21.7% initiation rate for 1971), with 43% exclusively breastfeeding.[72] From 1990 on, breastfeeding initiation has steadily risen. While exclusive breastfeeding and duration have also increased, these rates have not jumped at the same pace as initiation.[73] At the turn of the twenty-first century, approximately 69% of women tried breastfeeding, about 46% did exclusive breastfeeding, and an estimated 17% exclusive breastfeeding at 6 months.[74] A decade later, the national initiation rate was 75%, with 43% breastfeeding at 6 months, and only 13.3% exclusively breastfeeding at that time.[75]

Surprisingly, as breastfeeding was dramatically increasing in the 1970s, discussions of infant feeding, including nursing, were nearly absent from *Parents* magazine in the late 1970s and 1980s. More articles assumed that mothers would try to breastfeed, mentioning only breastfeeding or breastfeeding first before bottle-feeding. For example, the 1980 article "All About Breastfeeding, 25 Vital Questions and Answers" offered advice on a range of breastfeeding topics, from breast size to vegetarianism, followed by a short paragraph on bottle-feeding.[76] Likewise, Nissa Simon wrote "Why Breast-feed?" in 1984, touting its benefits.[77]

Yet, a few articles recommended supplementing, weaning or only address formula feeding. In "Starting Solids" (1982), Robert B. McCall included a section entitled "When breast milk isn't enough." The bolded headline and paragraph conveyed that breastmilk could be nutritionally inadequate.[78] The 1988 "Is Breast is Best?" article recommended supplementing premature babies (preemies) with formula because mother's milk may not be "nurtritionally sufficient for preemies."[79] For example, the "Doctor on call" article "Switching Formulas" (2001) outlined types of formula, with no breastfeeding mentioned.[80] Pictures of bottles or bottle-feeding also appeared during this time, for example, accompanying the 1988 article "Food to Grow On."[81] Mothers were also discouraged from extended nursing during this time, as illustrated in a reader question section in a 1989 article "Too Old For Breastfeeding?," in which the author stated that babies should wean to cow's milk after a year, otherwise breastfeeding may "interfere with normal independent development."[82]

In the 1990s, *Parents* featured more breastfeeding articles than bottle-feeding ones. In May 1992, a lengthy article explains how mothers can succeed with nursing while working, offering information on preparing to return to work and pumping.[83] The "day in the life" type articles also featured breastfeeding as a regular part of having a baby. A caption for the May 1993 article on a single mother's "diary" read "Sam loves my kitty more than anything else in life, except for me and my breasts."[84] Similarly, the May 1998 article "New Breastfeeding Guidelines" emphasized the importance of early breastfeeding initiation, exclusivity, and longer duration.[85] A 2003 article conveyed breastfeeding as the "norm," stating, "More moms are nursing their infants than ever before. A recent report found that in 2001, nearly 70% of mothers breastfed at birth (either exclusively or in combination with formula)."[86] Other articles present both breast and bottle-feeding as "choices," such as the September 1992 article "Parents Guide: Breast & Bottle Feeding," accompanied by a baby nursing and a man bottle-feeding a baby.[87] Even with the parallel title, the article was more focused on breastfeeding, suggesting nursing positions, books, and advice on overcoming obstacles to help with breastfeeding.[88]

Articles conveying breastfeeding experiences of "real" women became popular in the 1990s. At this time, more articles used readers' experiences and advice to each other—mostly household tips and humorous anecdotes. For example, readers offered tips in the series "From Our Readers: Can you help?" on a variety of subjects, such as using ice cube trays for freezing breastmilk, using the dishwasher to clean bottles, or wearing a camisole for easy nursing access. Readers also shared humorous stories in a monthly column entitled, "How embarrassing!" and "From our readers: I can't believe I did that! Parents confess to their most embarrassing moments." One tired mother wrote in explaining how she was so exhausted that she accidentally tried to nurse her toddler's doll, instead of her infant.[89] These tips and humorous stories primarily referred to breastfeeding, but sometimes mentioned bottle-feeding.

Most articles used a light-hearted tone and addressed easy-to-fix obstacles or situations. Only one article conveyed that the pressure to breastfeed has caused feelings of guilt for women who could not or chose not to breastfeed. In an article entitled, "Bottle-feeding Guilt" a mother lamented, "I breastfed my baby for 3 months while on my maternity leave. But once I returned to work, I couldn't keep up with the pumping, so I switched to formula. Now I feel horrible. Have I harmed my baby?"[90] The writer quoted Dr. Will Wilkoff, stating, "Pat yourself on the back for being among the roughly 65% of mothers who nurse at all. Though the American Academy of Pediatrics recommends that new moms breastfeed for at least 6 months, sticking with it for even 3 months provides a newborn with significant health and nutritional benefits."[91] While the "pat on the back" may have comforted the reader, the doctor reinforced the guilt associated with weaning by referring to the breastfeeding recommendations.

The many articles on embarrassing stories and domestic breastfeeding tips reflected the upward breastfeeding trends of the 1990s and 2000s. Photos accompanying the stories indicated that more women were breastfeeding. At the same time, since these (mostly reader) contributions primarily focused on trivial concerns or situations, their inclusion may have glossed over common real-life hindrances to successful breastfeeding, such as fears of insufficient milk, sore nipples, infection, and adjusting to working and breastfeeding. Furthermore, if expectant mothers were already worried about embarrassment or difficulty breastfeeding, these shared experiences may have contributed and magnified the readers' fears.

"Experts" in Infant Feeding

As with *LHJ* in the late 1800s and early 1900s, medical experts and medical research supporting dominant methods of infant feeding have been a staple part of *Parents* magazine throughout the 70 years studied. Beginning with Dr. Clara Davis in January of 1930, physicians and nurses contributed numerous articles on infant feeding. Psychoanalysts, anthropologists, therapists, and behavioral specialists also offered advice on infant feeding. This expert advice followed the general trends identified in this magazine—supporting bottle-feeding in the early years, citing the "difficulty of breastfeeding" and then promoting breastfeeding in later years. From the 1970s on, physicians regularly had monthly health pages in the magazine, in which readers could write-in questions for the doctors. In the late 1990s and 2000s, medical doctors responded to readers' health questions in regular health columns in the magazine. For example, a medical doctor answered readers' health questions in the monthly column "Dr. Nathanson on call." Readers asked for advice on reducing infant spit-up, if it was normal for babies to sweat while nursing, and many other health-related questions. This use of experts suggested that infant feeding was and continued to be considered within a medical framework throughout the time period studied.

Between 1968 and 2007, writers used medical research to encourage women to breastfeed, conveying its health benefits. According to *Parents* articles, breastfeeding helps the uterus contract,[92] provides antibodies used to ward off infection,[93] supplies all necessary nutrients for an infant,[94] helps to mature the intestinal tract, protects infants born without thyroid hormones, helps destroy parasites,[95] can increase intelligence,[96] and can reduce the risk of obesity.[97] No articles included medical research that addressed reasons not to breastfeed. In cases in which medical experts did not author the magazine story, writers often quoted doctors for their medical opinions. For example, the story about a mother's guilt, quoted a doctor's advice and in the column, "Health Q & A," in which a reader asked "Should I stop breastfeeding if I have a really bad cold?" the writer quoted Dr. Jane Morton, who advised the woman to continue nursing.[98] It is notable here that "experts" in the magazine had changed their perceptions toward breastfeeding, as weaning would have been recommended for illness and other obstacles in the early years studied.

The use of "experts" and scientific evidence has been a constant in this magazine, even as perceptions of which means of infant feeding have shifted. From a public health framework, it is positive that *Parents* magazine conveyed the benefits of breastfeeding, especially when it was new knowledge that breastmilk improved the health of babies. From a Feminist perspective, however, the division between women sharing lighthearted, mundane stories and the "experts" touting benefits leaves a gap in the discourse. Women's real breastfeeding experiences are missing here, including narratives about overcoming individual and institutional obstacles. This magazine also lacks diversity in its breastfeeding women, which may contribute to disparities across ethnic groups.

The Rise of Breastfeeding in Medical Journals

The significant increase in medical journal articles on breastfeeding over the twentieth and twenty-first century establishes the "experts'" growing interest in breastfeeding. To better understand the quantitative trends, a search on "breast-feeding," was conducted for the *New England Journal of Medicine* (*NEJM*) and *Journal of the American Medical Association* (*JAMA*) online databases. These journals mark two of the oldest and most popular medical journals in the United States.[99] As discussed in Chap. 2, in the early 1900s, the medical profession focused on concocting milk substitutes. Illustrated in Table 3.1, only one article that references breastfeeding appeared before 1900. Between 1900 and the 1970s, *NEJM* only averaged 8.25 articles on breastfeeding per decade. *JAMA* published an average of 12.5 articles. In other words, these prominent medical journals devoted only one or two articles on breastfeeding per year until the 1970s.

Fitting with *Parents* ideological shifts in infant feeding and United States breastfeeding rates, in the 1980s, the number of articles on breastfeeding significantly increased. *NEJM* published 50 articles related

Table 3.1 Frequency of Breastfeeding Articles in Medical Journals, 1883–2016

Year	*NEJM*	*JAMA*
1880s	0	0
1890s	0	1
1900s	6	7
1910s	24	13
1920s	14	24
1930s	5	17
1940s	1	3
1950s	2	13
1960s	5	13
1970s	9	10
1980s	50	34
1990s	112	81
2000s	139	17
2010–August 2016	102	7

to breastfeeding, compared to only nine the decade before. Similarly, *JAMA* moved from 10 articles in the 1970s to 34 in the 1980s. The numbers kept climbing. Across the two journals, 193 breastfeeding articles appeared in the 1990s and 156 in the 2000s. Since 2010, 109 articles on breastfeeding have been published in *NEJM* and *JAMA*. This rise in breastfeeding articles in medical journals demonstrates the growing recognition of breastfeeding as a public health issue, reflecting efforts established by the Code, the *Innocenti Declaration*, and other actions toward increasing rates. At the same time, this medical interest in breastfeeding is reminiscent of the physicians' role and interest in developing artificial food in the early 1900s and the continued presence of the "scientific motherhood." While the prevalence of breastfeeding studies reported in *JAMA* and the *NEJM* certainly helps raise public awareness of benefits and encourages health professionals to encourage breastfeeding, this medical frame also reinforces a dependency on experts and not on experience and intuition.

Conclusion

This chapter incorporated analysis of mothering manuals from the early 1900s and 77 years of magazine articles to explore ideological shifts in infant feeding and the constant role of the "scientific motherhood." From this study, it is clear that popular media reflected and perpetuated changing tides of infant feeding, with the steady use of experts and science to support the prevailing opinions. And yet, couched in a sea of bottle-feeding ads, articles started to encourage breastfeeding even before the rates began to change. "Experts" consistently advised women, regardless of the message. The fluctuation of breastfeeding articles in medical journals correlated both with breastfeeding rates and with the ideological shifts noted in *Parents* magazine. This study of media also demonstrates what was omitted from mainstream publication. Women of color are largely absent from this magazine. Moreover, fathers and partners are rarely mentioned, as *Parents* magazine largely means "mothers' magazine." This product mostly ignored unconventional family structures, infant feeding in Lesbian, Gay, Bisexual, Trans and Queer (LGBTQ) couples, people with disabilities raising children, and other underrepresented groups. Like the mothering manuals, the audience appeared to be a very specific demographic. Although breastfeeding is presented as the "typical" experience by the 1990s, it was only "typical" for a narrow group of mothers: middle-upper socio-economic class, able-bodied, light-skinned, heterosexual, and married—thus reinforcing class and race disparities in breastfeeding images and text. And, as stories and advice columns mainly focused on individual problems and experiences, institutional and cultural barriers to breastfeeding were overlooked. No mention of the Nestlé boycott or International Code of Breastmilk Substitutes appeared in any of the issues studied, even though other social justice concerns were covered. Moreover, this absence of the Nestlé boycott and macro-implications of breastfeeding for society presented and continues to present breastfeeding as a choice for individuals, with individual consequences. And, as the following chapters illustrate, these messages are not unique to this magazine or this medium alone, but are consistently conveyed through other media outlets and during contemporary times.

Notes

1. Hirschman and Butler, "Trends and Differentials in Breast Feeding."
2. Apple, *Mothers and Medicine: A Social History of Infant Feeding*; Apple, "Constructing Mothers," p. 162.
3. Apple, "Constructing Mothers."
4. Wolf, *Don't Kill Your Baby: Public Health and the Decline of Breastfeeding in the 19th and 20th Centuries.*

5. Scovil, *How to Bring Up a Baby: A Hand Book for Mothers*, p. 3.
6. Ibid., p. 36, 23.
7. Ibid., p. 14.
8. Ibid.
9. Coolidge, *The Mothers' Manual: A Month By Month Guide for Young Mothers*, p, 13.
10. Ibid., p. 21.
11. Ibid.
12. Ibid., p. 68.
13. Ibid., p. 166.
14. Apple, *Mothers and Medicine: A Social History of Infant Feeding*.
15. Ibid.
16. Greer and Apple, "Physicians, Formula Companies, and Advertising."
17. Van Esterik, *Beyond the Breast-Bottle Controversy*.
18. Wolf, *Don't Kill Your Baby: Public Health and the Decline of Breastfeeding in the 19th and 20th Centuries*.
19. Ibid.
20. Fomon, "Infant Feeding in the 20th Century."
21. Hirschman and Butler, "Trends and Differentials in Breast Feeding"; Ryan, Wenjun, and Acosta, "Breastfeeding Continues to Increase Into the New Millennium."
22. Greer and Apple, "Physicians, Formula Companies, and Advertising"; Apple, *Mothers and Medicine: A Social History of Infant Feeding*.
23. Greer and Apple, "Physicians, Formula Companies, and Advertising."
24. Ibid.
25. Ibid.; Apple, *Mothers and Medicine: A Social History of Infant Feeding*.
26. Greer and Apple, "Physicians, Formula Companies, and Advertising."
27. Ibid.
28. Apple, *Mothers and Medicine: A Social History of Infant Feeding*; Starr, *The Social Transformation of American Medicine*.
29. Starr, *The Social Transformation of American Medicine*; Tesh, *Hidden Arguments : Political Ideology and Disease Prevention Policy*.
30. Tesh, *Hidden Arguments : Political Ideology and Disease Prevention Policy*; Starr, *The Social Transformation of American Medicine*; Foss, *Television and Health Responsibility in an Age of Individualism*.
31. Apple, *Perfect Motherhood*; Apple, *Mothers and Medicine: A Social History of Infant Feeding*.
32. Mindich, *Just the Facts*.
33. Forde and Foss, "The Facts—the Color!—the Facts."
34. Schudson, *Discovering the News: A Social History of American Newspapers*.
35. Marchand, *Advertising the American Dream : Making Way for Modernity, 1920–1940*.

36. Ibid.
37. Schlossman, "Perils of Popularization."
38. Ibid., p. 66.
39. Odland, "Unassailable Motherhood, Ambivalent Domesticity"; Fox, "Selling the Mechanized Household."
40. "PARAAMStatement.pdf"; "Parents Magazine—Encyclopedia of Children and Childhood in History and Society."
41. "Parents Magazine—Encyclopedia of Children and Childhood in History and Society."
42. Newton, "Psychologic Aspects of Lactation."
43. Greer and Apple, "Physicians, Formula Companies, and Advertising." Newton, "Psychologic Aspects of Lactation."
44. Collins, "Fatherine by Touch."
45. Lepore, "Baby Food: If Breast Is Best, Why Are Women Bottling Their Milk?"
46. Woody, "Feeding the New Baby."
47. "Ample Supply of Bottles, Nipples."
48. Corbin, "How to Prepare the Baby's Formula."
49. Ibid.
50. Caulfield, "How Baby Care Has Changed."
51. Ehrenreich and English, *For Her Own Good: 150 Years of the Experts' Advice to Women.*
52. Tomkins and Slater, "Five Important Rules for Feeding Baby."
53. Wolf, *Deliver Me from Pain.*
54. Ibid.
55. Ibid.
56. Ibid.; Apple, *Mothers and Medicine: A Social History of Infant Feeding.*
57. Apple, *Mothers and Medicine: A Social History of Infant Feeding.*
58. Greer and Apple, "Physicians, Formula Companies, and Advertising."
59. Pyrex, "For Your Baby."
60. Carnation Milk, "This Gold Age for Babies."
61. Foss and Southwell, "Infant Feeding and the Media: The Relationship between Parents' Magazine Content and Breastfeeding, 1972–2000."
62. Bernath, "A Bottle for Baby with Love."
63. Montagu, "What Babies Need Most."
64. Goldreich, "Facts and Fallacies about Cesarean Births."
65. Kaminetzky and Meilach, "When Another Baby Is on the Way."
66. Ryan, Wenjun, and Acosta, "Breastfeeding Continues to Increase Into the New Millennium."
67. Wolf, *Deliver Me from Pain.*
68. Ibid.; Wright and Schanler, "The Resurgence of Breastfeeding at the End of the Second Millennium."

69. Brimdyr, "Lactation Management: A Community of Practice"; Wright and Schanler, "The Resurgence of Breastfeeding at the End of the Second Millennium." Chetley, *The Politics of Baby Foods.*
70. Mitchell, "Hospital Hints."
71. Ryan, Wenjun, and Acosta, "Breastfeeding Continues to Increase Into the New Millennium."
72. Ibid.
73. Ibid.
74. Ibid.
75. "Breastfeeding Report Card–United States, 2010."
76. Olds, "All About Breastfeeding, 25 Vital Questions and Answers."
77. Simon, "Why Breast-Feed?"
78. McCall, "Starting Solids."
79. Evans, "'Is Breast Best?' Q & A," p. 45.
80. Nathanson, "Doctor on Call: Kids' Health & Safety: Noted Pediatrician Laura Nathanson Tackles Your Tough Question: Switching Formulas."
81. Karlsrud and Schultz, "Food to Grow on."
82. "Too Old for Breastfeeding?"
83. "How Working Moms Can Breast-Feed."
84. Lamott, "And Baby Makes Two."
85. Schaaf, "New Breast-Feeding Guidelines."
86. "Breastfeeding Boom."
87. "Parents Guide: Breast & Bottle Feeding."
88. Ibid.
89. Lightfoot, "Sleepless and Showing It."
90. "Bottle-Feeding Guilt."
91. Ibid.
92. Shainess, "The Fine Art of Mothering."
93. Krugman, "What Does a Baby Need Most?"; Simon, "Why Breast-Feed?"; "Germs and Babies."
94. Wessel, "Ask Dr. Wessel: Why Give Vitamin Supplements?"; Karlsrud and Schultz, "Food to Grow on."
95. Simon, "Why Breast-Feed?"
96. Graham, "A Smart Start"; Dublin, "Boost Your Baby's IQ."
97. "6 Ways to Fat-Proof Your Child."
98. "Health Q & A."
99. "About NEJM Past and Present"; "About JAMA."

CHAPTER 4

Breastfeeding Promotion, Formula Marketing and the Role of Health Professionals

An obviously pregnant woman climbs up on a mechanical bull. The crowd cheers and the woman yells, "Woohoo!" as the bull picks up speed, tossing her around. Cut to a title slide with "You wouldn't take risks before your baby's born." The expectant mother falls off the bull. "Why start after?" The woman jumps up to applause. We see "Breastfeed exclusively for six months," as the voice-over states, "Studies show that babies who are breastfed are less likely to develop ear infections, respiratory infections, and diarrhea. Babies were born to be breastfed" (paired with a hotline and website from the U.S. Department of Health and Human Services).[1]

In the early 2000s, the Ad Council created a series of public service announcements (PSAs) for the Department of Health and Human Services' campaign to improve national breastfeeding rates.[2] As the bull-riding PSA demonstrates, these videos were unique in that, instead of emphasizing benefits, they highlighted the health risks of not breastfeeding.[3] Fearing the effectiveness of these messages, formula company executives so heavily protested that only a few of the PSAs aired, and those that did were greatly modified from the original content.[4] Breastfeeding advocates perceived this outcome as one more indication of the political clout of the formula industries and a move away from progress.

This controversy highlights not only the powerful force of formula marketing dollars, but also the difficulty in creating effective breastfeeding promotion. Scholar Joan Wolf, who has raised questions about breastfeeding research, argued that the risk-message approach used in

K.A. Foss, *Breastfeeding and Media*,
DOI 10.1007/978-3-319-56442-5_4

the Ad Council's PSAs was exploitive, faulty, and guilt-inducing for formula-feeding mothers.[5] While most breastfeeding advocates likely would not agree, Wolf's points may explain resistance to these persuasive strategies. Most breastfeeding discourse, at least in developed countries, has emphasized the benefits of breastfeeding, not the risks of bottle-feeding.[6] However, such presentation establishes breastfeeding as the alternative to bottles, not the default means of feeding a baby. This framework may also explain why breastfeeding campaigns have been far more successful in developing countries, as their messages stress the dire consequences of not breastfeeding.[7]

Campaigns and news media have successfully conveyed that breastmilk is nutritionally superior. Most people, including those without children, are well-aware that the benefits of breastfeeding far outweigh those of formula. Yet promotion has not resulted in raising initiation and duration enough to meet national breastfeeding objectives. Just as important, many women do not succeed in meeting their own breastfeeding goals.[8] Breastfeeding success depends on knowledge, resources, support, and an array of other factors—all of which have been and can be undermined by the tactics of formula corporations, which have positioned their products as a "fail-safe" for "insufficient" milk, and other reasons for early weaning. Factoring into the effectiveness of both breastfeeding and formula promotion is the endorsement and roles of hospitals, the health care system, and health professionals. This chapter examines the tug-of-war between breastfeeding promotion, infant formula corporations, and the health professionals that often serve as primary determinants for the mode of infant feeding. A look at the resources available in one town helps to illustrate how these relationships often play out, as well as the often limited information that expectant and new parents may receive as they decide how to feed their babies.

The Influence of Health Professionals and the Health Care System

From the initial appointment that confirms pregnancy through to delivery, a woman with a healthy pregnancy sees a health care provider an average of 11–15 times.[9] In addition to monitoring blood pressure, sugar levels, fetal heart rates, and overall health, these appointments also prepare the woman for birth and infancy, including infant feeding decisions. The extent to which health professionals support breastfeeding has been shown to heavily influence breastfeeding initiation and success.[10] Lu and colleagues found that when health care providers recommended breastfeeding, women were more than four times as likely to breastfeed, regardless of their racial/ethnic and social backgrounds.[11] Unfortunately, most physicians and nurses are woefully undereducated in this area, lacking knowledge and clinical training on helping mothers succeed at breastfeeding.[12] In a survey of the Fellows of the American Academy of Pediatrics (AAP), many physicians indicated that they would not support the continuation of breastfeeding in cases of an infant's low weight gain or jaundice, mastitis and nipple problems, despite little evidence that these conditions inhibit breastfeeding.[13] Similarly, Freed and colleagues found that 30% of practicing physicians surveyed chose inappropriate methods for helping mothers with low milk supply.[14] Breastfeeding education can have a significant impact on health professionals and their patients' success. In a study measuring this effect, medical residents exposed to breastfeeding in their curriculum exhibited more knowledge and confidence about breastfeeding.[15] Women who delivered at institutions with lactation curriculum were more likely to be exclusively breastfeeding at 6 months.[16]

Furthermore, many physicians underestimate the benefits of breastmilk over formula.[17] One study indicated that when physicians expressed "no preference" toward breastfeeding or formula, mothers were less likely to breastfeed beyond 6 weeks.[18] Likewise, Taveras and others found that women were less likely to be exclusively breastfeeding if their physicians recommended formula supplementation or did not regard breastfeeding duration as important.[19] Indeed, women cited diagnoses of "insufficient milk supply" or problems with an infants' weight gain as common justifications for early weaning, when in fact, most women produce enough milk to nourish a baby.[20] Mothers may also be influenced by the clinics they attend for prenatal appointments. Formula companies sometimes advertise their products in the waiting rooms or offer mailing cards for which parents can send in for free samples.[21] Such practices, according to Howard and colleagues, attaches a medical endorsement to the brand and formula feeding itself.[22]

Health professionals also control and shape the first breastfeeding experiences, determining interventions during birth, if a newborn is allowed to immediately nurse, the extent of lactation support, and the overall hospital experience. The doctors and nurses' actions, combined with hospital policies, set the foundation for the breastfeeding relationship. A woman's laboring and birth experience can impact breastfeeding success. Mothers who deliver vaginally have higher rates of breastfeeding initiation and duration, as do those who have healthy babies at birth.[23] While most contemporary health care providers would not encourage the "heavily drugged deliveries," known as twilight sleep,[24] or other outdated practices, the neutrality toward infant feeding remains for some physicians and nurses. Formula supplementation in the hospital still occurs regularly. In an analysis of the 2010 birth cohort of the National Immunization Survey, Perrine, Chen, and Scanlon noted that 24.2% of babies had received formula within the first 2 days.[25] These infants were less likely to be breastfed at 3 months.[26] Even mothers who had intended to breastfeed had babies with high rates of supplementation. In another study, Chantry and colleagues studied a diverse cohort of women intending to exclusively breastfeed.[27] Despite the mothers' intentions, 47% of the newborns were given formula, with "insufficient milk" as the most common justification.[28] These babies were three times as likely to be weaned by 60 days, compared to the exclusively breastfed newborns.[29] These correlations are not surprising, as supplementing hinders the establishment of a mother's milk supply, can cause nipple confusion, and can damage a woman's confidence in her ability to successfully breastfeed.[30]

Breastfeeding education for health professionals and lactation support can dramatically reduce the likelihood of supplementing with formula, thus increasing rates. At an institutional level, the Baby-Friendly Hospital Initiative (BFHI), created by WHO and UNICEF, sets up women for breastfeeding success.[31] To achieve the BFHI designation, hospitals must comply with the *Ten Steps to Successful Breastfeeding*, by mandating breastfeeding training for health professionals, routine rooming-in, nursing on demand, not offering pacifiers, refraining from supplementation unless absolutely necessary, and providing breastfeeding support groups.[32] As of 2015, 280 hospitals in 47 U.S. states had achieved the Baby-Friendly status.[33] Between 2009 and 2015, the number of births in "Baby-Friendly" facilities grew from 2.9 to 13.14%.[34] Although BFHI has been a big step towards increasing breastfeeding, even "Baby-Friendly" hospitals are not always in compliance. Nickels and colleagues discussed how discharge bags and pacifiers continue to be distributed at some "Baby-Friendly" hospitals, which exhibited lower breastfeeding duration rates than "Baby-Friendly" hospitals in-compliance, demonstrating the importance of adhering to the guidelines.[35] And, as Harris F. Koenig pointed out from his experience as the president and CEO of a Baby-Friendly community hospital, to improve breastfeeding rates at hospitals, it is not enough to change policies to be more conducive to breastfeeding (i.e., make rooming-in mandatory).[36] These changes must be paired with breastfeeding education opportunities for hospital staff.[37]

After the hospital stay, additional factors influence whether or not mothers will continue breastfeeding. The extent to which the new father or partner supports breastfeeding has been shown to be the most influential variant in duration. Maycock and colleagues found that mothers were much more likely to be breastfeeding at 6 weeks if their partners had attended a breastfeeding class and support group for fathers.[38] Another study showed that breastfeeding initiation was signficicantly higher for women whose partners had attended a class on breastfeeding.[39] The social support of family and friends also strongly impacts infant feeding decisions and outcomes, especially for women who are less educated and/or of a lower socio-economic status.[40]

Local Breastfeeding Resources[41]

Health professionals also serve as gatekeepers of information, in which certain authorities decide what messages are filtered through to the public.[42] In health care settings, providers often set the agenda, laying out what is relevant for the current visit. For example, Marvel and colleagues audio-recorded 300 appointments with family physicians to explore the extent to which patients shaped the topics addressed in their visits.[43] They discovered that doctors redirected patient concerns to their own agenda in less than 30 s of their appointments.[44] With breastfeeding, this agenda-setting means that physicians less familiar with breastfeeding (or who think it is less important) would be less likely to ask about it, encourage it, or fully listen to patients' concerns with breastfeeding obstacles.

Exploring the availability and visibility of breastfeeding resources in one town helps to shed light on how new mothers may access infant feeding information and support. It is also a good demonstration of the pervasiveness of formula marketing. In a mid-sized Tennessee city of just over 100,000 people, one might expect a wealth of resources.[45] However, Tennessee has the ninth lowest breastfeeding rate in the

United States, with only 74.9% of mothers ever breastfeeding.[46] Outside of LLL meetings, breastfeeding is an uncommon sight in this town. The availability of breastfeeding resources reflect this invisibility. Of course, the number of resources available to expectant and new mothers can vary dramatically by town. This example, though, demonstrates possible explanations to varied breastfeeding success as the materials and information about infant feeding reflect and reinforce these abysmal rates. It also adheres to this book's presentation of different sites for new mothers and the general public.

The city's hospital is part of a larger health care organization, consisting of several hospitals in the state, none of which have earned the "Baby Friendly" designation. Midwives are not part of labor and delivery at this hospital. However, free lactation consultants visit new mothers to help with breastfeeding initiation. And before discharge, the hospital requires all new mothers to go through a brief class (or a binder of materials) on caring for infants that provides an equal balance of bottle-feeding and breastfeeding advice. The town also has a local WIC office, which is part of the county health department, and numerous health clinics. For this case study, conducted with Dr. Reyna Gordon, infant feeding materials available for the public were collected from the hospital's lactation boutique, the county health department and WIC office, the local chapter of LLL, and five of the primary pediatrics clinics. We visited each site, examining walls and counter spaces for infant feeding promotional material. We also requested the typical infant feeding materials distributed for patients—the standard "kit" and materials offered upon request. Infant feeding references in "Well Baby Check-up" forms for ages 2 weeks to 18 months were also examined.

At the WIC office, lactation boutique, and LLL meetings, there was a wealth of breastfeeding information available in English and Spanish. The local WIC office displayed several pro-breastfeeding posters and provided pamphlets on benefits and basic breastfeeding instructions. A breastfeeding class and videos were also available for WIC recipients. The hospital lactation boutique offered numerous breastfeeding handouts, all of which were sponsored by the breastfeeding product company Medela. La Leche League provided handouts and breastfeeding books for free check-out, in addition to in-person support on personal nursing challenges.

On the contrary, the local clinics were much more neutral toward infant feeding. No breastfeeding posters or brochures were displayed in any of the waiting rooms. In contrast, other health and safety topics were promoted, with posters and fliers of proper car seat use. One clinic had a book with testimonies about the dangers of not vaccinating. Of the five clinics (all of which included pediatrics as part of their care), only one routinely distributed breastfeeding information as part of a regular baby wellness visit. Breastfeeding handouts emphasized its benefits, rather than the risks of formula feeding. Two offices offered complementary "for breastfeeding moms" packages, sponsored by Enfamil, which included brief descriptions of breastfeeding benefits, with formula samples and coupons. As numerous scholars have established, these marketing packages can be detrimental to breastfeeding.[47]

There was a lack of coordination between local resources: most printed materials did not inform the reader of where to find an International Board Certified Lactation Consultant (IBCLC), LLL meetings or other in-person breastfeeding help and support, even though all of these resources exist in this community. Wellness sheets (used to gather information from parents about their children's habits) revealed a neutral agenda about breastfeeding in the first few months, and extended breastfeeding was absent from the agenda. Parents fill out these forms prior to the check-up to provide background health information for the visit. For the "Well Baby Check-up" forms, no reference to breastfeeding appeared after the 9-month form (absent at the 12, 15, and 18 month check-ups), conveying the false perception that breastfeeding is no longer relevant after 9 months.

The dearth and poor quality of information at the pediatricians' offices was alarming, given that postpartum support and information dramatically influences breastfeeding success.[48] Such mixed messages can lead to confusion and ambivalence for women, leading to early weaning, especially among populations with already lower breastfeeding rates.[49] The absence of breastfeeding materials and the willingness of the health professionals to display formula coupons may indicate resistance in the local health care community to become more breastfeeding friendly.[50]

The scarcity of breastfeeding materials may give insight into the low breastfeeding rates in Tennessee. In the community, the pediatricians and other health professionals serve as gatekeepers of the breastfeeding information—particularly when patients must specifically request brochures and other materials. This gatekeeping function becomes more apparent when the lack of breastfeeding information is paired with the abundance of resources on other health issues. Furthermore, as wellness sheets set the agenda for clinical visits, the neutrality of these forms toward infant feeding early on presents breastfeeding as a comparable health choice to formula, discouraging conversation about breastfeeding obstacles. And, the absence of breastfeeding from the forms past age one ignores the notion of extended breastfeeding, possibly causing women to feel ashamed or abnormal if they choose to nurse past this point.

The Promotional Clash Between Breastfeeding and Formula Companies

How do you persuade women to breastfeed, especially when local support is inadequate? As with any health campaign, effectiveness depends on the ability to not only reach the intended audience, but also persuade them that adopting the healthy behavior is both attainable and worth overcoming the existing barriers, which include social perceptions and environmental obstacles. According to the Health Belief Model, a popular theory in health promotion, people must perceive themselves (or in this case, their babies) at risk of poor health, have confidence that they can adopt the desired behavior, and think that working through the obstacles will be worth the effort.[51] Additionally, perceptions of social norms also influence the probability of the healthy behavior.[52] Breastfeeding promotion, then, must convince women that breastfeeding will significantly improve their babies' health—so much so that they will be willing to seek help and overcome latching difficulties, supply problems, mastitis, thrush and other challenges. Just as important, promotional efforts must pair information about benefits (or risk messages of not breastfeeding) with lactation guidance and other support so that mothers believe they can successfully breastfeed. Self-efficacy is the best predictor of successful breastfeeding: however, this confidence can be difficult to achieve, particularly if friends and family, health professionals, formula advertising, and other forces undermine that confidence.[53] Finally, to help increase duration, breastfeeding needs to be normalized so that family and friends perceive it as the typical way of feeding babies. Regional variations in breastfeeding rates highlight this difference. Nursing mothers are more likely to feel comfortable and confident if they believe that everyone around them also breastfed and/or supports breastfeeding.

Following the adoption of the International Code of Breast Milk Substitutes in 1981, some countries began to pass legislation to restrict or ban formula marketing, while organizations launched localized and global efforts to improve breastfeeding rates.[54] In Haiti, for example, Dr. Bette Gebrian successfully led an extensive breastfeeding campaign through the Haitian Health Foundation (HHF) in the 1980s and 1990s.[55] The campaign was carried out in a series of steps. First, Gebrian and the public health workers used easily-recalled slogans to persuade people that newborns needed colostrum, not a purgative typically given.[56] With local health workers, the HHF members educated communities on breastfeeding benefits and provided lactation support with home visits, and nursing bras and supplies for milk expression.[57] The HHF campaign also strongly included men in the education and celebration of breastfeeding—fathers were even given celebratory t-shirts when their partners had nursed for 6 months.[58] Gebrian and her team were widely successful, raising breastfeeding rates from less than 1% of mothers exclusively breastfeeding in 1987 to 80% in 2010.[59] This success demonstrates several essential components of effective campaigns: understanding the culture and community and their unique obstacles or resistance to breastfeeding, combining education with support, and incorporating everyone in the intervention efforts to make the transformation a societal one.

Overall, campaigns have yielded significant success in raising breastfeeding initiation and duration at least in certain geographic regions.[60] In addition to the WHO Code, global and national advocacy groups have worked to raise awareness, restrict formula marketing, and celebrate breastfeeding with breastfeeding training for workers in developing and other countries, the *Innocenti Declaration*, World Breastfeeding Week, and other important actions.[61] In developing countries like Haiti, promotional efforts have resulted in exclusive breastfeeding (EBF) increases as high as six times the previous EBF rate in developing countries.[62] Part of this success can be attributed to modifying support to account for cultural and language barriers. For example, instead of verbally inquiring about specific obstacles, cards with illustrations of common problems can be an effective tool for health care workers to help mothers identify and then overcome problems.[63]

In the United States, breastfeeding rates have also increased, but not to the extent of other countries. As mentioned, the creation of the Baby-Friendly Hospital Initiative and designation has established measureable standards and guidelines for establishing an environment conducive to breastfeeding. National and local campaigns have aimed to create breastfeeding awareness and improve attitudes. In 2003, the U.S. Department of Health and Human Services launched the National Breastfeeding Awareness Campaign, using media messages and community-based demonstration projects (CDPs) to raise breastfeeding visibility.[64] The Ad Council and the Office of Women's Health ran TV, radio, magazine, newspaper, billboard and Internet ads, along with ads in bus shelters, conveying the campaign's slogan: "Babies were Born to be Breastfed." And, as mentioned earlier, the Ad Council's PSAs that used risk messaging were largely pulled from the air, but the campaign overall garnered widespread attention. Media messages were combined with breastfeeding advice and support through phone-lines and its website. Follow-up surveys assessed the extent to which non-WIC and WIC participants knew about the ad, determining that 34.8% of those enrolled in WIC were aware of the ads, compared to only 22% of those not enrolled.[65] Yet, even with the campaign messages and their reach, approximately 40% of mothers still believed that formula and breastfeeding were equal, demonstrating the need for further intervention beyond media dissemination.[66]

Statistically, low-income women, including WIC recipients are typically less-likely to breastfeed. In 1997, the United States Department of Agriculture (USDA) specifically encouraged WIC recipients to breastfeed with their Loving Support Makes Breastfeeding Work campaign.[67] This program addressed breastfeeding awareness at the individual and society levels, attempting to increase support from partners, family, friends, and the overall community through peer counseling, training kits, community leader materials, and other tools to create a breastfeeding-friendly environment. Women who breastfed were also granted expanded food allowances. In addition to individual benefits, financial incentives were also added for states with high breastfeeding rates. This campaign, in conjunction with other efforts, helped to raise breastfeeding initiation for WIC mothers from 41.5% in 1998 to 59% in 2008.[68]

Breastfeeding education efforts have also targeted specific groups. For example, Horodynski, Calcatera, and Carpenter studied breastfeeding attitudes and perceptions in six Native American communities.[69] Focus groups with local health paraprofessionals and Native American mothers highlighted unique obstacles within their community, including issues of trust, the importance of addressing older generations in breastfeeding education, and differences in beliefs about the introduction of solid foods.[70] This suggests that promotional efforts may be more successful when they are tailored to individual groups and cultures. Howell and colleagues measured the effects of behavioral education intervention on initiation and duration for African American and Latina women.[71] Those who received breastfeeding educational materials (designed with language and culture in mind) and a 2-week post-delivery call to address needs and challenges breastfed for a median of 12 weeks, compared to only 6.5 weeks for mothers who were not part of the intervention group.[72] This study demonstrated the importance of education and support, particularly through messages and methods that fit with the culture.

Peer counseling can especially help women that demographically are less likely to breastfeed (lower socio-economic status, single, younger, and/or African American), by offering support individualized to their reasons for breastfeeding cessation.[73] Campaigns may also be more effective when they utilize newer forms of technology. For example the local WIC program in Santa Barbara, California successfully uses text-messaging, apps, and online videos for support and advice for its new mothers.[74] At 1 month, the rate for exclusive breastfeeding for participants in the program was approximately 84%, compared to the average EBF rate of about 73% for non-participants.[75]

Of course, it is crucial that intervention efforts also target health care providers. Breastfeeding-focused education has shown to improve rates for the patients of medical residents, nurses, and other health professionals.[76] Education for nursing students is also important to make sure nurses can encourage and support breastfeeding.[77] Such education can also help create a climate open to achieving the "Baby Friendly" hospital status and reduce resistance from health professionals and administrators.[78] While efforts have certainly improved breastfeeding awareness and overall rates, unfortunately, formula marketing has diluted and derailed many of the efforts.

Formula Marketing: Past and Present

Breastfeeding campaigns can hardly compete with the multi-million dollar formula industry. The powerful influence of this industry has been recognized since the early 1900s, when U.S. formula companies (under pressure from physicians) voluntarily ceased advertising directly to consumers.[79] In the 1930s, formula companies had begun expanding their promotion to developing countries. This extensive marketing led to steeply declining breastfeeding rates in these areas. For example, between 1940 and 1974, breastfeeding rates in Brazil went from 96 to 39%.[80]

Singapore's breastfeeding rates decreased by 50% over 20 years.[81] Similar patterns occurred in other countries, with devastating consequences. The lack of clean water, income to provide enough formula and adequate supplies, and knowledge to safely prepare the food had tragic consequences as many babies became sick from malnutrition and diarrhea.[82] Mortality rates for artificially-fed infants in developing countries were significantly higher than breastfed babies.[83] In some countries, formula-fed babies died at three times the rate of breastfed ones, with an even higher incidence of malnutrition and poor health.[84] Bottle-fed babies in impoverished communities in the United States and other developed countries also faced greater rates of infection and death.[85]

As early as 1939, one doctor, Dr. Cicely Williams, remarked on the high mortality rates from breastmilk substitutes in Singapore at a Rotary Club meeting.[86] However, this tragedy went largely unnoticed by the general public for decades. Physicians and advocacy groups became involved in spreading awareness of the formula marketing practices in the late 1960s and early 1970s.[87] Then in 1974, a development agency, War on Want, published journalist Mike Muller's report, *The Baby Killer*, detailing evidence about the corrupt practices of the formula companies in developing countries and their tragic effects.[88] In this document, Muller used first-hand testimony to explain how formula company representatives, specifically Nestlé and Cow & Gate (a British company) masqueraded as health professionals and then persuaded mothers to bottle-feed.[89] This description was accompanied by morbidity and mortality statistics of artificially-fed babies, demonstrating the dire impact of formula marketing.[90]

Muller's report was widely translated and distributed, garnering extensive media coverage. The Nestlé corporation responded by suing for libel, winning a meager sum. Even more important than the outcome was the publicity of the case. This attention spurred action for both advocacy groups and the general public. In 1977, the Infant Formula Action Network (INFACT) spearheaded a boycott against Nestlé products on the basis of its formula marketing, using multiple media channels to encourage people to avoid Nestlé.[91] The campaign was successful, as Nestlé sales dropped dramatically. At the same time, the boycott and its publicity led to the 1979 WHO/UNICEF meetings that would produce the WHO International Code of Marketing for Breastmilk Substitutes in 1981.[92] Countries that adopted this document agreed to provide cautionary labels of the risks on breastmilk substitute packaging, ban the promotion or distribution of free formula in health care facilities, and prohibit formula companies from offering financial incentives for health professionals.[93] Additionally, the Code mandated monetary contributions from formula companies to conferences and research, and other tenets to restrict formula marketing from hindering breastfeeding, especially in developing countries.[94] When the World Health Assembly voted to adopt the Code, only the United States delegate voted against its adoption.[95] While the United States eventually adopted the Code, no action has been taken to implement the Code in the United States, according to a 2011 UNICEF report.[96] Globally, though, the Code's recommendations and resolutions were effective in raising awareness of formula marketing corruption and prompting many countries to create laws regulating formula marketing.[97] The Code also set a standard for evaluating breastmilk substitute promotional practices. That said, research on the Code's implementation has shown that international breastfeeding rates are still not meeting expectations, likely due to formula marketing, cultural barriers, and other factors that undermine the Code's tenets.[98]

It should be noted that the voluntary ban against direct-to-consumer formula marketing that started in the early 1900s in the United States has not existed for decades. In 1989, formula companies reversed their more than 50 year-old practice of not advertising directly to consumers.[99] The Nestlé-Carnation Corporation was the first to go against the industry's self-regulation when it launched its Good Start brand commercials on television.[100] Soon after, Gerber Baby started advertising formula on TV and widely distributing free samples and coupons.[101] Commercial formula is now regularly advertised in consumer publications. Amy Koerber analyzed rhetorical strategies in infant feeding controversies, concluding that "the discourses that formula companies are currently using to promote their products derive from bits and pieces borrowed from the scientific discourse that promotes breastfeeding."[102]

Supporting this notion, a contemporary study of parenting magazines found that formula was repeatedly advertised and used unsupported "health" statements in attempts to persuade consumers of their desirability.[103] These claims extend to the products themselves. Blamarich, Bochner, and Racine studied the product labels on 22 major formulas, finding that 13 claimed to resolve specific health issues, including "lactose sensitivity," and colic, despite a dearth of scientific evidence to support the claims.[104] The authors demonstrated how such false claims could undermine breastfeeding promotion efforts, encourage consumers to spend additional money on specialized formula, and may cause difficulties with WIC recepients.[105] In other words, formula marketing is even more prevalent now than in the 1800s period of no regulation, constantly bombarding people with largely unsolicited health messages that may hinder breastfeeding decisions, initiation, and duration. Its messages and pervasiveness have been shown to undercut efforts to support the Code by hindering maternal confidence, normalizing bottle-feeding, presenting conflicting health information, and, to some extent, inferring with pro-breastfeeding policies.[106]

The Influence of Formula Marketing

The promotion of breastmilk substitutes has had profound effects on the awareness, attitudes, and success of breastfeeding. Studies have shown that mothers almost universally agree on the prevalence of formula marketing, including in social media, yet many have difficulty identifying popular breastfeeding campaigns.[107] In a survey of formula-feeding mothers, 84.3% received formula information through print ads, while 72% got their formula information from television or radio.[108] Approximately 56% had received free formula in the mail. This prevalence of formula marketing campaigns has been shown to shorten breastfeeding duration.[109] This impact is even more profound with specific groups of women, including WIC recipients and mothers of ethnic groups with already lower breastfeeding rates.[110] The all-encompassing strategies of formula companies attempt to not only convince people to formula-feed, but also create a brand preference. Formula-feeding parents have indicated that hospital and physician recommendations of specific brands, followed by formula advertising, influenced their brand choice.[111]

Studies have demonstrated that formula samples given in clinics and hospitals have devastating effects on breastfeeding success. Rosenberg and colleagues found that women in Oregon who had received commercial hospital discharge packs were more likely to have weaned by 10 weeks postpartum.[112] Howard and collaborators conducted an experiment with more than 500 participants, measuring the effect of formula-sponsored hospital discharge bags on breastfeeding initiation and duration.[113] While sponsorship had no significant effect on initiation, women who received the formula pack were much more likely to stop breastfeeding before leaving the hospital, with 12%, compared to only

1% of mothers who were given generic educational materials.[114] The breastfeeding success rate at 2 weeks was also much lower for those with the formula-sponsored bags, especially for women who had set vague breastfeeding goals.[115] Dungy and others also found that breastfeeding duration was much higher for women who received only a manual breast pump compared to those who were given formula along with the pump.[116] A study of formula marketing interpretations found that hospital discharge bags given for "breastfeeding" mothers (sponsored by the makers of Enfamil and Similac) can make women question the superiority of breastfeeding over formula due to the messages about formula and the free coupons and samples included in the bags.[117] In addition, the messages in the bags caused many nursing mothers to doubt themselves.[118] The researchers concluded that these interpretations suggest that discharge bags may undermine confidence in one's ability to breastfeed, especially when recommended by health professionals.[119] Other aspects of formula marketing have also been shown to have deliberately confusing messages. For example, the use of the WIC acronym in formula marketing may suggest endorsement by WIC for formula, undermining the message that WIC promotes breastfeeding.[120] Despite these negative effects, formula-sponsored bags are still frequently distributed. According to the Infant Feeding Practices Study II, 89% of formula-feeding mothers had received a "gift pack" at the hospital, most of which contained formula samples.[121] Most of the mothers were still using the same brand of formula given by the hospital at 1 month postpartum.[122]

In addition to traditional advertising, social media and the Internet have created new outlets for formula advertising. Using "cookies," formula marketers can tailor messages to individual consumer's Internet habits. Therefore, a person searching "breastfeeding" might receive a number of formula ads as sidebars or pop-ups. Some may even be disguised as breastfeeding advice. With social media, people also willingly spread formula advertising, through *Facebook* "shares" of clever formula commercials (like the Similac "Mother 'Hood") or distribute formula coupons to other consumers. Considering the seemingly endless advertising budget of these corporations to create such videos, it is hard for breastfeeding advocates to establish an equal presence online, particularly because there is no product to sell. While some advocacy groups and others have had some success utilizing social media for breastfeeding promotion, it pales in comparison to the commercial formula corporations.[123]

Conclusion

One might wonder how formula marketing in the United States complies with the International Code of Breastmilk Substitutes. In short, it does not. As the Code is only a recommendation, not the law unless specifically adopted into legislation, formula companies do not have to legally meet its requirements. However, several steps have been taken to curb some of their influence. Recognizing the impact of health professionals on infant feeding, educators have expanded the curriculum to include more instruction on breastfeeding. And, hospitals that have earned the "Baby-Friendly" label do not provide discharge bags sponsored by formula companies. Some legislation has been passed to help nursing mothers. Most states have laws protecting the right to breastfeed in public.[124] Under the Affordable Care Act, employers must provide nursing mothers with time and space to pump (with exceptions for small businesses). Insurance companies are now mandated to provide breast pumps, free of charge, as well as lactation counseling and support.[125]

Unfortunately, these efforts are not enough unless a community and societal commitment to breastfeeding exists. Restrictions on formula marketing and health professionals' own commitment to encourage breastfeeding would dramatically improve resources and support for nursing mothers. At the same time, significantly increasing the pervasiveness of breastfeeding promotion, in a way that highlights the risks of not breastfeeding (like the "bull-riding" PSA) would raise awareness of the health need to breastfeed. Campaigns should more frequently utilize emerging technologies to reach the target audience and improve communication, employing many of the formula companies' social media strategies. This approach could especially be effective in connecting with groups with low-breastfeeding rates, such as adolescent mothers. Finally, changing the culture to be more breastfeeding-friendly would heighten the success of the promotion efforts. The following chapters address the important role of media in shaping public perceptions of breastfeeding through books for new parents, fictional and reality television, and online groups and social media.

Notes

1. "National Breastfeeding Campaign 'Ladies Night' TV Advert."
2. Wolf, "What Feminists Can Do for Breastfeeding and What Breastfeeding Can Do for Feminists."

3. Ibid.
4. Ibid.
5. Wolf, "Is Breast Really Best?"
6. Stuebe, "The Risks of Not Breastfeeding for Mothers and Infants."
7. Imdad, Yakoob, and Bhutta, "Effect of Breastfeeding Promotion Interventions on Breastfeeding Rates, with Special Focus on Developing Countries."
8. Stuebe, "Enabling Women to Achieve Their Breastfeeding Goals."
9. "Microsoft Word—Prenatal_visit_pattern.doc—Prenatal_visit_pattern.pdf."
10. Arora et al., "Major Factors Influencing Breastfeeding Rates"; Taveras et al. "Opinions and Practices of Clinicians Associated With Continuation of Exclusive Breastfeeding."
11. Lu et al., "Provider Encouragement of Breast-Feeding."
12. Schanler, O'Connor, and Lawrence, "Pediatricians' Practices and Attitudes Regarding Breastfeeding Promotion"; Freed et al., "National Assessment of Physicians' Breast-Feeding Knowledge, Attitudes, Training, and Experience."
13. Schanler, O'Connor, and Lawrence, "Pediatricians' Practices and Attitudes Regarding Breastfeeding Promotion."
14. Freed et al., "National Assessment of Physicians' Breast-Feeding Knowledge, Attitudes, Training, and Experience."
15. Feldman-Winter et al., "Residency Curriculum Improves Breastfeeding Care."
16. Ibid.
17. Schanler, O'Connor, and Lawrence, "Pediatricians' Practices and Attitudes Regarding Breastfeeding Promotion"; Freed et al., "National Assessment of Physicians' Breast-Feeding Knowledge, Attitudes, Training, and Experience."
18. DiGirolamo, Grummer-Strawn, and Fein, "Do Perceived Attitudes of Physicians and Hospital Staff Affect Breastfeeding Decisions?"
19. Taveras et al., "Opinions and Practices of Clinicians Associated With Continuation of Exclusive Breastfeeding."
20. Ibid.; Lewallen et al., "Breastfeeding Support and Early Cessation"; Wolf, *Don't Kill Your Baby: Public Health and the Decline of Breastfeeding in the 19th and 20th Centuries.*
21. Howard, Howard, and Weitzman, "The Physician as Advertiser."
22. Ibid.
23. Zanardo et al., "Elective Cesarean Delivery"; Prior et al., "Breastfeeding after Cesarean Delivery"; Al-Sahab et al., "Prevalence and Predictors of 6-Month Exclusive Breastfeeding among Canadian Women."
24. Wolf, *Deliver Me from Pain.*

25. Perrine, Chen, and Scanlon, "Early Formula Supplementation and Breastfeeding Duration (131.4)."
26. Ibid.
27. Chantry et al., "In-Hospital Formula Use Increases Early Breastfeeding Cessation Among First-Time Mothers Intending to Exclusively Breastfeed."
28. Ibid.
29. Ibid.
30. Sears and Sears, *The Breastfeeding Book.*
31. Cadwell, *Reclaiming Breastfeeding For The United States.*
32. "The Ten Steps to Successful Breastfeeding."
33. "Find Facilities."
34. See note 32.
35. Nickel et al., "The Extent That Noncompliance with the Ten Steps to Successful Breastfeeding Influences Breastfeeding Duration."
36. Koenig, "Breastfeeding Education for Healthier Babies. Baby-Friendly Designation Improves Infant, Mother and Community Health."
37. Ibid.
38. Maycock et al., "Education and Support for Fathers Improves Breastfeeding Rates A Randomized Controlled Trial."
39. Wolfberg et al., "Dads as Breastfeeding Advocates."
40. Khoury et al., "Breast-Feeding Initiation in Low-Income Women"; Meedya, Fahy, and Kable, "Factors That Positively Influence Breastfeeding Duration to 6 Months"; Barona-Vilar, Escribá-Agüir, and Ferrero-Gandía, "A Qualitative Approach to Social Support and Breast-Feeding Decisions."
41. This case study of breastfeeding resources was conducted in partnership with Dr. Reyna Gordon in 2012–2013 and presented at the 2013 Breastfeeding & Feminism Symposium as "We just have this one breastfeeding brochure" (sponsored by Enfamil): Exploring breastfeeding resources and agenda-setting in pediatrics' offices, WIC, LLL, and the community hospital. It is possible that materials have changed.
42. Shoemaker and Vos, *Gatekeeping Theory.*
43. Marvel et al., "Soliciting the Patient's Agenda."
44. Ibid.
45. "Murfreesboro, Tennessee (TN) Profile: Population, Maps, Real Estate, Averages, Homes, Statistics, Relocation, Travel, Jobs, Hospitals, Schools, Crime, Moving, Houses, News, Sex Offenders."
46. "Breastfeeding Report Card: United States, 2014 - 2014 breastfeedingreportcard.pdf."
47. Rosenberg et al., "Marketing Infant Formula Through Hospitals"; Howard et al., "Office Prenatal Formula Advertising and Its Effect on

Breast-Feeding patterns1"; Dungy et al., "Effect of Discharge Samples on Duration of Breast-Feeding."

48. DiGirolamo, Grummer-Strawn, and Fein, "Do Perceived Attitudes of Physicians and Hospital Staff Affect Breastfeeding Decisions?"; Taveras et al., "Opinions and Practices of Clinicians Associated With Continuation of Exclusive Breastfeeding"; Freed, Fraley, and Schanler, "Attitudes of Expectant Fathers Regarding Breast-Feeding"; Littman, Medendorp, and Goldfarb, "The Decision to Breastfeed The Importance of Fathers' Approval."
49. Kaufman, Deenadayalan, and Karpati, "Breastfeeding Ambivalence Among Low-Income African American and Puerto Rican Women in North and Central Brooklyn."
50. Brodribb, "Barriers to Translating Evidence-based Breastfeeding Information into Practice."
51. Pechmann, "A Comparison of Health Communication Models"; Becker et al., "The Health Belief Model and Prediction of Dietary Compliance"; Janz and Becker, "The Health Belief Model."
52. Janz and Becker, "The Health Belief Model."
53. de Jager et al., "The Role of Psychosocial Factors in Exclusive Breastfeeding to Six Months Postpartum"; Meedya, Fahy, and Kable, "Factors That Positively Influence Breastfeeding Duration to 6 Months"; Kools et al., "The Motivational Determinants of Breast-Feeding: Predictors for the Continuation of Breast-Feeding"; Khoury et al., "Breast-Feeding Initiation in Low-Income Women."
54. Cadwell, *Reclaiming Breastfeeding For The United States.*
55. Gebrian, "Bottles to Breastfeeding in Rural Haiti."
56. Ibid.
57. Ibid.
58. Ibid.
59. Ibid.
60. Haroon et al., "Breastfeeding Promotion Interventions and Breastfeeding Practices"; Imdad, Yakoob, and Bhutta, "Effect of Breastfeeding Promotion Interventions on Breastfeeding Rates, with Special Focus on Developing Countries."
61. Cadwell, *Reclaiming Breastfeeding For The United States.*
62. Imdad, Yakoob, and Bhutta, "Effect of Breastfeeding Promotion Interventions on Breastfeeding Rates, with Special Focus on Developing Countries."
63. Manjilalal, Februhartanty, and Basuki, "Assessment of Breastfeeding Problems Experienced by Mothers in the First Six Months Postpartum."
64. "2004.06.04: Public Service Campaign to Promote Breastfeeding Awareness Launched."

65. Haynes, “Evaluation of the National Breastfeeding Awareness Campaign.”
66. Ibid.
67. Whitacre and Moats, “Updating the USDA National Breastfeeding Campaign—Workshop Summary.”
68. Ibid.
69. Horodynski, Calcatera, and Carpenter, “Infant Feeding Practices.”
70. Ibid.
71. Howell et al., “An Intervention to Extend Breastfeeding among Black and Latina Mothers after Delivery.”
72. Ibid.
73. Rozga, Kerver, and Olson, “Impact of Peer Counselling Breast-Feeding Support Programme Protocols on Any and Exclusive Breast-Feeding Discontinuation in Low-Income Women.”
74. Beard, ““Bfed” Texting Program and “ Breastfeeding.”
75. Ibid.
76. Feldman-Winter, “Evidence-Based Interventions to Support Breastfeeding”; Davis, Stichler, and Poeltler, “Increasing Exclusive Breastfeeding Rates in the Well-Baby Population.”
77. Vandewark, “Breastfeeding Attitudes and Knowledge in Bachelor of Science in Nursing Candidates.”
78. Semenic et al., “Barriers, Facilitators, and Recommendations Related to Implementing the Baby-Friendly Initiative (BFI).”
79. Greer and Apple, “Physicians, Formula Companies, and Advertising.”
80. Chetley, *The Politics of Baby Foods.*
81. Ibid.
82. Ibid.
83. Muller, *The Baby Killer.*
84. Ibid.
85. Chetley, *The Politics of Baby Foods.*
86. Ibid.
87. Ibid.
88. Ibid.; Muller, *The Baby Killer.*
89. Muller, *The Baby Killer.*
90. Ibid.
91. Van Esterik, *Beyond the Breast-Bottle Controversy.*
92. Ibid.
93. Shubber, *The WHO International Code of Marketing of Breast-Milk Substitutes.*
94. Ibid.; Cadwell, *Reclaiming Breastfeeding For The United States.*
95. See note 93.

96. "National Implementation of the International Code of Marketing of Breastmilk Substitutes*—State_of_the_Code_by_Country_April2011.pdf."
97. Ibid.
98. Piwoz and Huffman, "The Impact of Marketing of Breast-Milk Substitutes on WHO-Recommended Breastfeeding Practices"; McFadden et al., "Spotlight on Infant Formula"; Rollins et al., "Why Invest, and What It Will Take to Improve Breastfeeding Practices?"
99. Greer and Apple, "Physicians, Formula Companies, and Advertising."
100. Ibid.
101. Ibid.
102. Koerber, *Breast or Bottle? : Contemporary Controversies in Infant-Feeding Policy and Practice*, p. 82.
103. Stang, Hoss, and Story, "Health Statements Made in Infant Formula Advertisements in Pregnancy and Early Parenting Magazines A Content Analysis."
104. Belamarich, Bochner, and Racine, "A Critical Review of the Marketing Claims of Infant Formula Products in the United States."
105. Ibid.
106. Piwoz and Huffman, "The Impact of Marketing of Breast-Milk Substitutes on WHO-Recommended Breastfeeding Practices."
107. Parry et al., "Understanding Women's Interpretations of Infant Formula Advertising"; Huang et al., "Association of Health Profession and Direct-to-Consumer Marketing with Infant Formula Choice and Switching."
108. Huang et al., "Association of Health Profession and Direct-to-Consumer Marketing with Infant Formula Choice and Switching."
109. Stuebe, "The Risks of Not Breastfeeding for Mothers and Infants"; "GAO-06-282 Breastfeeding: Some Strategies Used to Market Infant Formula May Discourage Breastfeeding; State Contracts Should Better Protect Against Misuse of WIC Name—d06282.pdf."
110. "GAO-06-282 Breastfeeding: Some Strategies Used to Market Infant Formula May Discourage Breastfeeding; State Contracts Should Better Protect Against Misuse of WIC Name—d06282.pdf."
111. See Notes 108.
112. Rosenberg et al., "Marketing Infant Formula Through Hospitals."
113. Howard et al., "Office Prenatal Formula Advertising and Its Effect on Breast-Feeding patterns1."
114. Ibid.
115. Ibid.
116. Dungy et al., "Effect of Discharge Samples on Duration of Breast-Feeding."

117. Parry et al., "Understanding Women's Interpretations of Infant Formula Advertising."
118. Ibid.
119. Ibid.
120. See Notes 110.
121. See Notes 108.
122. Ibid.
123. Asiodu et al., "Breastfeeding and Use of Social Media Among First-Time African American Mothers"; Abrahams, "Milk and Social Media Online Communities and the International Code of Marketing of Breast-Milk Substitutes"; Anstey, MacGowan, and Allen, "Five-Year Progress Update on the Surgeon General's Call to Action to Support Breastfeeding, 2011."
124. "Breastfeeding State Laws."
125. "Breastfeeding Benefits | HealthCare.gov."

CHAPTER 5

"So You're Going to Have a Baby?": Breastfeeding Messages in Parenting Guides and Children's Books

At the gift-opening portion of most baby showers, the expectant mother is surrounded by mounds of pastel gift bags and boxes, adorned by tulle bows and cutesy cards. While this event offers celebration and support for the pregnant woman, it also represents the commodification of infancy, paired with the bombardment of information. Among the onesies, burp cloths, and rattles, there is at least one present containing parenting books. Usually gifted by veteran moms eager to rapidly offer their own unsolicited advice, these books provide an extension of their own attitudes and philosophies toward baby wearing, sleep "training," and most prominent, breastfeeding. And yet, the baby shower is not the only source of distribution for such parenting handbooks, which are also given at the "confirmation of pregnancy" appointments at the OB/GYN's office, sent unsolicited in the mail, and offered secondhand from well-meaning acquaintances. These books signify a bigger trend over the past century. As Chap. 2 demonstrated, we have moved from an era in which women's birth and lactation experiences were openly shared with other women, replacing them with so-called "experts" for help with child-rearing. This chapter explores this advice for the new mother (and her partner), addressing breastfeeding discourse in "new baby" books for parents and older siblings.

K.A. Foss, *Breastfeeding and Media*,
DOI 10.1007/978-3-319-56442-5_5

The Role of Parenting Books

For expectant parents, popular books on pregnancy and childrearing are not just light reading before the baby comes—they help shape and confirm parenting philosophies and behaviors, including the decision to breastfeed. Arora and colleagues (2000) surveyed mothers about their infant feeding choices, finding that 78% of those that bottle-fed had decided to do so before pregnancy or during the first trimester.[1] After family, media ranked as the second main source of information about feeding, even more so than friends, medical professionals, or prenatal classes. Other studies have corroborated this conclusion. In an analysis of the Infant Feeding Practices Survey II, Chen, Johnson, and Rosenthal noted that 64.1% of respondents listed media (defined as newspapers, TV, books, newsletters, radio, and websites) as their primary source of breastfeeding information, a higher percentage than health professionals, friends, or support groups.[2] Survey participants with media as a main source had better duration rates than those who had relied on health professionals for information, but shorter breastfeeding periods than mothers who reported learning about breastfeeding from classes or support groups.[3] Furthermore, as Parry and colleagues demonstrated, infant feeding messages greatly influence both knowledge and confidence about breastfeeding, particularly when they are produced by formula corporations.[4] These mixed messages disseminated by news and entertainment media, breastfeeding promotion, and formula advertising can be especially problematic. In Arora's study, over 90% of bottle-feeding mothers said they would have been more likely to breastfeed if they had received more positive information from magazines, books, or television.[5]

As discussed in earlier chapters, breastfeeding and parenting advice have always been an abundant component of women's magazines, reinforced by ads conveniently marketing products addressed in the articles. Related to these magazines have been the parenting manuals and books, which continue to be widely popular, despite the demise of print books in nearly every other subject area. Many of the popular books on parenting have sold millions of copies and have produced multiple editions. For example, *What to Expect When You're Expecting*, first published in 1984, has over 14.5 million copies in circulation and is in its fourth edition.[6] Even with the steep decline in overall book sales, pregnancy and childrearing books remain widely popular. Nearly 50,000 books on pregnancy are available for purchase on Amazon.com. A search for "breastfeeding," yields over 4000 results. There appears to be a book, with "experts," on nearly every possible parenting situation, from adoption, to breastfeeding triplets. Furthermore, new baby books for older siblings dominate children's book genres. The popularity of these books exemplifies a continuance of the "scientific motherhood," of our reliance on "experts" to guide us in decisions that used to be part of conventional wisdom passed down through generations. With expectant and new parents relying on these books as supplements (or in lieu of) their health professionals, the advice inside has the potential to be very influential. Examining a sample of the prenatal and parenting books, as well as the "new sibling" children's books, can not only reveal the prevailing ideologies about infant feeding in the era in which they were published, but also provides an idea of the messages that new parents and children receive about infant feeding.

Advice for Expectant Parents

Most expectant parents begin with pregnancy advice books, which are often distributed at prenatal visits. These books are geared toward a mainstream audience and are saturated with "scientific" evidence phrased in layperson's terms. Many of these books incorporate the opinions of "medical experts" or are written by them, and aim to be prescriptive and informative. For example, the 2008 edition of *What to Expect When You're Expecting* begins with "Foreword to the Fourth Edition," in which Dr. Charles J. Lockwood recommends the book, stating, "It's packed with information and useful advice, the kind you would hear from your favorite doctor or midwife."[7] This introduction reinforces and demonstrates the role of these books—as advisers, experts, and supplements to the doctor. Without questioning who the authors are or the personal or institutional bias of the text, we accept these books as part of the ritual into parenthood, including their information on infant feeding. In addition, while most pregnancy books have been traditionally written for women, a new subgenre of the pregnancy books has emerged in recent years: advice for dads.

For this section, I analyzed the messages about infant feeding in popular pregnancy and childrearing books. Here, the objective was to collect as many popular books that may address infant feeding as possible. Background literature suggested that books on pregnancy, early childrearing, and sleep-training would likely offer infant feeding advice. To identify the books, an *Amazon* search was conducted in the above categories. The *Amazon* "best-seller" list was consulted for the "top" books in each category, combined with a search on the bookstore Barnes & Noble website, and blog lists of popular parenting books. Next, a textual analysis was conducted on the books themselves, examining advice relevant to infant feeding (for the list of books, see Table 5.1). Books specifically on breastfeeding were used as background information for analyzing the parenting books. The following sections outline the themes identified in the different books.

Breast or Bottle: A Choice?

The breast "versus" bottle decision (or sometimes labeled as a "controversy") is a staple part of pregnancy books. Each of these texts follows similar format: presenting the either/or of these methods, briefly acknowledging the health benefits of breastmilk, and then moving to the advantages/disadvantages of each one. In *What to Expect When You're Expecting*, which moves chronologically through the months of pregnancy, Heidi Murkoff and Sharon Mazel first mention breastfeeding in "The Eighth Month" chapter under "All About Breastfeeding."[8] They offer a brief history of how breastfeeding "went out of favor" and then returned in contemporary times. The section "Why Breast is Best," states, "Your human milk is the perfect meal for your human newborn." They offer a detailed overview of the benefits to the baby and mother, with contact information for LLL. The positive tone toward breastfeeding switches with the next section: "Don't feel guilty about choosing the bottle over the breast" and then negates all of the positives they have just listed about breastfeeding with bottle-feeding advantages.[9] This lengthy justification undermines the breastfeeding benefits, with subheadings explaining that formula-feeding offers "Fewer dietary restraints," "Less embarrassment for the modest," "Less stress," and other caveats that frame formula as the practical feeding solution, including "advantages" that could easily also work for breastfeeding.[10] Likewise, Vicki Iovine's *The Girlfriends' Guide to Pregnancy* (2007) discusses breast- and bottle-feeding as equal options.[11] Later, in the chapter on common complaints in the postpartum period, she includes a section "I Hate Nursing." She acknowledges societal pressure to breastfeed, but offers practical advice, with "Try it. If you like it, keep doing it. If you don't like it, you have our permission to quit."[12] The neutrality toward breastfeeding in these

Table 5.1 New Parent Books Studied

Author	*Year*	*Title*	*Type of Book*
	2011	*Mayo Clinic: Guide to a Healthy Pregnancy*	Pregnancy
Iovine, Vicki	2008	*The Girlfriends' Guide to Pregnancy*	Pregnancy
Murray, Hennen, Scott	2005	*The Baby Center Essential Guide to Pregnancy and Birth*	Pregnancy
Murkoff, Eisenberg, & Hathaway	2002	*What to Expect When You're Expecting*	Pregnancy
Brott, Armin & Ash, Jennifer	2015	*The Expectant Father: The Ultimate Guide for Dads-to-Be*	Partner pregnancy
Pfeiffer, John	2011	*Due, You're Gonna Be a Dad!*	Partner pregnancy
Brott, Armin & Ash, Jennifer	2010	*The Expectant Father: Facts, Tips, and Advice for Dads-to-Be*	Partner pregnancy
Port, David & Ralsont, John	2006	*The Caveman's Pregnancy Companion*	Partner pregnancy
Pearl, Michael & Debi Pearl	2015	*To Train Up a Child: Training for the 21st Century*	Childrearing
Shelvov, Steven P. & Hannemann, Robert E.	2005	*The Complete and Authoritative Guide Caring for Your Baby and Young Child, Birth to Age 5.*	Childrearing
Sears, William & Martha Sears	2001	*The Attachment Parenting Book: A Commensense Guide to Understanding and Nurturing Your Baby*	Childrearing
Pearl, Michael & Debi Pearl	1994	*To Train Up a Child*	Childrearing
Ezzo, Gary & Bucknam, Robert	2012	*On Becoming Babywise*	Sleep-training
Karp, Harvey	2012	*The Happiest Baby Guide to Great Sleep*	Sleep-training
Waldburger, Jennifer & Spivack, Jill	2007	*The Sleepeasy Solution*	Sleep-training
Ferber, Richard	2006	*Solve Your Child's Sleep Problems*	Sleep-training
Sears, William & Martha Sears	2005	*The Baby Sleep Book: The Complete Guide to a Good Night's Rest for the Whole Family*	Sleep-training
Pantley, Elizabeth	2002	*The No-Cry Sleep Solution*	Sleep-training
Cuthbertson, Joanne & Schevill, Susanna	1985	*Helping Your Child Sleep Through the Night*	Sleep-training

widely popular books undermines all of the positive statements, equating breastfeeding to other baby decisions—like which crib to buy or whether or not to make your own baby food.

The expectant father-type books also present the breast/bottle choice. *The New Father* (1997) and *The Expectant Father: Facts, Tips, and Advice for Dads-to-Be* (2010) contain sections that parallel both means of feeding—acknowledging that breastmilk offers more benefits, but swiftly introduce formula as an alternative. In *Dude, You're Gonna Be a Dad!* (2011) for example, under "Bottle vs. Breast," Pfeiffer begins with "Experts agree that breastmilk wins, hands down," lists a few benefits, then shifts to explaining that formula-feeding is acceptable and that it is the woman's choice.[13] In *The Caveman's Pregnancy Companion* (2011), David Port and John Ralston provide a similar overview, then advise expectant parents to decide "what's best" for their child.[14] And Armin Brott and Jennifer Ash (2010) advise purchasing formula for the mother who plans to breastfeed "just in case," even if "some breastfeeding experts" advise against having formula, in their book *The Expectant Father: The Ultimate Guide for Dads-to-Be* (2015).[15] These books also offered mixed messages on supporting new breastfeeding mothers. While *The Expectant Father* encouraged new parents to use lactation consultants, *Dude, You're Gonna Be a Dad!* is firmly against outside help. Pfeiffer offers what is supposed to be a humorously stern warning about LLL, devoting almost an entire paragraph to his intense dislike for the group. He warns fathers that if someone from LLL attempts to help:

> Be afraid. Be very afraid. It's unconfirmed that these people are the modern offshoot of the Nazi party. *Do not* by any means leave your partner alone for this experience. These people are only slightly less dedicated to breastfeeding than suicide bombers are to their cause. They will use *any* means necessary to achieve their goal, which is to get the mother of your child to breastfeed... Take their information for what it's worth, and if they get too aggressive, leave a carbon footprint on their ass as you kick them out of your room."[16]

Even if the author had a previous negative experience, this oddly-intense warning is not only frightening, but fiercely dissuades partners from encouraging breastfeeding mothers to seek support from other women, reinforcing an unfortunate stereotype that is not the norm of every group. Furthermore, this inappropriate advice degrades the importance of peer counseling, LLL, and other support that plays a significant role in breastfeeding success for many women.[17]

Even books endorsed by medical professionals are relatively neutral in their discussion of infant feeding. For example, the *Mayo Clinic: Guide to a Healthy Pregnancy* (2004) includes a section entitled, "Decision Guide—The breast or the bottle."[18] It begins with "Do you plan to feed your baby with breast milk or formula?"[19] Dr. Richard Harms explains in two sentences that breastfeeding is popular, followed by, "For a variety of reasons, other women choose to feed their babies with formula. Today's commercial formulas ensure that babies can be well-nourished with bottle-feeding."[20] Likewise, *The Complete and Authoritative Guide: Caring for Your Baby and Young Child, Birth to Age 5* (endorsed by the American Academy of Pediatrics (AAP)) begins its feeding section with "Should I Breastfeed or Bottle-feed?"[21] The book states that the AAP encourages breastfeeding, yet "while not identical to breastmilk, formulas do provide appropriate nutrition. Both approaches are safe and healthy for your baby, and each has its advantages."[22] Similar statements appear in the newest print edition of the book.

In *The Mayo Clinic* book, the chapter on infant feeding offers a rationale for both methods of feeding babies. Despite having the endorsement of the medical profession, the health benefits of breastfeeding are skimmed over and undermined, with words like "may help," "may be less likely," and "may offer a slight reduction" attached to the benefits.[23] The authors then highlight a few advantages, paired with a lengthy list of the possible challenges of breastfeeding, followed by a page on health reasons for not breastfeeding. The final pages of the feeding chapter explain the safety of commercial formula with, "If you can't breast-feed or choose not to, you can be assured that your baby's nutrition can be met."[24] This statement is supported by a lengthy section on the advantages of formula-feeding (seven pages), which exceeds the section on breastfeeding.[25] Again, given that this book is often distributed at OB/GYN offices as the medical reference for pregnancy, this seemingly neutral perspective is alarming.

Breastfeeding: Not Conducive to Working Outside the Home?

These pregnancy books suggest that working is not compatible with breastfeeding (even though, of course, many women successfully breastfeed and work). Discussions of working and pumping milk are notably absent from the "breast vs. bottle" decision-making guides. Instead, authors gloss over the possibility of successfully breastfeeding and working, presenting bottle-feeding (presumably formula since milk expression is largely overlooked) as the only option for the working mother. For example, in the advantages of bottle-feeding section of *What to Expect*, Murkoff and Mazel list "More freedom" (as a subhead), stating that, "Bottle-feeding doesn't tie the mother down to her baby. She's able to work outside the home without worrying about pumping and storing milk, travel a few days without the baby, even sleep through the night—because someone else can feed her baby."[26] Although expressing one's milk is briefly discussed, it is not highlighted, nor is it offered as a suitable alternative for the working mother.[27] *The Girlfriends' Guide* indirectly conveys breastfeeding as overly time-consuming, as Iovine reflects, "Nursing forced me to neglect the meaningless busyness of my life and pay attention to the baby and me."[28] Yet, she fails to mention how to juggle breastfeeding and working. Even in books that address pumping, it is not connected to working.

The absence of working and breastfeeding advice is problematic. Approximately 66 million women are employed in the United States, making up 47% of the labor force.[29] According to the Bureau of Labor Statics, in 60.2% of families with married couples, both parents work.[30] More than 60% of mothers with children under 6 years old are employed, and, even with children under a year old, more mothers work (57%) than stay home.[31] These statistics confirm that most mothers work, at least part-time, yet the parenting books ignore this possibility and present the combination of breastfeeding and a career as an impossible mix. A more breastfeeding-friendly approach would be to assume that many women want to breastfeed and work. Therefore, in the "preparations" section of the pregnancy books, authors could advise that women investigate pumping spaces and policies at their workplaces (as protected under the ACA) and check with insurance companies on hospital-grade pumps. This encouragement would help support breastfeeding for working mothers—a group of women that especially need support given that working outside the home is negatively correlated with breastfeeding duration.[32]

Sexualizing Breasts

The sexualization of breasts has been given as one reason people are uncomfortable with breastfeeding and is perpetuated and exaggerated in pregnancy advice books. In *The Caveman's Pregnancy Companion* (obviously geared toward men), Port and Ralson introduce breastfeeding with "Besides obvious voyeuristic advantages for the caveman, breastfeeding offers tangible benefits to both mother and baby."[33] For expectant fathers, this attempt at humor reinforces the "male gaze" with the notion that breastfeeding is pleasurable for men to watch.[34] For pregnant women that may read this book, such a statement may discourage breastfeeding in the presence of others for fear of objectification. Moreover, Iovine describes the sensual feelings of breastfeeding for the woman, stating that "Nursing feels really, really good" and compares it to sex.[35] If a woman is already somewhat uncomfortable with using her breasts to nurse, this statement will do little to help put her at ease.

Breastfeeding is framed as a hindrance to intimacy in *What to Expect*, as one perk of bottle-feeding is (in a bolded subhead) "Potentially, more romance." Murkoff and Mazel argue, "For bottle-feeding couples, the breasts can play their strictly sensual role rather than their utilitarian one."[36] A teaser box on the same page supports their position with the heading "The Breast: Sexual or Practical," which discusses "different roles of the breast."[37] These headings, particularly under the "pro-bottle-feeding" section, imply that breastfeeding conflicts with sexual relationships for its duration. This myth is not solely perpetuated in this book. Women have expressed reservations about breastfeeding with the concern that it would interfere with intimacy, even stating that they feared nursing in front of their partners because it would desexualize their breasts.[38] A more breastfeeding-friendly framework would reassure women that their breasts are multi-purpose and that partners should support mothers in breastfeeding, not dissuade them from doing it.

The Polarization of Parenting Philosophies

Although it may seem tangential to breastfeeding, books on childrearing, including "sleep-training," can also have dire effects on breastfeeding success. Parenting advice books run the gamut, from the strict authoritarian, parent-led approach that encourages babies to "cry-it-out" to the flexible, child-led Attachment Parenting philosophy, which revolves

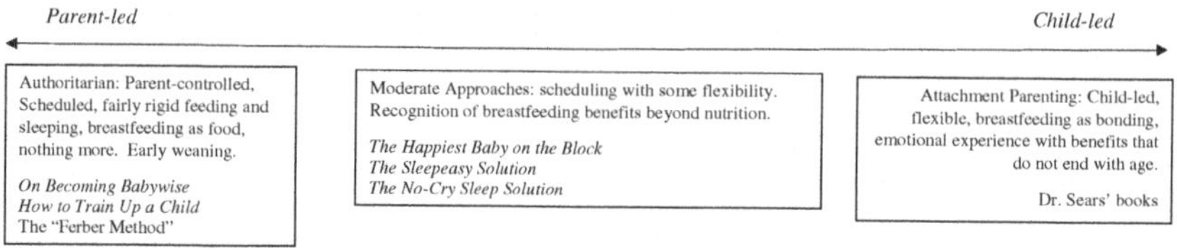

Fig. 5.1 Parenting philosophies and approaches

around children's comfort (see Fig. 5.1). Since these books often begin with infancy, breastfeeding is sometimes addressed. Therefore, popular childrearing books were examined for their infant feeding messages (see Table 5.1). In these texts, authors offer advice on every aspect of a baby's day in order to produce the "optimal" child, using a specific "method" (the money-maker for the book). Parents turn to these "experts" for advice on helping babies and toddlers sleep, when, what, and how to feed their children, and other topics on everyday life.

At the authoritarian end of the spectrum, authors prescribe a strict regiment for controlling babies, particularly for sleeping and eating. These authors suggest that past a certain point (which varies by book), babies should not wake up at night to nurse because it reinforces an instinct that is "wrong," "outdated," "inconvenient," or even "selfish." Furthermore, babies should not be fed on demand, but on regimented schedules determined by the parents. The end goal: the parent controls (or ignores) the baby's desire (need) to sleep and eat. This "objective" is accomplished by neglecting babies when they wake up at the "wrong" time and ending a breastfeeding session after a pre-determined length of time. However, perceptions of feeding on-demand, the prescribed age for night-weaning, and parental response vary by the severity of the approach.

Perhaps the most severe book in this genre is Michael and Debi Pearl's *To Train Up a Child* (1994), a text that uses scripture to justify beating young children into compliance.[39] Despite the heavy criticism for its use of corporal punishment, particularly in the early years, it certainly has a following. The Pearls advise "training" babies in infancy and beyond by striking them with willow branches. Breastfeeding is only mentioned once. The controversial book explains how to address biting during nursing sessions by pulling the baby's hair enough to cause pain.[40] And, instead of using breastfeeding to help with sleep, they recommend whipping babies with switches to subdue them.[41]

The more mainstream *On Becoming Babywise* adheres to a similar philosophy that parents need to control their children, including their eating and sleeping habits. Using a militant tone, Gary Ezzo and Robert Bucknam (2012) suggest that parents follow the formula:

Hunger Cue + Clock + PA (Parental Assessment) = Feeding Time

This "calculation" is supposed to help determine when to feed the baby.[42] Breastfeeding is recommended, but only for nutrition, and should always occur at their prescribed intervals.[43] They argue against nursing on demand and cluster feeding, insisting that scheduled feeding leads to breastfeeding success. Furthermore, they claim that breastfeeding after a year is unnecessary and "is done more out of Mom's preference than for a nutritional need."[44] Obviously, this statement ignores studies demonstrating the health benefits of extended breastfeeding and contradicts duration recommendations by the World Health Organization. Yet, it claims to have helped "six million parents," and is in its fifth edition, therefore many people are receiving (and heeding the advice of) this inaccurate information.[45]

Another popular "cry-it-out" philosophy is the "Ferber Method," coined by Richard Ferber in *Solve Your Child's Sleep Problems* (2006).[46] Ferber ardently criticizes feeding on demand and advises parents to "train" babies from infancy, declaring, "A full-term, healthy infant does not need hourly feedings, even if he seems hungry at these times and nurses when you offer the breast or bottle… It is unnecessary for the baby, and it interferes with the development of healthier sleepwake and feeding patterns."[47] Ferber offers a rigid feeding and sleeping schedule for parents for each month of the first year and advises night weaning by 5 months, explaining, "Basically no normal, healthy full-term babies still *require* a nighttime feeding when they are five months old, and you can certainly insist on stopping them altogether at that point if you want to."[48] Reminiscent of the "feeding experts" in magazines of the early 1900s, the authors of *Babywise* and Ferber do not directly scrutinize breastfeeding, but encourage restrictive feeding schedules and "scientific" approaches to breastfeeding that would likely destroy milk supply, leading to early weaning.

Most childrearing and sleep-training books are more moderate in their approach. For example, Harvey Karp's *The Happiest Baby on the Block*[49] (2012) recommends a flexible schedule for feeding and sleeping, based on the baby's age, needs, and feeding cues. Similarly, *The Sleepeasy*

Solution (2007) and *The No-Cry Sleep Solution* (2002) encourage feeding on demand, especially for the first 4 months.[50] Both texts recommend "gentle" approaches to sleep-training, including the delay of night weaning, which they say should be done slowly and only with older babies, ensuring that the milk supply does not dwindle.[51] Yet, even books that preach moderation may create troubles for nursing babies, as they sometimes suggest schedules and setting time-limits on nursing sessions, an approach that is counterintuitive to the supply and demand system of breastfeeding and ignores nursing for comfort.

At the other end of the spectrum, are advocates of the Attachment Parenting philosophy, an "instinctual, high-touch way of caring" for children, centered around babies' needs and wants.[52] William and Martha Sears, creators of this approach, encourage "birth bonding" through kangaroo care, breastfeeding, baby-wearing, and co-sleeping for parents and children in order to establish and maintain firm attachment.[53] Its proponents do not believe in "training" babies, but feeding on demand, keeping children close, and responding to their cues. For breastfeeding, Attachment Parenting works well, creating an ample supply and a closeness for mother and baby, especially with self-led weaning and co-sleeping that characterize this philosophy. However, critics of this philosophy argue that the child-centeredness leads to exhausted parents and is not practical for mothers who work.[54] Others have viewed the approach as an elitist and extremist practice in which its followers ridicule those who do not abide by the AP tenets.[55]

Regardless of the specific philosophy, all of these approaches exemplify parents' reliance on "experts" to instruct them on how to care for their children, with carefully laid-out steps to implement the plan. These "experts" strip power away from parents, encouraging them to ignore their instincts (and their babies) and instead follow a factory-model scientific approach to fight biological needs. From "Babywise" to "Attachment Parenting," these philosophies also polarize parents, distancing them from each other, thus instigating and fueling the so-called "Mommy Wars." Here, ridicule and blame for those who do not adhere to the specific approach are encouraged, as controversy boosts sales. And, instead of depending on family and friends for support, these books may take their place, and if strictly adhered to, could likely cause stress, fatigue, and trouble with achieving successful and pleasant breastfeeding experiences.

Infant Feeding Messages in Children's Books

Just as parenting books are given to new parents, the "new sibling" books are common gifts for older children. While these fictional books are not as prescriptive as the childrearing guides, they too make a statement predicting life with a new baby. These books are popular—https://www.amazon.com offers over 800 children's books on "new baby books for siblings." And, as children typically read books over and over, memorizing and internalizing the messages, these books have the potential to profoundly shape how children view infant feeding. Children's books also, of course, reflect and perpetuate dominant ideologies in society, including the default way to nourish a baby.

New baby/sibling books comprise their own genre at Barnes and Noble and other book stores. Amid the pregnancy and parenting books are colorful children's books with drawings of big brothers/sisters welcoming their new siblings. A list of 43 books was compiled from the "most popular" books on Amazon, books available at Barnes and Noble, and the books at the local library in attempts to mirror the books that expectant parents might obtain for the soon-to-be older sibling (see Table 5.2). While these books obviously vary somewhat by region, store, and library, collectively, they provide general patterns of infant feeding discourse. Across the books studied, although "new sibling" stories deviate slightly in their specific focus, they follow a similar narrative. The older sibling learns of the pregnancy and becomes concerned with his/her place in the family. Mommy assures the older sibling of her love. Baby arrives at home. Then a comparison of the older child and the baby follows, pairing eating, sleeping, toileting, and playing to demonstrate how different babies are from toddlers. Bright illustrations featuring animals or humans accompany the simple text, as most books are (presumably) written for toddler or preschool-aged children.

Omitting How to Feed the Baby

Sixteen of the 43 books analyzed do not address the feeding of a baby. Although all of these books focus on bringing home a new sibling, they cover other aspects of infancy: diaper changes, sleeping, playing, and bath time. For example, in *The Berenstain Bears and the New Baby* (1985), the storyline explains how Small Bear and his dad build a new bed for him so that the baby can have his old bed. The baby is introduced at the end

Table 5.2 Children's Books Studied

Author	*Title*	*Year*	*Feeding?*
Saunders, Katie	*Olive Marshmallow*	2015	Bottle
Capucilli, Alyssa Satin	*Henry is a Big Brother*	2014	Bottle
Capucilli, Alyssa Satin	*Hannah is a Big Sister*	2014	Bottle
O'Connor, Jane	*Lulu and the Witch Baby*	2014	Bottle
Bracken, Beth	*Henry Helps with the Baby*	2012	Bottle
Manushkin, Fran	*Big Brothers are the Best*	2012	Bottle
Manushkin, Fran & Richards, Kirsten	*Big Sisters are the Best*	2012	Bottle
Cole, Joanna	*I'm a Big Brother*	2010	Bottle
Cole, Joanna	*I'm a Big Sister*	2010	Bottle
Feiffer, Kate and Goode, Diane	*But I wanted a Baby Brother*	2010	Bottle
Landolf, Diane Wright	*What a Good Big Brother*	2009	Breast
Katz, Karen	*Best Ever Big Brother*	2006	Bottle
Sheldon, Annette	*Big Sister Now*	2006	Breast
Sears, William & Martha	*What Baby Needs*	2004	Both
Murkoff, Heidi	*What to Expect When the New Baby Comes Home*	2001	Both
Sears, William & Martha, Kelly, Christie Watts	*Baby on the Way*	2001	Breast
Berenstain, Stan & Jan	*And Baby Makes Five*	2000	Bottle
Civardi, Anne	*The New Baby*	2000	Breast
Harris, Robie H.	*Hi New Baby!*	2000	Breast
Rockwell, Lizzy	*Hello Baby*	1999	Breast
Langreuter, Jutta	*Little Bear is a Big Brother*	1998	Bottle
Henkes, Kevin	*Julius: The Baby of the World*	1990	Bottle
Rogers, Fred	*The New Baby*	1985	Both
Parish, Peggy	*Amelia Bedelia and the Baby*	1981	Bottle
Santomero, Angela C. & Jason Fruchter	*The Baby is Here! (Daniel Tiger's Neighborhood)*	2015	None
Simmons, Anthea & Georgie Birkett	*The Bestest Baby*	2015	None
Hood, Susan & Mary Lundquist	*Mission: New Baby*	2015	None
Dempsey, Sheena	*Bye-Bye Baby Brother*	2013	None
White, Kathryn	*Ruby's Baby Brother*	2013	None
Packard, Mary	*Little Bear's Baby Brother*	2011	None
Gaydos, Nora	*Now I'm Growing! I'm a New Brother*	2010	None
Gaydos, Nora	*Now I'm Growing! I'm a New Sister*	2010	None
Sullivan, Sarah	*Once Upon a Baby Brother*	2010	None

(continued)

Table 5.2 (continued)

Author	*Title*	*Year*	*Feeding?*
Woodson, Jacqueline	*Pecan Pie Baby*	2010	None
Regan, Dian Curtis	*Monster Baby*	2009	None
Saltzberg, Barney	*Cornelius P. Mud, Are you ready for baby?*	2009	None
Symes, Ruth	*Little Rex, Big Brother*	2009	None
Elliott, Laura Malone	*Hunter's Big Sister*	2007	None
Sarah, Duchess of York	*Michael and his New Baby Brother*	2007	None
Horse, Harry	*Little Rabbit's New Baby*	2006	None
Gliori, Debi	*Where Did That Baby Come From?*	2004	None
Wing, Natasha	*The Night Before the New Baby*	2002	None
Berenstain, Stan & Jan	*The New Baby*	1974	None

of the story, with no feeding mentioned. Other books skip the liquid-feeding stage and describe solid-feeding the new baby, with a drawing of a baby in the high chair covered in colorful food streaks.

Breastfeeding Only

Only six books studied exclusively mention or depict breastfeeding. In *Hi New Baby!* (2000), Robie H. Harris and Michael Emberley describe the fictional experience of the first days of having a new sibling from the perspective of the older child, explaining, "Mommy fed the new baby and ate a pickle. Then the new baby spit up."[56] The text here is accompanied by a drawing of the mother clearly nursing the baby, with the infant latched at the breast. Similarly, in *Hello Baby!* (1999), Lizzy Rockwell again writes from the point-of-view of the older child, stating, "Mommy nurses her in the rocker. Mommy's breasts make milk that is the perfect food for a baby. Soon Eliza falls asleep in her lap."[57] A drawing of the mother breastfeeding the baby complements this text. Anne Civardi's *The New Baby* (2000) also presents breastfeeding as the way to feed a baby. As with other books, Civardi provides an overview of what happens with a new baby, from labor to the mother and child coming home from the hospital. "When Susie is hungry, Mrs. Bunn feeds her with milk. Susie will need to be fed many times each day," paired with a drawing of the mother nursing the baby.[58] In *What a Good Big Brother* (2009), the older sibling asks why his new baby sister is crying. "'She's hungry,' his mom said. 'Do you know where the nursing pillow is?'" The big brother brings the pillow. The next page explains, "Cameron's mom tucked the nursing pillow around herself."[59] This narrative is illustrated with a drawing of the mother breastfeeding the baby using the pillow, while the brother happily watches.

The book *Baby on the Way* (2001), by Attachment Parenting gurus William and Martha Sears and Christie Watts Kelly, features a drawing of a woman nursing, with the text, "Tiny babies just sleep and nurse all day long—nursing is how babies get milk from their mommies' breasts."[60] This book ends with a page directed at parents that explains the philosophy of Attachment Parenting. A more subtle representation appears in Annette Sheldon's *A Big Sister Now* (2006). The text reads, "One morning I needed Mommy to get the bowl for my cereal. But Mommy was busy feeding Daniel."[61] The picture features an over the shoulder drawing of the mother, who seems to be nursing. The same drawing appears on the next page, as well. These books present breastfeeding as the means to feed a baby. In *What Baby Needs* (2004), William and Martha Sears even stress expressed milk for when mothers are absent, explaining that, "Baby nurses to get milk from your mommy's breasts," which is paired with a drawing of a baby nursing, latched on.[62] The next page states, "Or, when Baby is older, Baby might be fed Mommy's milk from a bottle if Mommy has to be away," illustrated with a drawing of a man feeding a baby a bottle.[63] Here, breastfeeding is emphasized, assumed, and conveyed as normal. The nursing mothers do not appear anxious or concerned, but calmly breastfeed their babies, without a blanket or other cover. Unfortunately, the breastfeeding-only messages do not dominate the new sibling books.

Breast or Bottle: "Equal" Options?

Some books present breast- and bottle-feeding as parallel in the images and text. For example, in *The New Baby* (1985), by the beloved children's television host Fred Rogers, the text explains, "Babies often get hungry. Sometimes they cry because they don't like to wait to be fed. How is your little brother or sister fed?"[64] Below this question are two photos: On the left, a mother is clearly breastfeeding, with the baby latched on and looking at his mother. In the right photo, Dad is bottle-feeding the baby. Likewise, Heidi Murkhoff's *What to Expect When the New Baby Comes Home* (2001) offers a similar comparison.

This book—the juvenile version of the pregnancy best-seller—answers the question "What do babies eat?" with "The milk they drink is a special milk that's just right for new babies.[65] It looks more watery and tastes a little strange to anyone who isn't a new baby. Mommies can make this special milk in their breasts, and new babies can drink it right from their mommy's nipples. That's called nursing or breast-feeding." The next section goes on to say "Or mommies can buy this special milk and put it in bottles for their new babies to drink. That's called bottle-feeding. Some new babies just bottle-feed, some new babies just nurse, and some new babies do both. Ask your mommy or daddy which way you ate when you were a baby."[66] The opposite page shows a drawing of two women feeding their babies on benches outside. The apparently Caucasian woman is bottle-feeding her child, while the African American woman is breastfeeding. Like many of the adult pregnancy books, this balance of breast- and bottle-feeding reinforces nursing as a choice, not a given or a second choice.

Bottles as the "Norm"

Overwhelmingly, bottles are presented as the "normal" means of feeding a baby. Fifteen of the 24 books that address feeding a baby only feature bottle-feeding. For example, in *Henry Helps with the Baby* (2012), by Beth Bracken, the fictional character, Henry, explains that his sister "likes sleeping, cuddling, and drinking milk," accompanied by a drawing of a baby sitting next to a half-full bottle.[67] The next page of this story depicts the mother holding the bottle and baby. And, toward the end of the book, the father is shown holding the bottle and baby. Even with the use of the word "milk," there is no indication of breastfeeding or the expression of breastmilk. This book is not alone in the multiple drawings and text perpetuating bottle-feeding. Joanna Cole's books *I'm a Big Brother* and *I'm a Big Sister* (both 2010), each include two pages with bottle-feeding images. For each book, the text reads, "Babies like to drink milk" with a picture of a bottle on a table.[68] And later, "Oh, it's time to change the baby's diaper. It's time for a bottle, too."[69] Again, bottle-feeding is the default, as it is with another sister/brother pair of books. Fran Manushkin's *Big Sisters are the Best* (2012) and *Big Brothers are the Best* (2012), state that "Little Babies drink bottles. Big sisters eat cupcakes!" or "Big Brothers eat cupcakes!," with a drawing of a baby drinking from a bottle, compared to a girl/boy holding a cupcake.[70] The

Big Sister book includes an additional bottle image, with the girl feeding a bottle to her baby doll. And in the big sister/brother books *Hannah is a Big Sister* and *Henry is a Big Brother* (2014) by Alissa Satin Capucilli, the texts reads, "Is Casey getting hungry?," which is accompanied by a drawing of a dad looking uncomfortable as he feeds baby a bottle.[71] Amelia Bedelia prepares a bottle for the baby that she babysits, with no mention of expressed milk. In *Olive Marshmallow* (2015), a bottle is pictured next to a carseat, as the big brother describes meeting his new sister.[72] Even though many of these books are contemporary, they still promote bottles as the default feeding method for babies.

Even in books that are not about human babies, bottle-feeding is depicted. Fictional animal characters are shown feeding their babies with bottles. In *Little Bear is a Big Brother* (2011), Little Bear tells his friends, "I'm already giving him his bottle, and I can burp him, too, and he hardly cries at all," paired with a drawing of a bear feeding a bottle to the baby bear.[73] A mouse carries a bottle for the baby in *Julius: The Baby of the World* (1990). In *Berenstain Bears: And Baby Makes Five* (2000), a half-empty bottle is on the side table. Even supernatural creatures use bottles, as opposed to other ways of nourishing their young. For example, in *Lulu and Witch Baby* (2014), the text reads, "Witch Baby had a bottle of brew. She was too little to eat pie. She was just a baby" (with a drawing of the baby drinking out of a bottle).[74]

These books overwhelming convey the message that feeding is not a central part of infancy. Many books exclude eating as part of the routine, while touching on diapering, sleeping, and other key activities in the early days of a baby's life. Furthermore, the families featured here are nearly all Caucasian, heterosexual couples, or animal characters. Only six books studied visibly include characters of other ethnicities. "New baby" books also mostly use illustrations, as opposed to photographs. The use of drawings may be problematic, particularly with breastfeeding images, as real photos could help children perceive breastfeeding as natural, not as something to hide or only depict through cartoons. When feeding is addressed, it is usually bottle-feeding, particularly as part of the background (with bottles on a table, for example). Breastfeeding seems to be more of a conscious choice by the writer—to make a point about breastfeeding or to compare it to bottle-feeding.

Why do these messages matter? Stories teach children about the world and about new experiences, helping to prepare them for significant life events. Here, by not presenting breastfeeding as the normal means of feeding a baby, these narratives suggest that bottle-feeding is more common, or the default, particularly when paired with toy bottles or stickers of bottles. And, aside from the absurdity of mammals feeding their young with bottles, the animal characters further reinforce the normalcy of bottles. These stories also influence more than just new siblings, as even in single-child families, these books are common. Bringing home a new baby is a common theme in children's literature—most popular book series include a new baby storyline: Mercer Mayer's Little Critter gets a sister in *The New Baby*, The Berenstain Bears add, not one, but two siblings in *The New Baby* and *The Berenstain Bears and Baby Makes Five*. Marc Brown's aardvark series also adds a sibling in *Arthur's Baby*. Many of these books also cross generations, with nostalgic parents purchasing their favorite children's books for their own children, meaning that outdated preferences for bottles continue to be disseminated through these books. Yes, children's books that feature breastfeeding do exist, but they are not in the mainstream. For example, *Mommy Feeds Baby*, *Milkies in the Morning: A Gentle Night Weaning Storybook*, and *You, Me, and the Breast* (2012), all feature breastfeeding. Yet, these books are on the periphery—clearly sought by families who are already very pro-breastfeeding and certainly not in the pile of books at the pediatrician's office or at the local library.

Conclusion

Overall, popular books on pregnancy, childrearing, and new siblings reinforce a bottle-feeding culture. These books generally give a nod to breastfeeding, but then center around and show bottle-feeding babies. Pregnancy books lack appropriate advice and support for breastfeeding. Popular books focused on breastfeeding model some tips, language, and tone that would drastically improve breastfeeding discourse in mainstream pregnancy books. First, pregnancy books could be reframed to assume that women will nurse—an approach used in the mainstream book *The Baby Center Essential Guide to Pregnancy and Birth* (2005). Unlike the other pregnancy texts targeting a mass audience, the feeding section of this book does not present breastfeeding as a parallel choice to bottle-feeding. Rather, "Breastfeeding" is the title of the chapter, which begins with *how* to breastfeeding, not *if* a woman should breastfeed.[75] In fact, formula and bottle-feeding are not addressed in any part of this chapter. This approach presents breastfeeding as normal, as it should be, without equating it as a mode of feeding to formula. Pregnancy books also need more images and illustrations of breastfeeding. Cutesy drawings of bottles accompany most of the infant feeding text in these books. Photos of real women breastfeeding, close-ups of good latches, and clear illustrations on common problems would strengthen advice about breastfeeding and remind readers that the sight of breastfeeding should be expected.

Books on childrearing vary in their breastfeeding-conducive recommendations. That said, all of these books share a commonality in their use of "experts" that instruct new parents. Why do we care if new parents pore over these books in quiet desperation to curb their babies' crying? First, as evidenced here, these books offer conflicting advice. Each author preaches that his/her "method" is superior, usually supported by "research" demonstrating the effectiveness of the "Baby Whisperer," or their "scientific" formulas to determine feeding time. For a new mother, some of the "advice" could permanently impede her milk supply. At the other end of the spectrum, parents may feel tremendous guilt if they cannot babywear their infants to work or become exhausted because bed-sharing just is not for them. The quantity and tone of these books also likely undermines the new mother's confidence in breastfeeding, as the "experts" lay the foundation for the "method" by establishing that a problem exists—that they are "bad" parents because their babies wake up at night (which is completely natural) or if they shudder at the notion of wanting personal space. Overall, the greatest concern with these parenting books is our dependence on them. In other words, the lack of information and support from the OB/GYN and pediatrician's offices forces new parents to rely on these books, including for breastfeeding advice.

Children's books also contain mixed messages about feeding babies. While one might dismiss their significance, these texts set the foundation for how children see the world, particularly if they do not have first-hand experience. Unlike most adults, children read their books repeatedly, poring over every detail until their stories become memorized. Thus, the text and images in these books become imprinted in their brains. These messages then help shape how children perceive and understand the world, impacting what they view as "normal" and "abnormal," and offer a prescription of how life should be. Moreover, children's books, along with the parenting advice books for adults, demonstrate what messages media disseminate about infant feeding, indicating that while progress has been made to increase breastfeeding knowledge, attitudes and the normalization of breastfeeding are still lacking.

Clearly, more pro-breastfeeding messages and pictures of a diverse group of nursing mothers are needed to improve the cultural climate. Just as importantly, we need to recognize the significance of partner and mother-to-mother support, even more so than relying on "experts" that have never met the babies firsthand. Such a community will also help to expose children to different mothers and families so that they can hopefully learn and see breastfeeding modeled in real people, as opposed to assuming a cartoon bear bottle-feeding her cub is the "normal" means of feeding a baby. As exemplified in the next chapter, these limited messages in books are not unique to the medium.

Notes

1. Arora et al., "Major Factors Influencing Breastfeeding Rates."
2. Chen, Johnson, and Rosenthal, "Sources of Education about Breastfeeding and Breast Pump Use."
3. Ibid.
4. Parry et al., "Understanding Women's Interpretations of Infant Formula Advertising."
5. Arora et al., "Major Factors Influencing Breastfeeding Rates."
6. "What to Expect When You're Expecting, 4th Edition (Description)."
7. Lockwood, "Foreword to the Fourth Edition."
8. Murkoff and Mazel, *What to Expect When You're Expecting, 4th Edition.*
9. Ibid.
10. Ibid.
11. Iovine, *The Girlfriends' Guide to Pregnancy.*
12. Ibid, p. 241.
13. Pfeiffer, *Dude, You're a Dad!* p. 169.
14. Port and Ralston, *The Caveman's Pregnancy Companion.*
15. Brott and Ash, *The Expectant Father.*
16. Pfeiffer, *Dude, You're a Dad!* p. 151.
17. Rossman, "Breastfeeding Peer Counselors in the United States"; Chapman et al., "Effectiveness of Breastfeeding Peer Counseling in a Low-Income, Predominantly Latina Population"; Rozga, Kerver, and Olson, "Impact of Peer Counselling Breast-Feeding Support Programme Protocols on Any and Exclusive Breast-Feeding Discontinuation in Low-Income Women."
18. Harms, *Mayo Clinic Guide to a Healthy Pregnancy by Mayo Clinic (2004) Paperback.*

19. Ibid, p. 363.
20. Ibid.
21. Shelov, *Caring for Your Baby and Young Child.*
22. Ibid, p. 23.
23. Harms, *Mayo Clinic Guide to a Healthy Pregnancy by Mayo Clinic (2004) Paperback.*
24. Ibid, p. 367.
25. Ibid.
26. Murkoff and Mazel, *What to Expect When You're Expecting, 4th Edition,* p. 334.
27. Ibid.
28. Iovine, *The Girlfriends' Guide to Pregnancy*, p. 242.
29. "Women's Bureau (WB)—Quick Facts on Women in the Labor Force in 2010."
30. "Employment Characteristics of Families Summary."
31. Ibid.
32. Al-Sahab et al., "Prevalence and Predictors of 6-Month Exclusive Breastfeeding among Canadian Women"; Thulier and Mercer, "Variables Associated With Breastfeeding Duration."
33. Port and Ralston, *The Caveman's Pregnancy Companion*, p. 77.
34. Mulvey, "Visual Pleasure and Narrative Cinema."
35. Iovine, *The Girlfriends' Guide to Pregnancy*, p. 242.
36. Murkoff and Mazel, *What to Expect When You're Expecting, 4th Edition.*
37. Ibid.
38. Nickerson, Sykes, and Fung, "Mothers' Experience of Fathers' Support for Breast-Feeding."
39. Pearl and Pearl, *To Train Up a Child.*
40. Ibid.
41. Ibid.
42. Ezzo and Bucknam, *On Becoming Baby Wise.*
43. Ibid.
44. Ibid, p. 77.
45. Amazon.com, "On Becoming Baby Wise: Giving Your Infant the GIFT of Nighttime Sleep: (Amazon Entry)."
46. Ferber, *Solve Your Child's Sleep Problems.*
47. Ibid, p. 55.
48. Ibid, p. 141.
49. Karp, *The Happiest Baby on the Block.*
50. Pantley and Sears, *The No-Cry Sleep Solution*; Waldburger and Spivack, *The Sleepeasy Solution.*
51. Pantley and Sears, *The No-Cry Sleep Solution*; Waldburger and Spivack, *The Sleepeasy Solution.*

52. Sears and Sears, *The Attachment Parenting Book.*
53. Ibid.
54. Jenner, "The Perils of Attachment Parenting."
55. Morrissey, "Attachment Parenting."
56. Harris, *Hi New Baby!*
57. Rockwell, *Hello Baby!*
58. Civardi, *Usborne First Experiences The New Baby.*
59. Landolf, *What a Good Big Brother!*
60. Sears, Sears, and Kelly, *Baby on the Way.*
61. Sheldon, *Big Sister Now.*
62. Sears, Sears, and Kelly, *What Baby Needs.*
63. Ibid.
64. Rogers, *The New Baby.*
65. Murkoff, *What to Expect When the New Baby Comes Home.*
66. Ibid.
67. Bracken, *Henry Helps with the Baby.*
68. Cole, *I'm a Big Brother*; Cole, *I'm a Big Sister.*
69. Ibid.
70. Manushkin, *Big Brothers Are the Best*; Manushkin, *Big Sisters Are the Best.*
71. Capucilli, *Hannah Is a Big Sister*; Capucilli, *Henry Is a Big Brother.*
72. Saunders, *Olive Marshmallow.*
73. Langreuter, *Little Bear Is A Big Brother.*
74. O'Connor, *Lulu and the Witch Baby.*
75. Murray et al., *The Babycenter Essential Guide to Pregnancy and Birth.*

CHAPTER 6

From the Milky Man Vest to Nursing on the Throne: Breastfeeding Representations in Fictional Television

In 1977, the children's show *Sesame Street* included a peaceful scene of a mother, Buffy, breastfeeding her baby. Big Bird asks, "What'cha doing, Buffy?" The mother answers, "I'm feeding the baby. See? He's drinking milk from my breast." Big Bird replies, "Hmm. That's a funny way to feed a baby." Buffy continues looking at her baby and nursing as she says, "Well, lots of mothers feed their babies this way. Not all mothers, but lots of mothers do. And he likes it because it's nice and warm and sweet and natural and it's good for him." She glances up at Big Bird, explaining, "And I get to hug him when I do it too." The scene concludes with Big Bird saying, "You know, that's nice."

This breastfeeding storyline was groundbreaking as one of the first to not only show breastfeeding, but to present it as positive and natural. Such depictions are an important part of normalizing breastfeeding, depicting nursing as the regular way to feed a baby. As previously stated, media messages have been identified as significant to creating a breastfeeding-friendly cultural climate.[1] Unfortunately, media products have showcased bottle-feeding, ignoring breastfeeding, or portrayed it as difficult, deviant, or humorous. Even *Sesame Street* has not consistently

---

A portion of this chapter first appeared as the article: Foss, K.A. (2013). "That's Not a Beer Bong, It's a Breast Pump!" Representations of Breastfeeding in Prime-Time Fictional Television. *Health Communication*, 28(4), 329–340. Reprinted with permission.

K.A. Foss, *Breastfeeding and Media*,
DOI 10.1007/978-3-319-56442-5_6

promoted breastfeeding. In recent years, the show has been criticized for primarily featuring bottle-feeding.[2]

Examining representations of breastfeeding over time can provide insight into the normalization (or lack thereof) of breastfeeding in the United States, highlight changing trends and perceptions, and explain why so many people are uncomfortable with seeing it.[3] This chapter explores portrayals of breastfeeding in television from the 1970s, when breastfeeding was first mentioned, through 2015. Fictional programs aimed at adults were studied for breastfeeding discourse. These programs were not necessarily for or about parents and vary in target audience and genre.

Censorship and Fictional Media

For much of early film and television, heavy censorship meant that anything focused on the body was not shown or discussed. In 1930, the Motion Picture Production Code, also known as the Hays Code, was adopted by the Motion Picture Producers and Distributors of America, Inc. and the Association of Motion Picture Producers, Inc.[4] Producers had to submit their films for approval by the Code's administration team since most studios refused to release movies that did not pass the board's recommendation.[5] The Code was very strict and specific, banning sexually suggestive scenes, references to homosexuality, vulgarity, profanity, "morally-objective" topics of religion and other subjects, depictions of certain crimes and obscenity.[6] While it did not explicitly prohibit verbal and visual references to breastfeeding, they were presumably covered under interpretations of the sex and obscenity sections of the Hays Code. Such censorship helps to explain why breastfeeding rarely appeared in films before the 1970s, according to an analysis by Sarah Rubenstein-Gillis.[7] Even after this point, breastfeeding was still limited in positive representations.[8]

When television emerged in the 1940s, it was just as censored, if not more censored than film. Perceived as entertainment for the whole family, television producers were exceptionally careful in the content they created for the medium.[9] For example, in the 1950s, the word "pregnant" was considered too vulgar for the small screen. When Lucille Ball became pregnant during *I Love Lucy*, the show used euphemisms to describe their impending arrival, never using the words "sex" or "pregnant."[10] Any hints of sexuality were strictly forbidden. For example, even married couples had two twin beds shown in their bedrooms, as seen in the 1960s program *The Dick Van Dyke Show* .[11] With the Civil Rights movement and the rise of counterculture, film and television eventually began loosening content restrictions. By the 1970s, *All in the Family* and other shows that followed greatly expanded what could be said and talked about on television, including racism and bigotry, sexuality and sexual orientation, and other socially-conscious topics previously considered too racy for television.[12] This shift in censorship, paired with the beginning of the resurgence of breastfeeding in the 1970s, opened the door for its depictions, even if it would be decades before breastfeeding would regularly appear in television.

The Impact of Entertainment

Research has demonstrated that fictional television is an effective tool for disseminating information, shaping public perceptions, and even changing behavior. For example, a 2008 Kaiser Family Foundation campaign used *Grey's Anatomy* to teach people the limited risks of HIV transmission through pregnancy.[13] Follow-up surveys showed an increase in knowledge by 46% points, with 61% of viewers correctly identifying the low risk of transmission.[14] Entertainment programming has also been used to teach people about emergency contraception, designated driving, reproductive health, and other issues.[15] Even fictional programming that is not a strategic part of a health campaign can influence viewers. In fact, Solange Davin found that people tended to trust the health information conveyed in medical dramas more than documentaries.[16] Fictional shows can also encourage people to adopt healthy behaviors. Sharf and Freimuth determined that a storyline about cancer in the program *Thirtysomething* prompted viewers to get preventative screenings.[17] Meanwhile, viewers who had experienced cancer identified with the characters and felt comforted by the narrative.[18]

Given the recognized influence of entertainment media, it makes sense that women and other people learn about infant feeding, including breastfeeding information, from magazines, websites, and television—an assumption that is supported by research. Pregnant women use media products to help make decisions about childrearing.[19] In addition, positive representations and more visibility of breastfeeding could help improve general public attitudes toward breastfeeding. By presenting breastfeeding as the normal means of feeding a baby, positive television representations also help shape cultural attitudes toward breastfeeding, normalizing the practice so that women feel comfortable nursing at home and in public. Furthermore, media stories that connect early weaning to hospital, business, and other institutional policies that inhibit breastfeeding could help garner support for Baby Friendly hospitals, pumping spaces at work, extended maternity leave, and other macro-level changes that are needed to drastically raise breastfeeding initiation and duration rates.

Exploring Fictional Television

This study analyzed verbal and visual depictions of breastfeeding on fictional television programming, exploring how entertainment television programs portray breastfeeding through all available fictional depictions. Since breastfeeding representations are infrequent, a purposive sample was used, compiled from Internet searches, websites, and social networks. Shows that aired for less than a season or were otherwise unavailable online or on DVD were excluded. The act of breastfeeding (regardless of a character's sex or biological link to the child), comments about breastfeeding, and other indicators that characters were breastfeeding were all explored, including expressing one's milk with a breast pump and the use of a Supplemental Nursing System (SNS). Only fictional programs that aired on television were examined. Unlike women's health magazines or breastfeeding literature, these programs target a mass audience, meaning that the messages reach a larger population than just pregnant women or nursing mothers, so people are more likely to be exposed to representations in prime-time television, even if they find such depictions "inappropriate."[20]

Breastfeeding on Television, 1974–2015

Eighty-two breastfeeding representations were analyzed in fictional programming from 1974 to 2015 (see Table 6.1). Of these 82 portrayals, 45 were only verbal references about breastfeeding, in which characters made remarks, but nursing was not shown. Only two representations showed nursing without relevant dialogue. In 24 depictions, characters talked about breastfeeding as it was shown (usually covered up). The use of a breast pump or supplemental nursing system appeared in five representations. Consistent with real-life breastfeeding rates, in recent years, breastfeeding representations in fictional shows have become

Table 6.1 Breastfeeding in Fictional Television

Program Title	*Year*	*Episode #*	*Episode Title*	*Verbal*	*Visual*	*Both*	*Pump Ver.*	*Pump Vis.*
Criminal Minds	2015	11.8	Awake	x				
The Big Bang Theory	2015	8.18	The Leftover Thermalization	x				
Archer	2014	5.13	Archer Vice: Arrival/ Departure			x		
Modern Family	2013	4.17	Best Men					
The New Normal	2013	1.15	Dairy Queen			x		
Parenthood	2013	5.3	Nipple Confusion				x	x
American Horror Story	2013	2.11	Spilt Milk			x		
Bones	2012	7.8	The Bump in the Road	x				
Bones	2012	7.8	The Bump in the Road	x				
Bones	2012	7.9	The Don't in the Do			x		
30 Rock	2011	5.16	It's Never Too Late for Now	x				
The New Girl	2011	1.8	Bad in Bed					x
Beavis and Butthead	2011	1.3	Holy Cornholio	x				
Game of Thrones	2011	1.5	The Wolf and the Lion		x			
American Dad!	2011	7.5	Virtual In-Stanity	x				
Bones	2011	7.5	The Twist in the Twister	x				
The Office	2010	6.18	The Delivery					
The Office	2010	6.22	Secretary's Day				x	x
The Big Bang Theory	2010	3.18	The Pants Alternative	x				
The Big Bang Theory	2010	3.17	The Precious Fragmentation	x				
Modern Family	2009	1.9	Fizbo	x				
The Secret Life of the Amer. Teen.	2009	1.23	And Unto Us, a Child is Born	x				
The Office	2009	5.14	Lecture Circuit, Part 1				x	
Ghost Whisperer	2009	5.1	Birthday Presence			x		
Criminal Minds	2008	4.6	The Instincts			x		

(continued)

Table 6.1 (continued)

Program Title	*Year*	*Episode #*	*Episode Title*	*Verbal*	*Visual*	*Both*	*Pump Ver.*	*Pump Vis.*
Bones	2008	3.12	The Baby in the Bough	x				
The Big Bang Theory	2008	2.1	The Bad Fish Paradigm	x				
30 Rock	2007	2.4	Rosemary's Baby	x				
The O.C.	2007	4.16	The End's Not Near, It's Here	x				
Two and a Half Men	2007	4.12	Castrating Sheep in Montana			x		
Two and a Half Men	2007	4.18	It Never Rains in Hooterville	x				
Scrubs	2007	6.3	My Coffee	x				
Scrubs	2007	6.5	My Friend with Money			x		
Gilmore Girls	2007	7.11	Santa's Secret Stuff				x	
Desperate Housewives	2006	2.17	Could I Leave You?	x				
Nip/Tuck	2006	4.4	Shari Noble			x	x	x
The Office	2006	3.8	The Merger				x	
The Sopranos	2006	6.1	Members Only			x		
Gilmore Girls	2006	7.10	Merry Fisticuffs	x				
Family Guy	2006	4.21	I take thee Quagmire			x		
Gilmore Girls	2005	6.9	The Prodigal Daughter Returns	x				
Law & Order: SVU	2005	6.21	Blood	x				
The Office	2005	1.6	Hot Girl	x				
Two and a Half Men	2005	3.2	Principal Gallagher's Lesbian Lover	x				
That '70 s Show	2005	7.18	Oh Baby We Got a Good Thing Goin'	x				
CSI: Crime Scene Investigation	2005	5.15	King Baby	x				
CSI: Crime Scene Investigation	2005	6.6	Secrets and Lies	x			x	

(continued)

Table 6.1 (continued)

Program Title	*Year*	*Episode #*	*Episode Title*	*Verbal*	*Visual*	*Both*	*Pump Ver.*	*Pump Vis.*
Charmed	2004	7.2	The Bare Witch Project			x		
ER	2004	11.3	Try Carter					x SNS
Two and a Half Men	2004	2.9	Yes, Monsignor	x				
House	2004	1.2	Paternity	x				
Friends	2003	9.11	… Rachel Goes Back to Work	x				
Law & Order: SVU	2003	4.14	Mercy	x				
Scrubs	2003	2.18	My T.C.W.	x				
Friends	2002	8.2	The One with the Baby Shower				x	
Friends	2002	8.24	The One where Rachel has a Baby	x				
Friends	2002	9.1	The One where No One Proposes			x		
Friends	2002	9.3	The One with the Pediatrician	x				
Gilmore Girls	2002	3.5	Eight o'clock at the Oasis		x			
Sex and the City	2002	5.1	Anchors Away		x			
ER	2001	8.4	Never Say Never	x				
ER	2001	8.2	The Longer You Stay	x			x	
ER	2001	7.19	Sailing Away			x		
Malcolm in the Middle	2001	2.25	Flashback	x				
ER	2000	7.9	The Greatest Gifts		x			
ER	2000	6.16	Under Control					x
Yes, Dear	2000	1.2	Weaning Isn't Everything					x
Law & Order	2000	10.12	Mother's Milk	x				

(continued)

Table 6.1 (continued)

Program Title	*Year*	*Episode #*	*Episode Title*	*Verbal*	*Visual*	*Both*	*Pump Ver.*	*Pump Vis.*
Family Guy	2000	2.8	I am Peter, Here Me Roar		x			
ER	1999	6.4	Sins of the Father	x				
ER	1999	6.8	Great Expectations	x		x		
7th Heaven	1999	3.15	It Happened One Night	x				
Everybody Loves Raymond	1999	4.1	Boob Job					
Chicago Hope	1998	5.4	The Best and the Brightest	x				x
Friends	1995	2.2	The One with the Breast Milk			x	x	
Married with Children	1994	9.5	Business Sucks, Part 1			x		
Married with Children	1994	9.6	Business Still Sucks			x		
Seinfeld	1994	5.16	The Stand-In			x		
Roseanne	1994	6.25	Altar Egos			x		
Seinfeld	1993	5.5	The Bris			x		
St. Elsewhere	1983	1.10	Hearts	x				
Little House on the Prairie	1974	114	The Lord is my Shepherd	x				

more common—69 of the identified portrayals appeared after 1998.[21] Multiple breastfeeding depictions were identified in several popular shows. For example, the program *ER* contained 10 portrayals. *Bones*, *Friends*, *Two and a Half Men*, *The Big Bang Theory*, and *The Office* also included multiple breastfeeding representations. Overall, the representations studied presented breastfeeding as mostly positive, but limited, as exemplified by the "typical" breastfeeding woman and experience, contrasted with the "atypical" or "deviant" breastfeeding act.

The Breastfeeding Woman

The breastfeeding woman in fictional television reflects a narrow group of women, defined by race, age, education, and occupation, and it is assumed that female characters who fit this type will breastfeed. For example, when Rachel is pregnant in *Friends*, she receives a breast pump as a baby shower gift. Upon receipt of the gift, she says, "Is that a beer bong for a baby?" Despite her lack of knowledge, Rachel goes on to successfully nurse her baby. In "Bad in Bed" of *The New Girl*, the character Schmidt wants to buy his boss a breast pump for her baby shower. Likewise, in *The Office*, manager Michael Scott remarks to a pregnant Karen, "Do you need to go pump?" She replies, "Not going to have to do that until after I have the baby." Michael's assumption (although incorrect), paired with Karen's response, suggests that both equate infant feeding with breastfeeding. Another episode of *The Office* insinuates that even childless women were considered future breastfeeders. In "Hot Girl," Dwight Schrute comments on the characteristics he finds attractive in a purse saleswoman, stating, "The purse girl hits everything on my checklist: creamy skin, straight teeth, curly hair, amazing breasts—not for me, for my children. The Schrutes produce very thirsty babies."

The characters who do breastfeed are usually older, educated, professional women, mirroring the real-life group with the highest rates,[22] and exemplified by the doctors in *ER*, Pam in *The Office*, Miranda in *Sex and the City*, and others. These women are also typically Caucasian,[23] with few exceptions, including Carla Espinosa in *Scrubs* and Dr. Jing-Mei Chen in *ER* (who then gives her baby up for adoption). Recent years offer more positive depictions with women of color. The Latina character Gloria Pritchett in the show *Modern Family* breastfeeds baby Joe. Jasmine Trussell-Braveman in *Parenthood* expresses milk for her infant son, while discussing breastfeeding. And in *Bones*, Angela Montenegro breastfeeds and pumps milk for her baby, with references about the experience over multiple episodes. These depictions incorporate diverse women who are equally main characters and experience similar obstacles to other breastfeeding characters. The representations are also narrow in that all breastfeeding characters are able-bodied and heterosexual, even when the programs contain characters with children outside this group.

For most characters who do not fit the archetype of the nursing woman, breastfeeding is presented as less likely and is not actually shown. The detectives in *Bones* are surprised to discover that a victim, a poor, single mother, breastfed her baby. In *Secret Life of the American Teenager*, 15 year-old Amy only breastfeeds her newborn when her own mother forces her to try (which is not shown). Finally, a Hispanic woman transmits drugs through her breastmilk in the *ER* episode "Under Control," accidentally causing her baby's death. None of these depictions include visuals of the mother breastfeeding, nor are they positive representations. In the *New Normal*, the only African American character, Rocky Rhodes, is the sole person against breastfeeding. All of the other protagonists, including Bryan and David (the same-sex couple on the show), their surrogate, Goldie, and her daughter all speak in favor of breastfeeding. Despite this, Rocky announces that she would not breastfeed because it would ruin her breasts—a statement followed by scene in which Rocky's breasts are long tubes. This difference between Rocky and the other characters illustrates and reinforces perceptions that African American mothers are less likely to breastfeed.[24] Such stereotypes may be discouraging to women of color who intend to breastfeed, as they may feel alone or unsupported.

Learning to Breastfeed

The image of the new (usually Caucasian, educated, and professional) mother learning to breastfeed was presented as the natural step after an infant was born and appeared most frequently. A short time after birth, the characters were depicted wearing hospital gowns, closely holding their infants. They often express uncertainty about how to breastfeed. For example, in the *ER* episode "Sailing Away," as Dr. Elizabeth Corday attempts to latch baby Ella to the breast, she says to her husband, "Mark, I don't think I can do this." At this point, a support person or expert guides the mother. In *ER*, Mark (also a physician) gently kisses his wife, reassuring her, "It just takes patience." In another *ER* episode, Nurse

Abby Lockhart helps Nurse Carol Hathaway on how to nurse, stating, "Wait until she opens her mouth really wide." Carol adjusts her breast over her gown and Abby says, "That's it. Yeah, make sure her mouth covers the whole areola. Yes, see her little jaw moving." The *Friends* episode "The One Where No One Proposes" includes a similar scene, in which a nurse helps a tearful Rachel latch baby Emma to the breast. In *Scrubs*, Turk takes his wife to see a team of lactation specialists.

The animated program *Archer*, "Archer's Vice: Arrival/Departure" adds a twist to the natural birth assistant. As Lana prepares to give birth at the airport, all are surprised to learn that CIA contractor/private investigator Archer also has training as a birth doula. He assists her natural, unconventional delivery and she breastfeeds with no issues. Likewise, in the 2010 episode "The Delivery" of *The Office*, character Pam has her baby and then wants to learn to breastfeed. To her husband Jim's surprise, the lactation consultant, Clark, is male. Although Pam is comfortable with Clark touching her breasts as he positions the baby, Jim clearly feels awkward about the situation. Clark helps Pam overcome her latch issues and, after practicing by accidentally feeding the wrong newborn, she succeeds in breastfeeding CeCe by the end of the episode. The appearance of lactation experts primarily in the hospital suggests that problems with nursing end after the initial breastfeeding session, despite the ongoing struggles that most women face.

The Benefits of Breastfeeding

Although it is assumed that pregnant characters will breastfeed, they seldom explain why they choose to breastfeed—likely because they fit the "typical" breastfeeding woman. When benefits are mentioned, it is in retrospect or to justify "deviant" breastfeeding behavior. In the *Bones* episode "The Baby and the Bough," the characters Seely Booth and Temperance Brennan allude to the health benefits when Brennan asks her partner if he was breastfed and then adds that she was. Likewise, in "The Bad Fish Paradigm" of *The Big Bang Theory*, the physics genius Dr. Sheldon Cooper mentions that he remembers the last time he was breastfed. Other episodes refer to Sheldon's brilliant friends Leonard and Howard also having been breastfed. Since all of these characters are known for their extraordinary intelligence, such references could reinforce the message that breastfeeding has been correlated with a higher IQ. Characters in *ER* and *Desperate Housewives* commented on the weight loss benefits for the breastfeeding mother. *The Secret Life of the American Teenager* conveyed that breastfeeding increases breast size. Finally, in the episode "Paternity" of *House, M.D.*, Dr. House briefly mentions that breastfeeding provides what he says is temporary protection against disease, in a lecture on the importance of immunization.

Other health benefits of breastfeeding are only used as justification for women outside the "norm" wanting to breastfeed—a baby about to be adopted, a baby needing surgery for extreme birth defects, and nursing a much older child. In the *ER* episode "The Greatest Gifts," Dr. Chen breastfeeds her son before giving him to the adoptive parents so that he can get the nourishment of colostrum, "which boosts their immune system." In *Nip/Tuck*, Sean McNamara encourages Julia to breastfeed, stating, "We need to think about his surgeries, Honey. His first one's in three months and breastfeeding helps him gain the weight he needs so that his immune system will be strong. Skin on skin contacts also make him secure so that he can handle the stress." And, in *The Desperate Housewives* episode "Could I Leave You?," Veronica lists the benefits of extended breastfeeding, including immunity and IQ-boosting properties of breastmilk. Storylines did not address other health benefits of breastfeeding for children, nor did they convey the impact of breastfeeding duration on health benefits. Long-term health benefits, such as reduced risks of breast cancer and osteoporosis, were absent from the representations studied.

A character takes breastmilk's benefits to the extreme in *The New Normal.* After nine year-old Shania learns that she was not breastfed as a baby, she is horrified and decides that she needs breastmilk to increase her intelligence. Unbeknownst to her mother, Goldie, Shania orders human milk online, from *Onlythebreast.com* (a real website). She shows her mother a large glass of the milk, telling Goldie that it is human milk from "a college professor named Katherine who doesn't smoke drink or read Stephanie Meyers." Goldie responds, asking her, "Do you know how stupid that sounds?" Shania becomes defensive and replies, "No, I don't because I wasn't breastfed so my feeble brain is underdeveloped." They struggle over the glass and the milk spills all over them. In the end, the episode concludes with Shania sharing her concerns about her mother's pregnancy and Goldie reassures her daughter. This depiction not only parodies how some perceive the benefits of breastmilk, but also exemplifies the only reference to purchased milk in the representations studied.

BREASTFEEDING OBSTACLES

The obstacles of breastfeeding were limited in these representations to initial problems with nursing and focused on individual problems. In the hospital and shortly after, characters faced latch issues with their babies, which were easily resolved with a little coaching from a nurse, partner, or lactation consultant. In the early days of breastfeeding, characters also complained of sore nipples. For example, in *Friends*, Rachel returns to work and finds her replacement, Gavin at her desk. He says, "Well, while you were on your baby vacation, I was doing your job." Rachel responds, "A vacation? My idea of a vacation does not involve something sucking on my nipples until they are raw." Gavin retorts, "Clearly you've never been to Sandals Paradise Island." In *Friends*, Carol (Ross's ex-wife) also states that breastfeeding hurts at first. And in *ER*, the character Chuck (using a Supplemental Nursing System) tells Dr. Carter about the pain of nursing. No remedies, other than time and practice, are recommended to ease the pain.

Characters also became emotional and upset because of nursing. In *ER*, baby Ella wakes up Elizabeth Corday and Mark, who then complains says that he has a shift in three hours. Elizabeth shouts, "What do you think I'll be doing in three hours? I'm the feeding trough!" Mark declares that he would nurse if he could. Elizabeth yells, "You take it! Take it all! The sore nipples, the rashes, the hemorrhoids, the leaking in your trauma gown, the public humiliation, the sleep deprivation, the incontinence, for goodness sake. Just take it. It's all yours!" Likewise, Carla, in *Scrubs*, weeps uncontrollably throughout the episode, even after her baby finally latches. In the *Nip/Tuck* episode "Shari Noble," the character Julia becomes emotional when she struggles to get her milk to let down. A lactation consultant attempts to help her, causing Julia more frustration. The woman advises her to drink a beer. Julia tells her she does not want beer, orders the woman to leave, and pumps her milk. Several more times, Julia attempts to nurse, but fails. In desperation, Julia contemplates using antidepressants so that she has to switch to formula. Finally, with the help of the male nanny and some informal counseling, Julia admits her guilt over her son's birth defect. Julia's admission, combined with a warm washcloth on her breasts, produces a milk let-down and her son is able to nurse. This storyline highlights the connection between emotion and lactation, along with offering some practical advice on helping let-downs, at the same time suggesting that

Julia's one milk let-down resolves all of her breastfeeding issues. These episodes conveyed that feeling emotional was part of breastfeeding and not necessarily indicative of postpartum depression.

Postpartum depression is only directly addressed in one breastfeeding storyline studied. In *Scrubs*, Carla is very emotional after giving birth. Over three episodes, her husband, Turk, and his best friend, J.D. notice that she cries easily, is reluctant to leave the hospital, and wants to be apart from her baby. They finally deduce that she has postpartum depression and eventually Carla agrees to get help after speaking with a female friend. Throughout this storyline, breastfeeding is connected to Carla's emotional state. She has difficulty latching at the hospital, prompting her to weepily declare, "I can't feed my baby!" Later, after the latching issues are resolved, Carla's unexpected let-down soaks her shirt, causing her to shed more tears. While no characters discuss the impact of postpartum depression on breastfeeding, it is clear that they are connected. And yet, we do not see exactly how Carla "gets help," if it affects breastfeeding, or how long she breastfeeds since the "diagnosis" episode is the last to address breastfeeding.

The episode "Nipple Confusion" of *Parenthood*, shows the parents' struggle to get their breastfed baby to drink from a bottle. It begins with a scene of Jasmine using an electric breast pump. We see the bottles fill with milk. Jasmine says, "I feel like a big old cow" and tells her husband, Crosby, that she needs their daughter to take a bottle. The baby starts to cry and Jasmine lifts her shirt to nurse her. Jasmine becomes increasingly discouraged and fatigued throughout the episode, while Crosby is very supportive. He discusses the problem with his father and even tries different nipples to help the baby take the bottle so his wife can rest. The episode concludes with Crosby successfully bottle-feeding the expressed milk to the baby. Although it shows the frustrations of breastfeeding, this storyline is very realistic—providing a breastmilk solution to her problem and depicting a supportive partner. This storyline could help prepare new parents for the difficulty in breastfeeding and offering them options for feeding babies when mothers need a break or must return to work.[25] Aside from the few obstacles mentioned, absent from the representations were other common physical obstacles faced by nursing mothers. No storylines addressed breastfeeding a premature, jaundiced, or tongue-tied newborn, mastitis, thrush, clogged milk ducts, inverted nipples, or other issues that can impede breastfeeding success. And since these issues were not part of the storylines, remedies for these obstacles were also missing.

Most institutional and other macro-level barriers were not addressed in the shows. However, breastfeeding presents some challenges for the fictional working mothers. While breastfeeding a newborn in the hospital is conveyed as natural and fairly easy, it becomes restrictive and unprofessional once the women return to work. For example, in *Friends*, while on maternity leave, Rachel visits her work, discovering her replacement. Fearing that she will lose her status in the company, Rachel wants to end her maternity leave early. Since she presumably has no pumped milk in reserve, though, Rachel heads home with Ross and Emma.

Breastfeeding poses issues for *ER*'s Dr. Elizabeth Corday when her breasts leak during surgery, forcing her to pump. In *The Office* episode "The Merger," a woman uses a double breast pump at her desk. All of the other employees stop working and stare at her—to the point at which she asks if one would like to take a picture. In both cases, the reactions of the other employees suggested that breastfeeding and pumping not only interfered with the nursing mother's work, but also hindered the productivity of those around her. And yet, while the individual women seemed embarrassed by the need to pump, having a place to pump or concerns about job security were not an issue, likely again because these women were in professional positions, not part of an assembly line.

Breastfeeding—Private or Public?

Most breastfeeding representations consisted of a mother calmly nursing her newborn, at home or in the hospital, covered by a blanket or clothing. No visual depictions of breastfeeding (even covered up) appeared until a 1994 episode of *ER*. The two representations before this time period are verbal references: In *Little House on the Prairie*, Dr. Baker advises Caroline to stop breastfeeding, which is not shown. And in *St. Elsewhere*, a nurse asks a new mother if she will breastfeed. She does not and ultimately abandons the baby at the hospital.

Representations of uncovered breastfeeding were uncommon, but appeared increasingly in contemporary times. *The Sopranos* episode "Members Only" (2006) begins with a close-up of the tattoo on Janice's breast and then pans to her baby nursing. As no characters interact with Janice, nor refer to breastfeeding, this scene serves as a calm moment in an otherwise chaotic episode. In the *Sex and the City* episode "Anchors Away" (2002), Miranda's baby is visibly latched on, as he suckles her breast in her apartment. It should be noted that the naked breasts of two other characters, Samantha and Charlotte, also appear in this episode. *Two and a Half Men* also contains a less covered-up image of breastfeeding, when Alan's date nurses during dinner. The animated show *Family Guy* features several breastfeeding sessions between Stewie and Lois. In *Archer* (2014), Lana openly nurses her baby after birth, in which you can see the baby latched on. Later in the episode, she breastfeeds as she talks with Archer. *The New Normal* and *Parenthood* also include uncovered breastfeeding. In these depictions, characters receive positive and supportive responses from the main protagonists—a progressive move toward normalizing breastfeeding.

With other representations, even with a cover, breastfeeding made other characters visibly uncomfortable. In the *Friends* episode "The One with the Breast Milk" (1995), when Carol nurses Ben, Joey and Chandler become ill at ease and walk over to the kitchen. Ross follows them, saying, "Look, will you guys grow up? This is the most natural, beautiful thing in the world." Joey replies, "Yeah, we know. But there's a baby sucking on it." Ross then explains, "This is my son having lunch, okay? It's gonna happen a lot so get used to it. Now if you have a problem with it, if you're uncomfortable, just ask questions. Carol's fine with it. C'mon." They return to the living room and began asking Carol bizarre questions, such as, "If he blows into one, does the other one get bigger?" At this point, Ross pushes them back into the kitchen. *The O.C.* characters Seth and Ryan also quickly leave when they learn Kristen is about to nurse. In *Gilmore Girls*, Lorelai complains about her friend, Sookie, breastfeeding at the dinner table, arguing that she and Luke should make Sookie and her husband as uncomfortable as they were. And Carrie, of *Sex and the City*, becomes noticeably uneasy when Miranda unlatches her nursing bra in preparation to nurse.

Only one depiction studied showed nursing in public as normal and part of life. At the end of the *Roseanne* episode "Altar Egos" (1994), Roseanne's sister, Jackie, has her milk let-down as she is preparing to walk down the aisle. In the next scene, she and the groom say their vows. When the minister announces, "You may kiss the bride," the camera zooms out and we see that Jackie is nursing her baby as she weds. She replies, "Just let me switch sides first." A guest says to Jackie's niece, "I suppose you're next, Darlene." Darlene pauses, then retorts, "Uh, no thank you. I drink my milk from a glass now." Here, the joke is not directed at Jackie and her nursing, but at Darlene's interpretation of the wedding guest's "you're next." Overall, this portrayal conveys that breastfeeding is normal, necessary, and can be done anywhere, at anytime.

In the other seven portrayals in which women nurse in public, their actions are heavily criticized and conveyed as inappropriate. In the *Gilmore Girls* episode "Eight O'Clock at the Oasis," Luke complains to Lorelai and Rory about a woman nursing in his diner, "Why? Why do they do this? It's a public place, people are eating here." Luke becomes very uncomfortable and continues, "When did that become acceptable? In the old days, a woman would never consider doing that in public. They'd go find a barn or a cave or something. I mean, it's indecent. This is a diner, not a peepshow." At this point, Luke asks Lorelai to get rid of them. She refuses, although she does not defend the nursing mother. In *Two and a Half Men*, Alan dates a single mom. As they are having dinner, she begins to breastfeed her baby. He is surprised and then has trouble eating. Breastfeeding also makes characters uncomfortable in *Seinfeld*. In "The Bris," Jerry and Elaine visit their friends in the hospital after the birth of their baby. When the mother starts to nurse (covered up, in her hospital bed), Jerry and Elaine grimace and squirm in their seats. The new father asks Jerry, "This doesn't make you uncomfortable, does it?" Jerry responds sarcastically, "Nooo, nooo. Uncomfortable? Not at all. My friend's wife's breast is sticking out. Why would that make me uncomfortable?" Similarly, in "The Stand-In," a friend of Jerry's scowls and shakes his head when he sees a woman nursing on a bench in the hospital, loudly exclaiming, "Oh, look at this. What? She's gotta breastfeed in public?!" Jerry replies, "Yeah, that's the last thing you want to see. Well, next to last" (referring to his friend's indecent exposure earlier in the episode).

Three storylines challenge the criticism of breastfeeding characters with public protests. The *Charmed* episode "The Bare Witch Project" begins with two of the main characters, Piper and Phoebe Halliwell, sitting at a café, while Piper nurses her son under an oversized blanket. Other customers snicker, prompting the manager to ask Piper to leave. Throughout the episode, public breastfeeding becomes a symbol for female progress, as the sisters help a conjured Lady Godiva return to her historic time. At the end of the episode, inspired by Lady Godiva, Phoebe rides naked on horseback to the café, where she publicly declares that the manager believes women "should be ashamed of breastfeeding, the most natural thing in the world. Well, shame on him. I'm not ashamed and neither should you be. It's a shame women have to take off their clothes to be heard. We shouldn't have to be exploited like this. Right?" At this point, Phoebe's speech convinces the manager to take down the "right to refuse service" sign. Despite the declaration about nursing in public, after the initial scene, no images of breastfeeding appear.

In "Business Sucks" and "Business Still Sucks" of *Married with Children*, the character Al becomes so uncomfortable with a woman breastfeeding in his women's shoe store that he asks her to leave. She returns the following day as part of a group of militant breastfeeding women. Al's neighbor, Marcie, leads the group, using a whistle to direct their marching. Later, Marcie challenges Al's refusal to allow the woman to nurse, declaring, "How dare you deny her her God-given right to nurse her baby whenever Mother Nature calls! Breastfeeding is a natural, biological function." Al responds, "So's peeing, but you don't see me doing that in public." The studio audience cheers as Marcie says, "Well, the last time I looked, the side of my garage was in public." Although Al eventually allows breastfeeding in his store to please his boss, his initial refusal, backed by the studio audience's groans, laughs, and applause, frames public breastfeeding as absurd and obscene—even in a show that aims to be obscene.

The New Normal also uses a breastfeeding protest for humor in the storyline. After the main characters, Bryan and David, learn of their friend's negative experience breastfeeding in a restaurant, Bryan stages a nurse-in. Bryan and the friend return to the establishment. The mother begins to breastfeed her baby, while Bryan sits waiting at another table. The manager predictably asks her to leave, stating, "It's just that what you're doing may make some of our patrons uncomfortable, so if you wouldn't mind." The mother declares, "Actually, I would mind. My breasts won't be silent and my breasts are not alone." Bryan turns on some music, as women appear, dancing around and then nursing their babies, singing the pop artist Kelis' song "Milkshake." However, the protest ends abruptly when Bryan tries to join in, mimicking breastfeeding with a doll and a nipple vest. His friend tells him that he turned the protest "into a joke." Bryan storms off and the scene ends with no results. With this storyline, the nurse-in is more of a silly celebration than a Lactivist event, particularly with Bryan's involvement, the pop song, and the lack of resolution. Its inclusion in the storyline exists as a humorous break, rather than a serious advocacy moment.

Sexualizing the Breast

One justification for concealing breastfeeding is that breasts are sexual objects, not meant to be publicly displayed. Many of the breastfeeding representations sexualized breasts, especially in programs geared toward men. In the *Married with Children* episodes, Al's disgust at the breastfeeding woman is then contrasted to his attraction to women's breasts. After he orders the nursing woman out of the store, he comments to his (male) associate, "What is happening to this country when a woman of the opposite sex can just waddle into your place of business, your holy sanctuary, and bare her breasts. It's disgusting." The other employee replies, "It's repulsive." They reach down and pick up magazines with the titles *Big 'Uns* and *Black Big 'Uns*, turn their magazines sideways, then exchange magazines. The *Charmed* episode with public breastfeeding ends with Phoebe riding naked on a horse to protest the ban, equating her nudity with breastfeeding. While no characters criticize Janice for breastfeeding in *The Sopranos*, this show as a whole frequently objectifies women, as Mob Boss Tony Soprano regularly conducts business in the Bada Bing strip club, where topless women parade around and are expected not to speak. The characters in *Archer* may not have reacted to Lana breastfeeding because most of the female characters wear very provocative clothing. In *Sex and the City*, the image of Miranda breastfeeding appears in a storyline about breasts, in which Carrie accidentally sees Samantha and Charlotte flash their breasts to men at a party. Likewise, in *Friends*, Joey and Chandler mention feeling uncomfortable with breastfeeding because they are used to viewing breasts as sexual.

We see this sexualization of breastfeeding in numerous other shows as well. In *Two and a Half Men*, Charlie struggles with intimacy with Lisa after he sees her breastfeed. Charlie says to Lisa, "I'm looking at the sexiest woman in the world and all I see is a thermos," implying that breastfeeding makes her less attractive to him. In another episode of this program, "It Never Rains in Hooterville," Charlie asks his brother to rewind a tape of home movies so that he can see Alan's ex-wife breastfeeding. And in a *Family Guy* episode about weaning, the hypersexualized Quagmire realizes his marriage is a mistake when he becomes aroused by Lois's engorged breasts. In another *Family Guy* episode, Peter is ordered to attend a Women's Sensitivity retreat after he makes sexist comments in the workplace. Peter returns, appearing ultra-feminine. This experience prompts him to breastfeed Stewie. In the next scene, Lois tries to arouse Peter, shaking her breasts. Breastfeeding is also sexualized in the *Beavis and Butthead* episode "Holy Cornholio." While at the hospital, Beavis and Butthead walk past a delivery room. Butthead tries to peer in and asks if the new mom is going to take out her "boob." He chuckles as she screams at him to leave. In all of these representations, the juxtaposition of breastfeeding with attraction reinforces the myth that breasts are sexual objects, and therefore do not belong in the public eye.

The "Boob Job" episode of *Everybody Loves Raymond* addresses breastfeeding in conversations about breast implants. As Raymond, Robert, and their father talk enthusiastically about a woman's augmentation, matriarch Marie becomes confused at their excitement, explaining that her sons should not be interested in breasts because, she says, "I never nursed them." Frank responds, "What the hell are you talking about?" Marie explains, "Everybody know that if you breastfeed boys when they're babies, they're going to grow up to be obsessed with breasts." While this supposed rationale exists for comic relief, it also falsely ties breastfeeding into sexual fascination, even though the men mock Marie's beliefs. Likewise, in *Yes, Dear*, after the character Jimmy praises the mother in the park for breastfeeding, his wife questions his declaration, stating, "You just wanted to get a free peek at her boobs." Jimmy reassures her, "It's a woman breastfeeding. There's nothing sexual about that." Then, just to his friend, Greg, Jimmy excitedly asks, "Did you see them?" Greg answers disappointedly, "A little. The kid's head was in the way." And later, Greg's wife, Kim, admits to nursing past her child's first birthday—not for the benefits, but, as she says, "for the boobs... I like having big boobs. Big, milk-filled boobs. I never had anything like these before and I'm not ready to give them back." In an attempt to get her husband's sympathy, Kim compares her lactating breasts to Greg temporarily having "a big penis." She adds, "It's like they have magic powers. Men see them and just go into a trance." Eventually, Greg convinces her that he will still like her body, even without her enlarged breasts. In this situation, Kim's honest justification for extended breastfeeding("boobs," not benefits), connected to the discussion of penis size, reinforces breastfeeding as sexual and for men's attention.

Breastfeeding as Deviant, Socially Unacceptable, or Harmful

The sample studied clearly suggested what were considered "normal" and "abnormal" breastfeeding activities. When mothers breastfed their new babies covered up in their homes, it was presented as beautiful and natural. As exemplified with Ross's encounter with Joey and Chandler, statements about breastfeeding reinforced this message, often accompanied by soft music and the peaceful faces of the nursing mothers. Characters criticized others who were uncomfortable.

On the other hand, storylines consistently portrayed other breastfeeding activities as unacceptable or deviant, as indicated by the other characters' responses. No programs visually portrayed women nursing more than one baby, even though Carol Hathaway gave birth to twins and breastfed. In the *Friends* episode "The One Where Rachel Has a Baby," the character Joey enters Rachel's hospital room and announces, "Hey, I just saw a woman breastfeeding both of her twins at the same time. It is like a freak show up here." In *7th Heaven*, the character Annie asks her daughter, Ruthie, for help in getting ready to breastfeed her twins. Ruthie expresses disgust and quickly leaves the room. The babies' feeding is not shown.

Only two storylines presented alternative means of breastfeeding a baby. The *ER* episode "Try Carter" involves the use of a supplemental nursing system, in which Dr. John Carter sees the character Chuck breastfeed his son using a Lact-Aid. Chuck has his shirt pushed aside, one nipple exposed with the system hooked up and baby Cosmo in the cradle position. At this point, Carter does a double take, then says: "Chuck, what are you doing?" Chuck responds, "Oh, it's a supplemental nursing device. What? You've never seen a father breastfeed his kid before?" Chuck pulls out the bottle attachment to show Carter and says, "These things are amazing. You know, it allows the father to bond with the child the same way that the mother does if you can get past the sore nipples. You want to give it a shot?" Carter looks puzzled and says firmly, "No," as he leaves the room. The absurdity of Chuck wearing the system, reinforced by Carter's reaction, emphasizes that this "abnormal" situation serves as comic relief for the medical drama. Similarly, in *The New Normal*, Bryan and David are using a surrogate so that they can have a child. Bryan's desire to bond with his new baby prompts him to purchase "The Milk Man," a vest with nipples for men to nurse babies. He wears it around, despite questions from his partner. However, Bryan loses interest when his friend and her husband buy a vest and the father uses it. Bryan tells David, "Now that I see it with an actual baby, it does look stupid." Like many aspects of this breastfeeding-themed episode, the Milk Man is just another device offered for comic relief. No benefits of it are discussed and even the lactation consultant at the breastfeeding store declares it "weird."

The depictions studied also conveyed clearly defined ages for "appropriate" breastfeeding. Women are pressured to wean when their babies get older and are ridiculed if they continue breastfeeding. In the *Yes, Dear* episode "Weaning Isn't Everything," the main characters openly gawk at a mother breastfeeding her preschooler at the park. Back at the house, they ridicule the woman (both for breastfeeding at the park and for the child's age).

Greg:	Call me old-fashioned, but I think a child is too old to breastfeed if he can unhook Mommy's bra with one hand.
Christine:	I mean the problem with breastfeeding that long is, I mean, how do you stop? I mean at that point, you got to do the whole 'don't worry, we'll still be friends' speech.
Greg:	One year, that's what most of the books said. Right, Kim?
Kim (holding her child's bottles):	Yeah, most of them said a year. Some said a little more or some said a little less, but a year was more than enough for me. I couldn't wait to stop. That woman's a freak.

Later, Greg discovers that his wife, Kim, is secretly nursing her older baby. As she nurses their son, Sammy, in a rocking chair, she yells, "Don't come in here! Get out! Get out!" Afterward, Greg tries to console Kim with, "I just want you to know that I don't think you're a bad mother," and, he adds, "not some sort of freak." Their dialogue confirms Kim's shame at waiting "too long" to wean.

Greg:	What do you think we should do about this?
Kim:	I guess tomorrow when he wakes up, we can try to give him a bottle.
Greg:	I think that would be best.

Without further discussion, Kim and Greg commence weaning the next night, which quickly becomes a miserable experience. The baby cries and cries when Greg attempts to feed him—so much that Kim must move into the guest house because it becomes too painful for her to hear. Ultimately, instead of nursing the baby, in desperation, Greg dons Kim's pink nightgown to do the night feeding. When Sammy finally drinks from the bottle, Greg exclaims, "My son's drinking from my breast!" While humorous, the *Yes, Dear* storyline only condemns nursing older babies (young enough to sleep in a crib, drink from a bottle, and wake up to feed at night), against WHO recommendations. This "cold-turkey" approach promoted in the storyline could also misguide viewers. As opposed to conveying gradual weaning, which can be much easier for mother and baby, this episode suggests that Kim's breastfeeding is so shameful that it must be curbed immediately, even if it is painful for her and her child.

The programs also presented extended breastfeeding as odd or even deviant. Older babies or toddlers were not typically shown breastfeeding. Instead, extended breastfeeding involved much older children and was presented as strange, inappropriate, and distracting. In *Desperate Housewives*, employees discover a coworker, Veronica, breastfeeding her five year-old in a conference room. Her coworkers agree that it is too "bizarre" and "distracting" for her to continue nursing, even if she breastfeeds in private. They insist that the only other female employee, Lynette, request that Veronica stops and then forces weaning by offering the child chocolate milk. An episode of *30 Rock* also paints extended breastfeeding as deviant when a strange and awkward man, named Donny, announces that he cannot be seduced by another woman's breasts because he was "breastfed until he was eleven." Even the medical comedy *Scrubs* mocks extended breastfeeding. In "T.C.W.," Dr. Cox advises painkillers for kidney stones to a female patient. As she holds a preschool-age child, the mother responds, "I can't take painkillers. Justin's still breastfeeding." Her child winks and gives the doctors a "thumbs up." Dr. Cox tells the boy, "Oh, you like milk, do ya? Huh. Why don't you get on your bike and go down to the store and get some?" Meanwhile, we hear J.D.'s inner monologue: "I think that at a certain point, breastfeeding becomes creepy." The shot jumps to J.D.'s imagination in which a teenage boy is bent over nursing, then stands up with a milk moustache. The episode's narrative does not return to the patient and her decision. Intead, the mockery of the extended nursing (as very extended, in the break in the show's reality), is a humorous distraction in the story's main narrative.

In the *Game of Thrones* episode "The Wolf and the Lion," a noble woman, Lysa Arryn, sits elevated on a throne, breastfeeding a child around six or so when her sister and a group of knights enter the castle. She continues clearly breastfeeding her child as she criticizes their actions. At one point, the child unlatches. Resting his cheek against her exposed breast, he says articulately, "Mommy, is that the bad man?" Lysa responds. The boy yells at the group and Lysa orders them to take away the prisoner. Throughout this scene, Lysa's breast is bare, yet no one comments or stares, nor do they remark on the boy breastfeeding or his age. While critics online interpreted the extended breastfeeding as a demonstration of Lysa's insanity, overall the lack of reaction from the other characters suggest that her behavior is not out of the ordinary or deviant.

Adult breastfeeding representations appear in several programs. Men who desire to nurse are conveyed as aberrant in numerous ways, not just in this one fetish. In the *CSI: Crime Scene Investigation* episode "King Baby," investigators discover that a powerful billionaire secretly dresses like a baby—wearing diapers, sleeping in a large crib, and blackmailing a "milk maid" to breastfeed him. The CSIs repeatedly express their astonishment at the situation, calling him a "freak." Ultimately, this behavior leads to his death as the milk maid drugs him, causing the man to jump off his balcony. Toward the end, we find out that the victim's mother refused to breastfeed him as a baby, because, as she says, "Suckle the baby, cuckold the man." In the final scene, the CSIs call the mother a "piece of work." Here, the mother is blamed for her son's extreme deviance and ultimately, his death.

American Horror Story also connects adult breastfeeding to fatal results. The episode "Spilt Milk" begins with a large-breasted African American woman arriving at a man's apartment. She introduces herself as "Pandora" and confirms that he is "Johnny."

Johnny: Just want to make sure. The pictures on the website don't show your beautiful face.

Pandora: Oh, you won't be looking at my face, not once these triple-Ds come out to play. And trust me, I haven't had one complaint yet.

He slips some money out of his pocket and gives it to her,

Pandora: I've been saving up all day, honey. Even gave my baby a bottle of formula so there's no way I'll run dry (squeezes her breasts). Oooh, they're so juicy right now. They're ready to burst (smiles at him).

He sighs and stares at her intensely. Later in the episode, a scene begins with Johnny vigorously suckling from the naked Pandora. He looks up and breathes heavily, as milk dribbles down his chin. She comments about "Mommy issues," prompting a flashback to Johnny's father's necrophilac behavior in a mental institution in the 1960s. When the scene returns to present time, Johnny nurses again as he sobs. His emotion escalates as Johnny jumps up and yells about his mother. Pandora attempt to calm him down, coaxing Johnny with "Now look at me. I have a rockin' body and a tittie full of milk. Let me help you forget about her." He becomes more upset. She tries to seduce him. Johnny reacts by strangling her as she yells for him to stop.

The 1960s flashbacks, including the final scene, offer some insight into Johnny's rage and milk fetish. Johnny is the son of the necrophiliac and a baby born from rape. In the episode's final moments, his mother is in the hospital, refusing to see her baby. The nurse begs the new mother to breastfeed Baby Johnny, pleading with "He's allergic to formula and he's been crying for seven straight hours... I thought maybe if he suckled, he might calm down." Reluctantly, the mother takes her baby, unbuckles her hospital gown, and lets the baby latch. As he nurses, she stares at the cross mounted on the wall above her bed. From her perspective, it is upside down on the wall, symbolizing the evilness of her rapist's baby suckling and foreshadowing Johnny's malevolent future.

Three representations studied portray adult interest in breastfeeding light-heartedly. In the sitcom *That '70s Show*, the character Fez is obsessed with a baby's bottles of pumped milk. Later in the episode, his friend, Kelso discovers that Fez has been drinking it and tells him, "You need help, man." Likewise, a strange orderly in *Scrubs* shows a surprising fascination with breastfeeding in "My Coffee." The episode begins with J.D.'s voice-over, stating, "Carla discovered that her baby wasn't the only one who loved breastfeeding," as a woman holds her baby in the hospital. She says to her fussing newborn, "Oh, are you hungry, Sweetie?" The hospital worker suddenly appears and shrugs with

"I could eat." He emerges several times later in the episode, including at a tough time for Carla. Believing she is alone, Carla tells Baby Isabella, "Ugh, my breasts are so sore. I wish I could just give you formula." She hears a low whisper (from the worker), "Formula is bad for the baby. Boob milk's healthier." Carla looks around, puzzled and the story is not concluded. A scene from the animated show *American Dad!* conveys a similar tone. In "Virtual In-Stanity," CIA Deputy Director Avery Bullock uses a virtual reality machine to transform himself into a swaddled baby avatar in a crib. He smiles and looks at the camera, then deliberately cries, prompting a woman with large breasts bound in a tight shirt to enter. She exclaims (as she reaches for the baby), "Another feeding! My, you have quite the appetite!" We see his point-of-view of the large breasts approaching him and he smiles. The scene is superfluous to the main storyline. It exists then to show the audience that of all the avatars he could make, he chooses a baby so he can nurse off a large-breasted woman.

Five representations conveyed that breastfeeding could be dangerous or even deadly. In the 1974 *Little House on the Prairie* episodes "The Lord Is My Shepherd," parts one and two, Caroline Ingalls gives birth to a son, Charles Jr. Within a few days, he becomes sickly and lethargic. The town physician, Dr. Baker, tells Caroline that his low weight gain may be attributed to the quality of her breastmilk, stating that it may not have the right "chemistry" for his body. Baker recommends cow's milk for the baby. Unfortunately, Charles Jr. continues to become more sick until he passes away. This storyline suggests that had Caroline not given the baby breastmilk, thus initiating his weakened state, he may have survived. It should be noted that this explanation for the baby's death was fictional, as Laura Ingalls Wilder herself did not go into detail about her brother's death in her autobiography.[26]

As previously mentioned, the *ER* episode "Under Control" conveys the dire consequences of drugs in breastmilk. In this storyline, a baby is rushed to the Emergency Room in cardiac arrest. The medical team desperately tries to revive the baby, but cannot save her. They determine that the baby died from amphetamines and Dr. Greene and Nurse Hathaway question the mother about the drugs.

Mother:	I work two jobs. Sometimes I get so tired, I take something to stay awake but I never bring drugs home.
Hathaway:	Are you nursing the baby? [The woman nods.]

Greene:	The drugs are in the breast milk.
Mother (cries):	I love my baby. I would never hurt her. I didn't know. Really, I didn't know.

In this storyline, breastfeeding leads to the infant's unintentional death. While obviously, it is good to convey that drugs can be passed through breastmilk, writers missed an opportunity here to address the factors that led to the fictional mother's amphetamine use (i.e., poverty, lack of support, etc.).

Breastfeeding is also used to show the disturbed mind of the "unsub" (or assailant). In the *Criminal Minds* episode "The Instincts," a woman breastfeeds her victims, believing each five year-old boy is her infant son. In the context of this show, breastfeeding is an act of torture, as the victims are forced to drink and slowly starve to death on breastmilk. The image of the serial killer attempting to nurse this large boy that is not hers, as the SWAT team prepares to surround her home, emphasizes the extreme psychosis of the woman and the deviance of breastfeeding. No positive representations of extended breastfeeding were identified in the study, despite the known benefits of this practice.[27]

Breastfeeding has dire consequences in the episode "The Breast and the Brightest" of *Chicago Hope*. The episode focuses on Dr. Diane Grad, who has just returned from maternity leave, and a tragic case in the Emergency Room. Early scenes in the episode show Grad pumping her milk and expressing distress about leaving her baby to go back to work. Suddenly, paramedics rush in, pushing a baby on a gurney. They shout, "Severely dehydrated!" "We lost the pulse on the ride!" His parents helplessly plead for the doctors to save their child. Grad questions the parents, determining that the baby is only seven pounds at six weeks old. Just then, the baby starts to flatline. The doctors shock his chest repeatedly, but cannot get a pulse. In a heart-wrenching moment, the doctors call "time of death," as the mother sobs uncontrollably.

Grad (to the sobbing parents):	What the hell did you do to this baby?
Father:	What?
Grad:	Keith (another doctor), it's obvious. He's six weeks old. Look at him.
Dr. Keith Wilkes:	We won't know anything until we wait for the autopsy.
Grad:	Autopsy? A first-year med student could figure this one out. This baby's been starved.

After the commercial break, Grad continues to blame the grieving mother for her baby's death, while Wilkes defends her, stating, "Maybe she wasn't producing enough milk. Some women don't." Grad retorts, "She should have paid attention to that. The baby was skin and bones" and demands that the mother be arrested for "criminal negligence." The baby's mother tearfully responds, "I did not neglect him! I was concerned and the nursing director told me I shouldn't supplement." The parents leave. Later, it is determined that the mother tried to get lactation help and was advised to breastfeed, not supplement, at all costs, causing the baby to starve to death. Because the hospital staff refused to recommend formula, they are ultimately blamed for the fatality.

Similarly, also in 2000, detectives arrest and convict a breastfeeding mother for starving her baby in the the *Law & Order* episode "Mother's Milk." Unlike the *Chicago Hope* storyline, the episode contains no visuals of breastfeeding or pumping, and in fact, no successful nursing mothers. The entire narrative is grim, from the blood-stained bassinet to the tiny arm and leg poking out from under a blanket on the autopsy table, to the graphic testimony of discovering the child's cold body by his mother, Amy. This episode paints Amy as a "bad mother," who smoked, ignored her baby's cries, and left him alone—poor parenting that extended to her breastfeeding failure. The hospital's Lactation Consultant (LC) repeatedly blames Amy, calling her "not one of the most receptive clients that I've worked with." Assistant District Attorney Abbie Carmichael then asks, "So why not have her just give the baby a bottle?" The LC responds, "No, breast milk is what's best for the baby. It's just a matter of getting the mother to put the effort into it." Carmichael reports back to the detectives, stating, "The lactation counselor says Amy was shown the right techniques to breastfeed, and the baby's sucking reflex was fine. She just resented putting in the effort." They take Carmichael's words as fact and decide to arrest Amy for the baby's death.

At the trial, the LC again faults Amy, explaining, "Her milk production seemed fine," and, "If she was putting in the effort, there's no question she would have been successful." Throughout the episode, the detectives and attorneys for both sides bring up the "unopened bottles and sealed cans of formula" found at the baby's residence, questioning why they were never used. Interviewing the baby's father on the stand, Amy's lawyer asks, "There was formula in that apartment. There were bottles. Ever think to feed your son?" The parents justify their decision by claiming that they signed a contract, promising to breastfeed, as they were led to believe that "giving him a bottle might be dangerous." During the trial, the Defense demonizes the LC, criticizing how she did not recommend a bottle due to "nipple confusion." She responds, "I use whatever methods I can to insure that the baby gets breast milk." Amy's lawyer continues with, "Yeah, and those methods often include threats and intimidation, don't they?" Their concluding exchange further scrutinizes the intention of the LC:

Defense:	Breastfeeding is almost a crusade with you, Miss Strickland, isn't it? That's not true. You lecture on the benefits of breast milk. You have written articles on the subject, haven't you?... Not that far, when you insist that a mother breastfeed her child exclusively, when it's obvious that a baby is in trouble.
LC:	You make it sound like breastfeeding is an unnatural process. Formula is what's unnatural. Children have difficulty digesting it, and it doesn't contain the same antibodies or immunities.
Defense:	But babies don't starve to death on it, do they?

In her closing argument, Amy's lawyer declares, "Only a woman can know the social pressure to breastfeed today. And only a woman can suffer the stigma of that failure." Ultimately, Amy is convicted of negligence and receives a year in prison. Throughout this episode, breastfeeding is conveyed as either "easy"—if you just "try hard enough"—or as so overly complicated that few women could succeed. On the other hand, formula is presented as the fail-safe rescue, reinforced by false statements about babies not starving from it (despite real-life mortality rates, especially when formula is tainted or mixed improperly). Moreover, the LC, with her hospital contract, is depicted as an extremist without the best interest of her clients, or their babies. Given the rarity of LC characters in television, this portrayal could suggest that those that support lactation in real-life will be demeaning, strict, and recommend actions that could even harm your baby.

The *Chicago Hope* and *Law & Order* episodes were loosely based on the 1997 Tabitha Walrond case, in which her 2 month-old son died of starvation after she attempted to exclusively breastfeed him.[28] According to *New York Times* coverage of the case, Walrod had undergone a breast reduction and did not know that it could negatively impact her milk supply.[29] Reporters also noted other details about Walrod—that she was an African American teenage, single mother without health insurance.[30] Prosecutors argued that she intentionally starved her baby, while the defense claimed that Walrod never received the lactation advice and support she needed.[31] Even considering her age, lack of accurate breastfeeding knowledge, and absence of support, Walrond was charged with second-degree manslaughter and ultimately convicted of criminally negligent homicide.[32]

Obviously, key information was changed for both fictionalizations. The mother in *Chicago Hope* is Caucasian, in her early 30s, middle-upper class, and married with strong partner support. She also presumably has health insurance, never had breast surgery, and visited the hospital's LC with concerns about her baby. In other words, other than the connection between exclusive breastfeeding and a baby's death, the *Chicago Hope* version strips away the complex challenges faced by the real-life breastfeeding mother. Additionally, the television parents are not held responsible, as the negligence case is dropped and, in fact, the parents sue the hospital for providing poor advice. Similarly, *Law & Order* writers changed the race of the parents to Caucasian and omitted the breast reduction surgey (an important detail). And yet, they included some of the Walrond case information—a lack of insurance, problems with Medicaid, the mother's young age, and her relationship problems, albeit in a misconstrued narrative that blames the mother, the LC, and breastfeeding as causes for the baby's death.

Scholars have used the *Chicago Hope* depiction as an example of media's distortion of real-life cases. Bentley, Dee, and Jensen noted that at the time of this broadcast, CBS was in a partnership with the Johns Hopkins School of Medicine and an organization that encompassed infant formula corporations.[33] Likewise, Jacqueline Wolf noted the mediated distortion of the actual case, arguing media overall missed an opportunity to address "the inadequacy and inefficiency of Medicaid... poor communication between doctors and patients... teen pregnancy and motherhood" and other issues, along with "the nonexistent public support network for pregnant and nursing mothers in the United States."[34] Thus, these episodes serve as examples of how television normalizes formula use, highlights and exaggerates breastfeeding tragedy, while bypassing the institutional, economic, and social obstacles that contributed to the real-life Walrond case.

Breastfeeding as Individual or Institutional?

Most representations studied focus on the individual mother and her breastfeeding experiences: Carla, Pam, and Rachel learning about latching. Frustrations with pumping at work for Dr. Corday and a minor character in *The Office*. Individual cases of restaurant and retail managers ridiculing mothers who are nursing in public. Seldom is breastfeeding contextualized within institutional or economic contexts. One exception is "The Leftover Thermalization" of *The Big Bang Theory*. As the main characters chat at dinner, astrophysicist Raj proposes that society may be approaching gender equality, as exemplified by Marvel Comics changing the superhero Thor to a woman. Neuro-biologist Amy Farrah Fowler quickly responds, "We won't know if there's equality until female Thor has a baby and the Avengers are cool with her pumping breast milk at work." The role of institutional contexts rarely appears in fictional television. In fact, the *Chicago Hope* episode in which the baby dies from starvation is the only episode studied to bring in any real-life breastfeeding policies and/or call to action. The episode begins with a regular meeting of the physicians and Chief-of-Staff. While the doctors wait for Grad to arrive, Dr. Keith Wilkes says impatiently, "Can we at least talk about this Baby-Friendly nonsense?" The ensuing conversation sets the foundation for the primary case of the episode:

Dr. Dennis Hancock:	What nonsense? It's a contract stating that the hospital feels breastfeeding's best for the child.
Dr. Lisa Catera:	Forcing women to nurse? It's a little Orwellian.
Hancock:	They're not forced. They're encouraged.
Wilkes:	We're not allowed to send them home with formula. That seems like some pretty heavy encouragement.
Hancock:	Are you challenging the obvious health benefits of breastfeeding?
Wilkes:	I'm not challenging anything.

At this point, other doctors at the meeting change the subject. While somewhat timely, this negative framing of the Baby-Friendly Hospital Initiative (BFHI) is a direct misrepresention of BFHI. It also eschews the facts of the actual case, which was not about contracts and the BFHI. It should be noted that Baby Friendly hospitals do not forbid health professionals from ever recommending milk substitutes, as is conveyed here.

Rather, Baby Friendly hospitals simply discourage widely supplementing and distributing free formula.[35] Overall, it is unfortunate that this one storyline is the sole reference to an effort that has been very successful in raising breastfeeding rates.[36] Just as important, no deaths from breastfeeding malnutrition have been connected to the Baby-Friendly Hospital Initiative.

Discussing Breastfeeding on Television

Overall, the representations varied in genre and target audience. Crime and medical dramas, sitcoms, and animated programs included breastfeeding references. Even with these differences, the representations studied consistently conveyed that for a certain group of women, in a private place, for a newborn, breastfeeding is natural, beautiful, and easy. However, outside this narrow definition of "normal," breastfeeding was presented as absurd, unnecessary, socially unacceptable, or deviant. The benefits and obstacles of breastfeeding largely focused on individual women, rather than many of the macro-level issues that influence breastfeeding (e.g., hospital practices that interfere with breastfeeding). These findings were consistent with previous literature that suggests that contemporary media tend to present breastfeeding positively, but as a difficult endeavor for the individual woman.[37]

Little diversity existed among the type of women shown breastfeeding, despite real-life comparisons. Statistically, educated, affluent, Caucasian women are more likely to breastfeed than those who are younger, less educated, and of a lower socio-economic class.[38] Hispanic and Caucasian women are more likely to breastfeed than African American women.[39] Although breastfeeding rates are highest with this type of person, the absence of other representations could discourage other women from nursing by failing to present them as the "normal" women who nurse, particularly if the macro-level reasons for the racial disparity in breastfeeding were addressed. Media can help challenge and dispel myths about breastfeeding and race. More representations of women of color would establish that yes, women of different ethnicities do breastfeed. Fictional storylines could also help bring in the history of hypersexualization of African American women (as discussed by Blum) to explain why, historically, a racial disparity has existed.[40] Furthermore, narratives of women of color breastfeeding successfully would also help transform inaccurate media messages that blamed individual women of color for the failure to thrive, as Hausman outlined.[41] Additionally, diversity in other ways is needed. For example, as this study shows, breastfeeding characters who are gay, lesbian, bisexual, and transgender characters are completely absent from television. With the addition of *The L Word*, *The New Normal* and numerous other shows with regular characters who are LGBTQ, there are opportunities for them to breastfeed—they have just been missed. In recent years, changes in who breastfeeds has started to occur. By having more diverse characters breastfeed without failure, these narrow definitions will continue to expand.

While it is encouraging that contemporary television programs typically address breastfeeding in a positive, albeit limited, approach, many opportunities to promote breastfeeding are missed. Most domestic comedies include a "new baby" storyline at one point. And yet, until the 1990s, breastfeeding was usually not mentioned. Even programs that begin a "new baby" storyline with the "learning to breastfeed" experience rarely refer to breastfeeding once the baby is home from the hospital. It would be easy to expand breastfeeding representations to include twins or premature babies, or nursing toddlers, and to insert positive breastfeeding storylines for diverse characters. In *ER*, which contains many breastfeeding portrayals, several women of color birth babies, and yet their breastfeeding experiences are not addressed. African American Dr. Peter Benton's ex-girlfriend gives birth to a premature baby. This storyline would have been an excellent opportunity to showcase an African American woman breastfeeding, as well as the challenges of pumping and feeding a preemie—a common event in real-life, despite little coverage in entertainment television.[42] Such representations could help improve breastfeeding rates and help to normalize breastfeeding for the types of women usually excluded.

Breastfeeding benefits were not typically addressed, especially the specific health benefits for children and mothers. Educating people on the numerous health benefits of breastmilk could help people realize that breastfeeding is a key determinant in future health and would save Americans money on health care if more women breastfed.[43] Furthermore, programs could outline the lesser known health benefits for nursing mothers, such as lower risks of breast cancer and hip fractures.[44] Knowledge about breastfeeding has been strongly correlated with a mother's confidence in breastfeeding.[45] And beyond the individual benefits, if media representations conveyed the positive impacts of breastfeeding on society, more people might be supportive of breastfeeding— for example, the productivity of nursing mothers in the workplace (because they take fewer sick days) or the billions of dollars saved in health care costs if the majority of the population breastfed.[46]

While characters mentioned certain challenges repeatedly, namely, latching issues and sore nipples, other common obstacles, such as engorgement, mastitis thrush and fear of a low supply, were never addressed. Research has shown that women's concerns about lactation issues and the baby's nourishment are given as the most frequent reasons for weaning.[47] These programs could help allay these fears, thus extending duration, by counteracting myths about "insufficient milk" and offering solutions to typical problems. Furthermore, such depictions could reassure viewers that these issues are normal and therefore not a reason to wean. Solutions could include dried breastmilk for sore nipples, medication for mastitis and thrush and pumping to boost supply. In addition to individual challenges, cultural obstacles could also be fictionalized in entertainment media to raise awareness, such as hospital practices that hinder breastfeeding, legislation or lack of public support, and other sites of resistance for the breastfeeding woman.[48]

Breastfeeding was presented as inconvenient and restrictive for working women. It was suggested that time away from work because of nursing could hinder one's career. No solutions were presented, even though in real-life, numerous societal changes could improve breastfeeding success for working women. Furthermore, no policy changes or legislation are addressed in the shows, even for those that appeared after the Fair Labor Standards Act of the Affordable Care Act, which positively impacts working mothers.[49] Fictional programs could address strategies to help working women breastfeed, including on-site child care, flexible working arrangements, sufficient pumping breaks, and extended maternity leave.[50] Such representations could alert potential employers to the needs of working mothers and garner public support for policies to protect them. Improving working conditions for breastfeeding is especially important given that working full-time has been shown to decrease breastfeeding duration by an average of 8.6 weeks.[51]

In the programs, breastfeeding often made other characters uncomfortable, even when the mother was covered up, reinforcing the idea that some consider breastfeeding to be indecent or obscene. Breastfeeding was only shown in *The Sopranos*, *Sex and the City*, *Two and a Half Men*, and animated in *Family Guy*. These programs also all contained storylines that sexualized breasts, therefore, may do little to change perceptions that breastfeeding differs from public nudity or indecent exposure. While it may be difficult for actors to mimic breastfeeding or for the act of breastfeeding to be aired on television, doing so would be a significant step toward normalizing breastfeeding. This step is especially important given that mainstream media as a whole rarely include images of real breastfeeding. Hausman (2003) argued that images of women breastfeeding (without covers) are much more likely to depict women in developing countries than "typical" American women (i.e., Caucasian and middle-upper class).[52]

Nursing in public was presented as negative and embarrassing. The few depictions of nursing in public conveyed that, while it is permitted by law, the nursing mother will likely be the target of disapproving looks and may be asked to leave—not very encouraging for a new mother who would like to venture out in public. A nursing mother would have a difficult time breastfeeding past a few months if she fears breastfeeding outside of her home. While the *Charmed*, *Married with Children*, and *The New Normal* episodes involve a protest of breastfeeding criticism, the storylines offered no practical advice on how to address concerns about nursing in public, such as support for lactation rooms or other facilities for nursing mothers.[53] Positive depictions of public breastfeeding could help women become comfortable with the notion prior to trying themselves, similar to the "safe" spaces that LLL provides for nursing mothers.[54] Repeated positive depictions could normalize public breastfeeding so that it no longer seems threatening to new mothers or offends onlookers.

Breastfeeding more than one child and the use of supplemental nursing systems were presented as deviant. The use of milk banks and using supplemental nursing systems to relactate or nourish adopted children were not seriously explored. These tools could be viable options for women who adopt or have difficulty breastfeeding, especially if their babies are premature or suffer from chronic illness.[55] Additionally, extended breastfeeding was conveyed as deviant, an alarming finding considering that the health benefits for mother and child dramatically increase with duration.[56] Instead of highlighting the abnormality of nursing an elementary school-aged child, programming could include more portrayals of breastfeeding older babies and toddlers, thus reinforcing breastfeeding recommendations of the World Health Organization (WHO) and the American Academy of Pediatrics.[57] The "deviant" storylines, which framed breastfeeding as dangerous, perpetuate what Hausman (2003) called the "Dead Babies" media discourse.[58] As breastfeeding promotion has become more prevalent, media backlash has highlighted extreme consequences of the "breast is best" message, with news stories of babies starving because their mothers refused to provide formula.[59] Media stories, including fictional ones, that present breastfeeding as normal could help counter these sensationalized cases, especially images of women breastfeeding healthy babies.

Finally, representations consistently emphasize and blame individual mothers for breastfeeding successes and "failures," ignoring institutional barriers and obstacles that relate to socio-economic class, racial bias, insurance status, and other complex factors. Furthermore, the only reference to the Baby Friendly Hospital Initiative paints a false picture of its intentions and impliementation. The Code, *Innocenti Declaration*, "The Surgeon's Call," and *Healthy People 2020* are absent from fictional television. Instead, television emphasizes the individual woman and her struggles. It should be noted that fictional television as a whole tends to eschew policy and political context as a whole. For example, at the height of the health insurance crisis, even the medical drama genre rarely addressed uninsured populations.[60] Yet, if there is a place in television's narratives for blaming individual women for breastfeeding "failures," comic protests that involve dressing as Lady Godiva or donning a milky-man vest, then such important issues can also be included, provided they are presented factually and not distorted by a "breastfeeding as choice" discourse.

Conclusion

The key to increasing breastfeeding rates in the United State is shifting overall public perceptions of breastfeeding—at the individual, interpersonal, and societal levels. Koerber argued that breastfeeding women often sought "competing alternatives" to the medical discourse that lacked breastfeeding information.[61] Media, then, can help provide the missing information—which plays an important role in women's decision to breastfeed.[62] Since the opinions of family and friends also influence breastfeeding success, normalizing breastfeeding on TV, while conveying the benefits of breastfeeding, may help people become more supportive.[63] Restaurant managers may be less likely to scold nursing mothers if they believe that breastfeeding is the normal means of feeding a baby. Employers might be more willing to grant pumping time to working mothers if they realize that breastfed babies experience less illness, resulting in fewer absences for the mothers. Overall, general support for breastfeeding would mean that more women would feel comfortable nursing, regardless of who may be watching.

Similar to the health campaigns promoting designated driving, immunizations, and contraception, fictional television could be used to promote breastfeeding.[64] Such campaigns could introduce breastfeeding terminology, such as Nursing in Public (NIP), engorgement, nursing strike, and exclusive or extended breastfeeding, into mainstream public discourse. Programs could also correct misconceptions about breastfeeding—for example, what conditions do and do not prevent women from breastfeeding. These shows could also teach women helpful remedies for common problems, like techniques to deal with biting during breastfeeding. Furthermore, since fictional programs (unlike news stories) can provide in-depth stories about breastfeeding, these shows could highlight many of the underlying macro-level issues that discourage breastfeeding, including maternal guilt about insufficient milk, the hypersexualization of breasts entrenched in culture, and the need for resistance for breastfeeding mothers.[65] Storylines could also address the shifts in society that have transformed women's roles and encouraged a dependency on experts, thus hindering women's abilities to rely on other women for breastfeeding advice.[66]

It has been established that television helps to define normative behavior. Cultivation studies have established that television dramatically impacts how people perceive the world.[67] While the numerous positive representations of nursing after birth indicate progress toward normalizing breastfeeding, the representations are limited in scope. By presenting extended breastfeeding, public breastfeeding, and other "deviant" behaviors as normal, media representations can help change attitudes toward breastfeeding, helping women to feel comfortable breastfeeding when and wherever their babies demand, without a fear of public scrutiny or police intervention. It is only when nearly all babies are breastfed in the United States that we can honestly claim that we are doing our best to protect our nation's health.

Notes

1. Gartner et al., "Breastfeeding and the Use of Human Milk"; ASH/OPHS, "The Surgeon General's Call to Action to Support Breastfeeding"; Brown and Peuchaud, "Media and Breastfeeding: Friend or Foe?"
2. Urban, "UPDATE: A Response from Sesame Street on Breastfeeding|Care2 Causes."
3. Li et al., "Public Beliefs about Breastfeeding Policies in Various Settings"; Foss and Blake, "'It's Natural and Healthy, But I Don't Want To See It': The Impact of Entertainment Television on Breastfeeding Attitudes."
4. "The Motion Picture Production Code of 1930 (Hays Code)."
5. Mondello, "Remembering Hollywood's Hays Code, 40 Years On."
6. "The Hays Code Brings Censorship To Motion Pictures."
7. Rubenstein-Gillis, "Reel Milk: Sexual? Maternal? Investigating the Portrayal of Breastfeeding in American Cinema."
8. Ibid.
9. "The Museum of Broadcast Communications - Encyclopedia of Television - Censorship."
10. Pondillo, *America's First Network TV Censor.*
11. "The Museum of Broadcast Communications - Encyclopedia of Television - Censorship."
12. Ibid.
13. Rideout, "Television As A Health Educator: A Case Study of Grey's Anatomy."
14. Ibid.
15. Brodie et al., "Communicating Health Information Through The Entertainment Media"; Winsten, "Promoting Designated Drivers"; Folb, "Don't Touch That Dial!"
16. Davin, "Healthy Viewing: The Reception of Medical Narratives."
17. Sharf and Freimuth, "Confronting Cancer on Thirtysomething."
18. Ibid.
19. Aaronson, Mural, and Pfoutz, "Seeking Information"; Lewallen et al., "Breastfeeding Support and Early Cessation."
20. Li et al., "Public Beliefs about Breastfeeding Policies in Various Settings."
21. "Breastfeeding Report Card: United States, 2014 - 2014breastfeedingreportcard.pdf."
22. Ibid.
23. Karen, in *The Office*, played by Rashida Jones, has a multi-ethnic background. However, she does not appear in the show after she has her baby.
24. Nommsen-Rivers et al., "Comfort with the Idea of Formula Feeding Helps Explain Ethnic Disparity in Breastfeeding Intentions Among Expectant First-Time Mothers."

25. Mozingo et al., "It Wasn't Working."
26. Wilder, *Pioneer Girl.*
27. Gillman et al., "Risk of Overweight Among Adolescents Who Were Breastfed as Infants"; Beyerlein and Kries, "Breastfeeding and Body Composition in Children."
28. Bernstein, "Mother Charged With Starving Baby Tells of Frantic Effort to Save Him."
29. Ibid.; Bernstein, "Trial Begins for Mother in Breast-Fed Infant's Starvation Death."
30. See note 28.
31. Bernstein, "Trial Begins for Mother in Breast-Fed Infant's Starvation Death."
32. Bernstein, "Mother Convicted in Infant's Starvation Death Gets 5 Years' Probation."
33. Bentley, Dee, and Jensen, "Breastfeeding among Low Income, African-American Women."
34. Wolf, *Don't Kill Your Baby: Public Health and the Decline of Breastfeeding in the 19th and 20th Centuries*, p. 201.
35. "Baby-Friendly Hospital Initiative."
36. Pérez-Escamilla, Martinez, and Segura-Pérez, "Impact of the Baby-friendly Hospital Initiative on Breastfeeding and Child Health Outcomes."
37. Brown and Peuchaud, "Media and Breastfeeding: Friend or Foe?"; Rubenstein-Gillis, "Reel Milk: Sexual? Maternal? Investigating the Portrayal of Breastfeeding in American Cinema."
38. Bolton et al., "Characteristics Associated With Longer Breastfeeding Duration"; Ryan, Wenjun, and Acosta, "Breastfeeding Continues to Increase Into the New Millennium."
39. Jones et al., "Factors Associated With Exclusive Breastfeeding in the United States"; Forste, Weiss, and Lippincott, "The Decision to Breastfeed in the United States"; Ryan, Wenjun, and Acosta, "Breastfeeding Continues to Increase Into the New Millennium."
40. Blum, *At the Breast.*
41. Hausman, *Mother's Milk.*
42. In 2009, Michelle Duggar (the mother in *19 Kids and Counting*, a reality show on the Learning Channel), breastfed her micro-preemie, Josie, until it was determined that Josie could not digest Michelle's breastmilk. An episode centered on the very ill Josie becoming much healthier after she is given formula.
43. Bartick and Reinhold, "The Burden of Suboptimal Breastfeeding in the United States."
44. Cumming and Klineberg, "Breastfeeding and Other Reproductive Factors and the Risk of Hip Fractures in Elderly Women"; Enger et al., "Breastfeeding History, Pregnancy Experience and Risk of Breast Cancer."

45. Chezem, Friesen, and Boettcher, "Breastfeeding Knowledge, Breastfeeding Confidence, and Infant Feeding Plans."
46. Bartick and Reinhold, "The Burden of Suboptimal Breastfeeding in the United States."
47. Li et al., "Why Mothers Stop Breastfeeding."
48. Koerber, "'You Just Don't See Enough Normal' Critical Perspectives on Infant-Feeding Discourse and Practice"; Koerber, "Rhetorical Agency, Resistance, and the Disciplinary Rhetorics of Breastfeeding"; Wolf, "What Feminists Can Do for Breastfeeding and What Breastfeeding Can Do for Feminists."
49. "Breastfeeding State Laws."
50. Fein, Mandal, and Roe, "Success of Strategies for Combining Employment and Breastfeeding"; Wolf, "What Feminists Can Do for Breastfeeding and What Breastfeeding Can Do for Feminists."
51. Fein, Mandal, and Roe, "Success of Strategies for Combining Employment and Breastfeeding."
52. See note 41.
53. Li et al., "Public Beliefs about Breastfeeding Policies in Various Settings."
54. Koerber, "Rhetorical Agency, Resistance, and the Disciplinary Rhetorics of Breastfeeding."
55. Newman, "Breastfeeding Your Adopted Baby or Baby Born by Surrogate/ Gestational Carrier."
56. See note 44; Gillman et al., "Risk of Overweight Among Adolescents Who Were Breastfed as Infants"; Beyerlein and Kries, "Breastfeeding and Body Composition in Children."
57. "WHO Breastfeeding"; Breastfeeding, "Breastfeeding and the Use of Human Milk."
58. Hausman, *Mother's Milk.*
59. Ibid.
60. Foss, *Television and Health Responsibility in an Age of Individualism.*
61. Koerber, "Rhetorical Agency, Resistance, and the Disciplinary Rhetorics of Breastfeeding."
62. Arora et al., "Major Factors Influencing Breastfeeding Rates."
63. DiGirolamo, Grummer-Strawn, and Fein, "Do Perceived Attitudes of Physicians and Hospital Staff Affect Breastfeeding Decisions?"; Freed, Fraley, and Schanler, "Attitudes of Expectant Fathers Regarding Breast-Feeding"; Littman, Medendorp, and Goldfarb, "The Decision to Breastfeed The Importance of Fathers' Approval"; Taveras et al., "Opinions and Practices of Clinicians Associated With Continuation of Exclusive Breastfeeding."

64. Brodie et al., "Communicating Health Information Through The Entertainment Media"; Glik et al., "Health Education Goes Hollywood"; Winsten, "Promoting Designated Drivers."
65. Blum, *At the Breast*; Hausman, *Mother's Milk*; Koerber, "'You Just Don't See Enough Normal' Critical Perspectives on Infant-Feeding Discourse and Practice"; Koerber, "Rhetorical Agency, Resistance, and the Disciplinary Rhetorics of Breastfeeding."
66. Foss, "Perpetuating 'Scientific Motherhood'"; Wolf, "What Feminists Can Do for Breastfeeding and What Breastfeeding Can Do for Feminists"; Hausman, *Mother's Milk*.
67. Gerbner and Gross, "Living With Television."

CHAPTER 7

Reality Television Programs and the Failure Narrative

> Hey! My name is Maci. I'm 16. I live in Chattanooga, Tennessee and I'm a total overachiever... All my friends are psyched for senior year, but I'm graduating early and moving in with Ryan because... *I'm pregnant.*

In 2009, this opening introduced MTV viewers to its new reality show: *16 and Pregnant*. Each week, the show featured the real-life pregnancy and childrearing experiences of a different teenage girl. Filled with the drama of adolescence, mixed with the unscripted surprises of a reality program, *16 and Pregnant* was an instant hit. More than two million viewers watched the finale of the first season in 2009.[1] The show has also been widely popular online. Over nine million streams of the first season were noted within a month of its online release.[2] The show and its spin-off series, *Teen Mom 1, 2, & 3* which follows the *16 and Pregnant* mothers, have thus far produced 15 seasons with 88 episodes.

This pregnancy/new baby reality format is not unique to MTV, nor did it originate on this channel. Pregnancy and infancy reality programs have dominated programming on The Learning Channel (TLC) and Discovery Health Channel (DHC) since the early 2000s, well before

A portion of this chapter first appeared as Foss, K. (2012). Breastfeeding in the Baby Block: Using reality television to effectively promote breastfeeding, Chapter 20. In P.H. Smith, B.L. Hausman, & M. Labbok (Eds.). *Beyond Health, Beyond Choice: Breastfeeding Constraints and Realities*. Rutgers University Press.

K.A. Foss, *Breastfeeding and Media*,
DOI 10.1007/978-3-319-56442-5_7

16 and Pregnant. Catering to a vastly different audience, in the reality shows *A Baby Story*, *Bringing Home Baby*, *Deliver Me*, and *Deliver Me: Home Edition*, cameras follow families through their experiences of labor, delivery, and the first days of infancy. Even with differences in demographics across these channels, these programs address many of the same topics, including baby showers and other preparations for the new arrival, depictions of prenatal appointments and childbirth, and the exhausting first nights of parenting. And, as infant feeding is an integral part of preparing and caring for a newborn, "breast or bottle?" discussions and depictions were and continue to be part of this "new baby" narrative, therefore perpetuating and normalizing infant feeding choices for "regular" people. This chapter examines messages about breast and bottle-feeding in the reality programs of MTV, TLC, and DHC, exploring the "real" experiences of feeding babies, as well how this genre could be used as a tool to promote breastfeeding. This chapter also addresses the product placement of formula marketing as it relates to the programs.

Background: The Rise of Reality Television

In the early 2000s, the genre of reality television boomed, featuring "real people" as they underwent makeovers, competed in talent contests, and remodeled their homes as America watched.[3] While this genre was not new to television, it had never been so popular, nor covered so many different areas until its resurgence at this time. From a production standpoint, reality programming makes sense, given the lack of scripting and paid actors. This genre is also ideal for product integration, as it is easy to incorporate commercial products and feature them in reality shows.[4] Since viewers can easily avoid traditional commercials through DVRs, *Youtube*, and online streaming, in recent years, product placement has become even more appealing and pervasive.[5] This approach has demonstrated effectiveness in creating brand recognition and in influencing consumer attitudes and purchase intentions towards the product.[6] The integration of formula marketing then not only normalizes bottle-feeding, but can also shape consumers' perceptions of infant feeding. As evidence of the potential effects of product placement, the integration of infant formula into television shows is prohibited in both the United Kingdom and France.[7] Yet, much like other damaging practices in the

United States, the product placement of infant formula into reality and fictional television is wholly allowed in American media.

The Influence of Reality TV

While people may disregard reality television as mere entertainment, this genre has and can significantly impact the viewing audience. Scholars have demonstrated that watching reality television has been correlated with attitude shifts about home repair, body image, and childbirth.[8] Studies have also suggested specific behavior changes. For example, viewers of "makeover" reality programs are more likely to go tanning than non-viewers.[9] In a survey of people seeking plastic surgery, many of whom identified as heavy viewers of cosmetic surgery reality shows, 80% reported that watching television encouraged them to have procedures done.[10] Exposure to weight-loss reality programs has been shown to negatively impact attitudes toward people who are obese, with higher viewer beliefs that people can control their weight.[11] And, as reality TV often casts people in terms of archetypes that they bring to the show, this genre reinforces stereotypes about Asian Americans, African Americans, people from Appalachia, and additional subpopulations.[12]

With the popularity of *16 and Pregnant* and *Teen Mom*, scholars have focused specifically on assessing the effects of these programs on adolescent perceptions and behaviors. Kearney and Levine correlated geographic viewing trends with pregnancy rates by region, determining that areas with the highest viewership also had lower teen pregnancy rates.[13] Furthermore, they noted an overall 5.7% reduction in birth rates 18 months after *16 and Pregnant* premiered.[14] Addressing this study, however McKinney argued that the birth rate possibly declined because of increases in diabetes and obesity, not as a direct effect from these programs.[15] Regardless of the birth rate impact, other attitudinal and behavioral responses have been noted. Kearney and Levine also examined Internet searches in conjunction with the programs, finding that tweets about birth control and abortion increased after episodes aired, as did Google searches of "birth control."[16]

Not all effects have been positive. Martins and Jensen surveyed high school students about teen pregnancy.[17] Compared to non-viewers, fans of *Teen Mom* and similar reality shows were more likely to envy the lives of teenage mothers, believing that they had a "good" quality of life, with ample free time, easy access to child care, and few struggles in completing high school.[18] The concern that these programs encourage teen pregnancy by creating celebrities out of ordinary girls has been expressed in popular media. Articles in *ABC News*, *Fox News*, *The Huffington Post*, *Time* magazine, and others have contended that these programs glamorize pregnancy. In a 2011 article in *CNN*, the series' creator, Lauren Dolgen, responded to concerns stating that she intended to bring the issue of teen pregnancy into the public eye and give a voice to this population.[19] Furthermore, these shows have become part of the National Campaign to Prevent Teen and Unplanned Pregnancy, which offers free copies of the series in the hope of encouraging sexual responsibility.

While little research exists on the effects of other reality pregnancy shows, it can be assumed that the programming of MTV, TLC and Discovery Health all impact viewers. These shows follow real people through their prenatal decisions and postpartum actions, including how they decide to feed their babies. An examination of breast and bottle-feeding in these programs, accompanied by any product placement, should provide a solid understanding of how reality TV talks about feeding. And of course, while *16 and Pregnant*, *A Baby Story*, *Bringing Home Baby*, *Deliver Me*, and *Deliver Me: Home Edition* are largely unscripted, we must remember that they were carefully filmed, edited, and packaged for cable television.

MTV's *16 and Pregnant*

Each episode of this one-hour (42 min without commercials) program follows a similar format. In a voice-over, the teen mom introduces herself, her lifestyle, and her family. Then, with a close-up of her bourgeoning belly, we hear, "And *I'm pregnant*!" The teen moms featured are almost all Caucasian, but vary in their family structure, coming from both single parents and dual-parent homes. Approximately half the episode focuses on the pregnancy, depicting the expectant teen mom's interactions with her friends, family, and the expectant father, including, at some point, a conversation in which the pregnant teen discusses her use of contraception—or lack thereof. Prenatal appointments, baby showers, and other "preparing for baby" moments are also typically shown. Themes of this show convey the internal struggles of "growing up too fast," demonstrated through the teen mom's parents' disapproval, the isolation of the "cheerleader turned stay at home mom," and the ill-fated teen romance leading to "Daddy desertion" shortly after childbirth. Messages about infant feeding are sometimes woven through these themes.

The first two seasons[20] of *16 and Pregnant* were analyzed, along with *Teen Mom* episodes for the mothers who were still breastfeeding at the end of the first series. In total, 16 episodes were analyzed for messages about infant feeding, as well as images of breast- or bottle-feeding. The appearance of specific breast- or bottle-feeding products was also noted.

THE "NORM" OF BOTTLE-FEEDING

Every baby in the 16 episodes of *16 and Pregnant* is bottle-fed at some point in the episode. For most of the teen moms featured, breastfeeding is not discussed or attempted. Rather, it is assumed that the new parents would bottle-feed their children. Maci, Amber, Whitney, Caitlynn, Nikkole, Valerie, Samantha, and Leah only formula-feed, without any discussion or attempt to breastfeed their babies. In the first episode of the series, immediately after Maci gives birth, the camera shows a close-up of the baby drinking from a pre-filled formula bottle. Seconds later, we see another person (not mom or dad) feeding the baby a pre-filled formula bottle. Teen moms Farrah and Amber also feed their babies pre-filled formula bottles at the hospital. A pre-filled formula bottle is next to Caitlynn's sleeping baby in the hospital bassinet. This bottle-feeding theme continues throughout *16 and Pregnant*, where mixing bottles is a standard part of the "getting up with the baby" montage that is typically part of each episode. After 2 weeks postpartum, no positive references or visual images of breastfeeding appear in this program.

FILMED PRENATAL DISCUSSIONS

In *16 and Pregnant*, teens often have conversations about childrearing with each other and their health professionals during the filmed prenatal appoints. Yet, the "feeding conversation" is only shown in two episodes. At her 24-week appointment, cheerleader Farrah announces to her doctor, "Um, I plan on not breastfeeding." She then adds, "I prefer not to do that." Farrah's doctor responds:

Doctor:	would say, gosh, if you could nurse for a week, 2 weeks, as long as you could, I think it's definitely going to benefit the baby. It'll help protect them against cold viruses, bacteria, things like that so it keeps them healthier. It's more natural—
Farrah (talking over her doctor):	What happens to your boobs if you breastfeed?
Doctor:	Nothing—
Farrah's mother interjects:	All I know is that women who have had a lot of babies, their boobs seem to get bigger and saggier. I don't know
Farrah:	Will that make your boobs more saggier if you breastfeed?
Doctor:	No. Pregnancy would do that to ya—

After birth, Baby Sophia is shown bottle-feeding.

Only one episode shows a breastfeeding discussion between the expectant parents, with expectant mom Lizzie and her (male) partner, Skylar. They sit on a couch casually discussing parenthood. Then Skylar asks, "So you plan on breastfeeding, right?" Lizzie replies, "As long as I can, yeah." He looks at her and says, "Good, cause it's better for the baby." She adds, "And it's cheaper." Skylar concurs, "Exactly, it's cheaper." But, despite their intentions, as described below, they wind up bottle-feeding their daughter.

Breastfeeding Experiences

16 and Pregnant presents breastfeeding as unusual, painful, inconvenient, embarrassing, and doomed to failure. Breastfeeding first appears in the fourth episode, with teen mom Ebony. At a few days old, the baby is home. During a voice-over, Ebony sits down in a chair, calmly unbuckles her nursing tank and easily latches on her baby. Yet, within the same week, Ebony feeds her a bottle and breastfeeding is not shown or addressed again.

Breastfeeding is only attempted or even mentioned at the hospital in two episodes. In the first episode of season two, a nurse gives new mom Jenelle a pep talk about how eating is a learned behavior. She comes over to Jenelle's hospital bed and asks, "What side do you want to try on first?" Jenelle's son Jace latches on and nurse says, "What a natural!" As part of the "new baby" montage, Nicole breastfeeds under a blanket, which she briefly lifts to show baby latched on. Yet, both Jenelle and Nicole only use bottles after these brief experiences.

Teen mom Chelsea wants to breastfeed her new daughter, who was born at 35 weeks, but is discouraged by the nurse because of the baby's prematurity. The nurse states, "I know you wanted to nurse, but she just doesn't have the strength to do that." In the next frame, Chelsea's boyfriend is using a breast pump on himself, as Chelsea jokes about nipple hair. Meanwhile, the baby is fed a pre-filled formula bottle. At home, Chelsea briefly attempts to breastfeed once (not covered up). She quickly becomes frustrated, announces that it hurts, switches sides, and quits. Her boyfriend barely glances up from his phone during her experience. Later in the episode, Chelsea scoops formula from a Similac can.

And even with the baby's father's support, breastfeeding seems to fail. After Lizzie's baby, Summer, is born, she attempts to nurse her, covered in a large blanket. Lizzie cries, "Ouch! She's been doing this for a like an hour." "Breastfeeding?" Skylar says. Lizzie whines, "Yes, I haven't gotten to eat my lunch yet or take a shower." No health professionals are in the room to guide Lizzie. At home, Lizzie speaks in a voice-over, "The first few attempts at feeding her were really painful, but breastfeeding is cheaper than buying baby formula so I'm going to keep trying." We see a brief shot of her nursing and then Lizzie hands the baby to Skylar, who immediately gives the baby back, telling Lizzie that she is still hungry. Reluctantly, Lizzie sits with her infant. And without using a nursing pillow or other support, latches her on. Lizzie loudly exclaims, "Owwww! Oh, girl, that hurts." In the next frame, Lizzie continues to wince in pain. Not surprisingly, Lizzie's next voice-over states, "Breastfeeding Summer at home isn't getting any easier. I think I'm going to switch to formula." At 2 weeks postpartum, partner Skylar confirms the switch, "Are you totally done with breastfeeding?" Lizzie responds, "Yes, I am. I don't think it's supposed to hurt like that."

Breastfeeding is also conveyed as private and potentially embarrassing. When new mom Kailyn has her teenage friends over, she tells them, "I have to breastfeed and you guys can't watch that." Her friend responds, "That's what pillows are for." Kailyn shyly replies, "Well I'm still getting like used to it and (pauses) I'm not producing regular milk yet." She then bottle-feeds her son, Isaac, who is then bottle-fed throughout the remainder of the episode. Following this exchange, we see Kailyn and other people repeatedly feed the baby bottles. Yet, Kailyn makes one reference to milk, when she becomes angry at the baby's father for leaving out a bottle. Other than this argument, breastfeeding is not addressed again, nor is it shown.

Overall, *16 and Pregnant* suggests to its (predominately) teenage viewers that bottle-feeding is the way to feed babies. It is conveyed as more expensive, but seemingly worth it, as breastfeeding is shown to be too difficult to sustain. All of the babies of the first two seasons are bottle-fed at some point, even for the mothers who had intended to breastfeed. This transition is not surprising. Breastfeeding is depicted as a hindrance to teen socialization, with the nursing mothers portrayed as alone in a corner, covered with blankets. With bottle-feeding, babies are passed around to numerous people, without a break in conversation. Formula-feeding is also portrayed as more convenient, as numerous people feed the new babies, including the new fathers, parents, grandparents, and friends, allowing the teen moms to attend school, go to work, and socialize with friends.

Why does this program only support bottle-feeding? True, teenage mothers do, on average, have lower breastfeeding rates. Approximately 67% of mothers under the age of 20 reported ever breastfeeding, compared to 73.6% of those aged 20–29 and over 84% of women older than 30.[21] Exclusive breastfeeding for teenage mothers is much lower than for older women. At 3 months, only 19.3% of mothers under 20 were exclusively breastfeeding, with 36.4% for women in their 20s and 45% of those over 30.[22] The disparity is clear. At the same time, these rates also tell us that most teenage mothers do breastfeed, at least initially, suggesting there is potential for improvement to increase exclusive breastfeeding and overall duration. For *16 and Pregnant*, teen breastfeeding rates indicate that this show dramatically underrepresents breastfeeding. Why do the teen mothers fail? Very little lactation support is shown in the episodes. No International Board Certified Lactation Consultants (IBCLCs) appear, no grandmothers offer support, and the only partner concerned with breastfeeding, Skylar, does not know how to help with baby Summer's painful latch. No one challenges or intervenes to prevent the seemingly inevitable need for early breastfeeding cessation by encouraging the new mothers, correcting improper latching, providing and supporting milk expression, or helping the nursing teens comfortably breastfeed around other people.

We should also consider the format and outlet of this program. Every minute of *16 and Pregnant* is intentionally filmed, edited, and packaged as a product of MTV. It is very possible that more of the teen mothers breastfed, at least part of the time. In fact, in interviews, teen mom Kailyn has spoken about her breastfeeding experiences, even posting to Instagram pictures of her nursing her second child.[23] Corporate sponsorship also likely played a role, as commercial formula brands were clearly shown in two episodes of the series. Regardless of the motives of MTV, the negative messages about breastfeeding, paired with the overwhelming normalization of bottle-feeding are alarming, particularly for this vulnerable audience. And, since this program and its spin-off *Teen Mom* series are part of MTV's "social responsibility" programming, its messages about breastfeeding should be prosocial, supporting a group of mothers who need extra encouragement.

"New Baby" Reality Programs on Other Channels

MTV is not the only channel to offer reality programming about pregnancy and parenting. The cable channels TLC and Discovery Health cater to a far different audience—viewers who are older and established, with primarily planned pregnancies, as the "new baby" reality shows feature older, more-established expectant parents (typically Caucasian, married, and middle-upper class). Given these demographics, their breastfeeding initiation and duration rates should be much higher than the teenage mothers of *16 and Pregnant*.

A case study was conducted on reality programming for two cable channels, exploring what messages are disseminated about infant feeding in this genre. One week of daytime programming was recorded, totaling 27.5 h of programming: 25 episodes of *A Baby Story*, 10 episodes of *Bringing Home Baby*, and 10 episodes of *Deliver Me: Home Edition* (*DMHE*) on TLC and DHC, all of which originally aired between 2003 and 2010. These programs follow real-life families as they experience labor, delivery, and caring for their new baby, including their childrearing decisions. The programs differ in some ways. *A Baby Story* (*ABS*) focuses on one couple in New York or New Jersey as they prepare for birth and experience childbirth. *DMHE*, a spin-off from *Deliver Me*, which follows a group of obstetrician-gynecologists, centers on the relationship between a pregnant woman and her doctor in California. *Bringing Home Baby* (*BHB*) follows the first 36 h after a baby is brought home from the hospital and uses a theme in each episode, conveyed in the episode's titles, such as "Panamanian Celebration" and "Stay at Home Dad." All three programs provide an update of the families within the baby's first year. Combined, these programs tell common stories of women prior to and during delivery, as well as an update a few months after birth. Since this process is documented, these programs often convey messages about breastfeeding initiation and duration—as indicated by the updates.

A textual analysis was performed on the episodes studied. The following questions guided the analysis: Is breastfeeding, bottle-feeding, or formula feeding verbally addressed? During the episode, is the baby breastfed or fed with a bottle? Is commercial formula mentioned or shown? What messages are conveyed about breastfeeding, by the narrator, parents or family of the baby? Is infant feeding addressed in the update for the show? Is the woman still breastfeeding?

Overall, 55 episodes of the three programs were studied. Ten episodes of *ABS* did not address any method of infant feeding. Instead, the update focused on other aspects of childcare, such as bathing or a walk in the stroller. Of the 45 episodes with infant feeding, 17 episodes visually and/or verbally depicted only breastfeeding. Eight episodes include both breastfeeding and an alternative (bottle and/or formula-feeding). Twenty episodes addressed feeding without verbally addressing or visually depicting breastfeeding.

The "Typical" Breastfeeding Experience

Nearly all of the breastfeeding images take place in the birthing center, hospital, or mother's home, conveying that breastfeeding is a private activity. For example, at the 4-month update of the *DMHE* episode "Connie Kawai," Connie sits in a rocking chair breastfeeding her baby in the cradle position on a Boppy pillow. This image is repeated with different women with most of the episodes with breastfeeding depictions. In fact, even in their own homes, most of the breastfeeding women sit alone with a blanket or discreet clothing to mask what they are doing. For example, in the *ABS* episode "Baby Frasca," the 1-month update shows the mother holding her baby at the kitchen table. It is only when she pulls her shirt down afterward that it is clear that she was breastfeeding. Rarely are women shown breastfeeding around guests or even their spouses. Episodes also convey that breastfeeding is limited to early infancy. The updates, which ranged from a few weeks to 10 months, seldom showed breastfeeding. Usually, babies were bottle-fed or feeding was not mentioned. For example, at the 10-month update of the *DMHE* episode "First-Time Mom," the baby drinks a bottle in the playpen as the parents give their interview. No episodes addressed extended or tandem breastfeeding, or the breastfeeding of premature babies, multiples, or adopted children.

Deviating from the Norm

"Abnormal" breastfeeding behavior only appears in episodes in which the show presented the family as different in another way. For example the only woman to breastfeed in public is featured in an episode entitled "Two Moms,"—at her lesbian partner's soccer game. It should be noted here, as labeled in the episode's title, the focus is on the couple's alternative lifestyle. Another episode suggests that a toddler breastfed until shortly before the new baby arrived. "The Family Bed" focuses on the family's alternative choices of co-sleeping, babywearing, and breastfeeding. At one point, the two year-old climbs onto the couch next to her mother and snuggles close. The mother asks: "Are you pretending to breastfeed?" The child mimics latching on, as the mother's voice-over explains, "She still is very into Mommy's milk. She's not breastfeeding anymore, but she would like to be." The child's behavior and the mother's statement implies that the toddler likely breastfed past infancy. As implied by the titles, difference is the theme for these episodes, so all behavior, including breastfeeding, is likely viewed in that frame.

Difficult, but Wonderful

Mothers in the programs describe their experience as transforming from initially difficult to a calm, wonderful activity. In *BHB* "Trainer's Baby," the mother admits, "Breastfeeding was really hard at first, but it's getting a lot easier. And the bonding experience with breastfeeding is just so amazing." Likewise, in "Two Moms," the mother says, "Breastfeeding was my biggest concern. It was harder for us to learn to breastfeed than it was to actually deliver her." The mother breastfeeds as she continues, "We toughed it out and she learned to suck and it's like, it's the best feeling in the world." In the *DMHE* episode, "Rachel McDermott," she reflects, "My all-time favorite bonding experience is actually breastfeeding. I think that it's an automatic time-out during my day." At this point, the camera shows her breastfeeding her daughter as she gently strokes the baby's hair. McDermott continues:

> To just spend time with her and it's something that I can give her. I love the fact that I can just hold her and look at her and she'll stay still. That's been one of the greatest things throughout my time with her so far is being able to have that time everyday to breastfeed her. It's amazing.

While mothers often mentioned the obstacles of early breastfeeding, no specific challenges were discussed. Also, no women address how and why breastfeeding became easier.

Justifications for Quitting: Sponsorship and the Weaning Episodes

The most problematic depictions appear in what could be referred to as "the weaning episodes." While some episodes show mothers or couples using bottles or formula, infant feeding decisions are only addressed if mothers attempt to breastfeed during the episode. In these cases, mothers, their partners, or the program's narrator explained why the woman chose to wean. The use of cleverly placed commercial formula brands may help explain why these women ultimately do not succeed at breastfeeding.

The *BHB* episode "Single Mom" features a 21 year-old woman, Laura, who lives with her single mother. The father is on house arrest and, therefore, has limited visits. Soon after they arrive home, Laura bottle-feeds the baby. Grandma tells the camera, "Laura's milk is coming down, but it's very painful for her to breastfeed." Laura adds, "Feels like she has teeth and she's like biting me, you know." Moments later, Grandma is outside her room and admits, "I want to get in there and show her how, but I can't. She has to learn that for herself the same way I learned it for myself so now we're doing the bottle and we're trying to give her breasts a break." Later, Laura explains, "I was breastfeeding her more in the hospital at first, you know. She was trying to latch on pretty good, but man, she hurt me." The camera shows a close up of the baby drinking a Similac pre-filled formula bottle. Laura continues, "They're feeling really sore, I mean. That's why I have her on the bottle right now." Another close up of the Similac bottle is shown. That evening, Laura takes a shower to ease her engorged breasts and decides to give up breastfeeding, saying, "It's too much for me." Then Laura feeds the baby out of a pre-filled Similac formula bottle.

Likewise, in "Stay at Home Dad," the narrator explains, "Since Ariana's breast milk hasn't come in yet, she gets some formula to give to Baby Aidan, whose weight is still a concern." The mother, Ariana, gives the baby premixed Similac. Later in the episode, the parents set up a breast pump and close the door. Afterward, the father, Eli, tells the camera that she failed to express milk so the baby will have to drink formula. Ariana does not attempt to breastfeed him. In the update teaser, the narrator asks, "Will Aidan switch to breastmilk now that he's had nothing but formula since birth?" accompanied by a close up of Aidan getting a bottle. Not surprisingly, the answer is no. At the 8-week update, Ariana justifies why she switched to formula, "I tried to breastfeed him and he wouldn't latch on. He took a bottle like that was what he was meant to do," as she bottle-feeds the baby.

In two episodes of *BHB*, doctors recommend parents supplement with formula to help with a baby's jaundice. In "Headstrong Parents," the father mixes bottles as the narrator explains, "Because of the jaundice situation, the couple is feeding the baby a combination of breast milk and formula." In the interview, the mother admits, "It's disappointing to have him supplemented with formula because I wanted to do exclusively breastmilk because it's best for him for the first couple of months, but now, because the formula is so easy for him, it seems that's all he really wants. So, he's still latching on to the breast, but it's almost like he's using it as a pacifier to put himself to sleep. He really just wants the formula. But, he'll work through that. He'll be fine." In the 10-week update, the father feeds the baby a bottle. Breastfeeding is not mentioned. Similarly, in "Amber's Miracle," over the phone, a doctor advises giving the baby formula for 24 h. Despite the support of a lactation consultant, the 10-week update shows the baby drinking formula.

The clear product placement in these episodes indicate that the "feeding decision" storylines were likely devices to focus on the Similac bottles, especially because some of the products are also advertised during commercial breaks. The purpose of American television is to sell products. And, because of increasingly fragmented audiences and technology allowing people to skip commercials, this form of marketing is rapidly growing. "The baby block" is not unique in its product placement. *Survivor*, *American Idol*, *The Apprentice*, and other reality programs have included blatant product placement.[24] *Bringing Home Baby* does not hide its product placement—links on the show's webpage lead to an online marketplace in which viewers can learn more about the products.

That said, why promote formula, especially for real women who are struggling to breastfeed? A more breastfeeding-friendly approach would be to advertise Medela or other breastfeeding products. At the very least, formula product placement should be limited to women who have no intention of breastfeeding, not the vulnerable ones who are wavering in their decisions. For example, in the case of single-mom Laura, she tells the camera that breast pain is hindering her breastfeeding experience and so she bottle-feeds, using Similac. Why not offer her other free child-care products, like Pampers, which is marketed in other episodes and/or structure the episode around getting her help? The juxtaposition of the storyline with product placement of commercial formula in these programs sends three clear messages to women: 1. Breastfeeding is too difficult for most women/look how much easier formula is. 2. Doctors often recommend supplementing/here's the brand they recommend. 3. Formula must be fine for babies because these real women are giving it to their children on supposedly baby-friendly networks (certainly, these channels would never advertise anything unhealthy for children, right?).

Applying the "Social-Ecological Model" to Reality TV

The "social-ecological model," identified by the Centers for Disease Control & Prevention (CDC) and WHO,[25] can illuminate the potential impact of media messages about breastfeeding, such as those in the "baby block." At the *individual level*, women who lack information about breastfeeding from other resources may learn about infant feeding from these programs. First, one might gather that only a certain type of child should be breastfed, one who is a singleton, full-term, and has a biological relationship to the mother and only in early infancy. This false information obviously ignores the numerous health benefits for multiples, premature babies, adopted infants, and older children. Second, one might gather that breastfeeding should be done in private, therefore, by choosing to breastfeed, a woman binds herself to the home—not a practical (nor enjoyable) choice for most women. These programs miss an opportunity to promote nursing in public, a far easier and more convenient choice than hauling around bottles and powered formula.

Next, viewers might believe women have a universal breastfeeding experience—a static picture of a lonely woman with her Boppy-boosted baby, cradled at the breast. Breastfeeding experiences vary by woman and child and change as the baby ages, birth scars heal, and breasts deflate. And, not all women prefer the cradle position, require a Boppy (support pillow), or shroud the infant's head in a flamboyant tent. On television, babies breastfeed calmly without reaching up to insert tiny fingers in Mommy's nose or unlatching to smile, coo, or pass gas. We do not see a 6-month old chomp down on the nipple as she experiments with her new teeth or a thrashing older baby trying to crawl away as his mother puts him to the breast. Because these experiences are not familiar to most women, mothers may be surprised when their babies do not behave like the ones on television and may be inclined to wean, believing that their babies are ready.

These programs provide very little information about breast feeding. Several women mention generic benefits of breastfeeding, although no episodes state specific benefits. Even with narrators and featured experts on these programs, little practical advice is given about breastfeeding. Only two episodes address the process of breastfeeding. A mother in one episode discusses eating additional calories and a doula explains how colostrom changes into mature milk. While many mothers mention the difficulty of early breastfeeding, no specific obstacles, like thrush or mastitis, are addressed. From these programs, viewers would learn little about how to breastfeed and solutions for common obstacles. Even when women voice specific questions, no answers are provided. For example, in the episode "Circle of Life" of *BHB*, the mother wonders, "I just still am a little confused about how long to nurse him for. Like, he'd stay on for the whole day if I just sat here." Despite the numerous specialists and experts that appear in other episodes to resolve more mundane issues, such as childproofing a house (before the baby is born?), experts are rarely consulted for breastfeeding questions.

More information is provided for justifications to wean. In the teen reality shows, mothers supplement so soon after initiating breastfeeding that we really do not see a weaning process. According to the "baby block," women should wean, or at least supplement, while waiting for their mature milk to come in, if they are engorged or experience sore nipples. Despite the appearance of lactation consultants, no episodes addressed pro-breastfeeding solutions to these obstacles, such as dried breastmilk for sore nipples, hand expressing to relieve pressure, and increased breastfeeding to bring in mature milk. With this advice, nearly all women would believe that they needed to supplement, which of course, has been proven detrimental to long-term breastfeeding.[26] Babies were also given formula for jaundice, despite research indicating that supplementing is unnecessary.[27] In one of the episodes, the mother confers with a lactation consultant about maintaining supply while supplementing. Yet, like the doctor, she does not instruct the mother to breastfeed. Redesigned as a pro-social tool, these programs could acknowledge the challenges faced by nearly all women and then teach new mothers how to overcome common issues. These programs could also instruct women to seek breastfeeding help from other mothers, breastfeeding-friendly doctors or lactation consultants.

At the interpersonal level, these programs convey that breastfeeding can hinder bonding between the non-breastfeeding partner and baby. In "Two Moms," a primary concern is that the non-breastfeeding lesbian partner will not be able to share in the experience of caring for the newborn. Before the baby is born, the mother, Cathy, explains how her partner will be able to help by changing diapers or bringing the baby over to breastfeed. And yet, during the baby's first night home, the partner argues, "With Cathy breastfeeding, it's hard. I can't relieve her if the baby is hungry." When Cathy refuses to give the baby formula, the partner storms away and does not help for the remainder of the night. With other couples, the tension appears to be resolved by letting the partner or spouse bottle-feed the baby. A more breastfeeding-friendly approach would be to include images of partners supporting the breastfeeding women, by performing other infant care tasks, such as bathing, changing diapers, or rocking the baby.

While most episodes depict the mother breastfeeding alone in a dark room, not all women share this experience. In "A Doula's Help," the mother calmly breastfeeds as she chats with family members about her new baby. More representations like this one could help debunk myths that breastfeeding causes the new mother to feel alone and isolated from others. And as one episode suggested, breastfeeding can strengthen relationships. For example, the "Circle of Life" episode shows a woman and her sister breastfeeding their babies next to each other. They mention how their other sister is also breastfeeding. Depictions of strong relationships with breastfeeding women could help skeptical family and friends understand the importance of support for the breastfeeding mother.

These messages suggest that bottle-feeding is more common, formula is a suitable alternative, and breastfeeding should be done privately. At the organizational, community, and public policy levels, the dominant messages in these texts imply breastfeeding is an individual issue and therefore, no structural changes are needed. If more women addressed personal obstacles, these shows could acknowledge that many women face similar obstacles, some of which are created by social norms and policies that hinder breastfeeding.

If more obstacles were voiced, it may be more likely that Feminist organizations would place more attention on breastfeeding as a women's rights issue. The "baby block" limits breastfeeding to the home, suggesting that women must choose between venturing in public and breastfeeding their babies—attitudes that lead to public humiliation of women who dare to feed their babies in public. Women who are unsuccessful with breastfeeding are shown calling their doctors when trouble arises, conveying that women should not rely on other women, but should depend on health care providers to advise them on breastfeeding issues. Similar to the medicalization of childbirth, this reliance on "experts" shifts agency away from women and women's networks to physicians, who are typically male and ill-informed about breastfeeding.[28]

The recognition of breastfeeding as a Feminist issue could lead to further support for breastfeeding and structural changes. Communities could add inexpensive or free breastfeeding classes or support groups. Episodes that covered the challenges of breastfeeding and working could help prompt employers to adopt more breastfeeding friendly policies (i.e., pumping breaks, places to pump, and refrigeration for expressed milk). And, ultimately, if pro-breastfeeding messages could help policy makers understand that this is a public health issue, more laws could be passed, protecting mothers from advertising and free samples that hinder breastfeeding success and enforce existing legislation protecting mothers nursing in public. Similar legislation to that in the United Kingdom could remove the product integration of formula in television, akin to the tobacco bans of the 1970s. As argued by Charlotte Faircloth in a report for UNICEF UK, the National Childbirth Trust, and Save the Children UK, this marketing undermines breastfeeding and leads consumers to believe formula is as safe as breastfeeding.[29] If the low breastfeeding duration rates were truly recognized as a public health issue, such legislation is necessary, as evidenced by the abundance of product placement in the reality programs.

Conclusion: Manipulating Reality

Overall, while it is positive that some women breastfeed on reality television, the messages about breastfeeding are limited, vague, and, in some cases, blatantly erroneous. The premise of these programs make them ideal for promoting breastfeeding, yet they are currently falling short of their potential. Reality programs are constructions of reality, shaped by a production process designed to create profits for the networks. Furthermore, Katherine Sender argued that the audience readily buys into this false reality, displacing enough disbelief to enjoyably consume the programs.[30] Even with some awareness of the production of reality TV, viewers are still impacted by its messages, relating emotionally to participants and to the "unscripted" storyline.[31] With these "new mom" shows, we know that parts of their lives are not shown, yet assume that the important moments are edited into create the constructed narrative.

Obviously, these programs depict real women. When casting agents choose a pregnant woman to film, they cannot predict whether or not she will successfully breastfeed. And yet, because a reality program is a contrived media product, packaged for television, the producers, editors, writers, and other people involved can shape the messages about breastfeeding. As suggested by Brown and Peuchaud, media producers have the potential to positively impact breastfeeding perceptions and rates.[32] At each step of production, changes could be made to promote breastfeeding. In the screening process, casting agents can ask about infant feeding choices and select women who intend to breastfeed. During filming, the interviewers can ask mothers about breastfeeding. If they express concerns, lactation consultants can be provided (the visit could then be part of the show—which is not uncommon).

The editing of the programs also could have featured more breastfeeding. In *16 and Pregnant*, several of the teen moms were shown breastfeeding at home, without footage of them initiating at the hospital. Rather than editing out their first time latching, including these breastfeeding experiences would convey to viewers that teenagers can and do breastfeed. Furthermore, at least one teen mom later spoke about her commitment to breastfeeding, yet her episode did not include video of her nursing. These reality programs are highly influential in their modeling of pregnancy and early motherhood. Showcasing successful breastfeeding would help normalize it for teen mothers and establish breastfeeding as the default means of infant feeding for viewers overall.

The reality programs also missed opportunities to include breastfeeding in other ways. Many episodes across the programs feature special events or outings, such as painting pottery or taking a birthing class. And, instead of providing commercial formula as part of product integration, producers can seek out breastfeeding-friendly products, such as Medela breast pumps or the My Brest Friend pillow. For the final package, footage could be edited to highlight successful breastfeeding and include more women talking about their experiences. Finally, the voice-over could support breastfeeding. In the episodes studied, narration only addressed breastfeeding if it was unsuccessful. Positive voice-overs could inform viewers about solutions to obstacles and reinforce success, stating something like, "Wanda treated her Thrush with Oregano Oil. Now, their breastfeeding relationship is back on track."

Such actions would not take away from the programs, nor dampen the "reality" of the final products. It would not be difficult to alter the casting or editing of these shows to encourage all women, regardless of age, paired with supportive partners. Even small changes in the framing of breastfeeding in media could lead to significant progress toward creating a breastfeeding-friendly society, in which most babies drink straight from the tap—without the help of Similac.

Notes

1. Cancel Bear, "MTV's Season Finale of '16 & Pregnant' Hits Series High 2.1 Million Total Viewers Thursday - Ratings."
2. Ibid.
3. Mittell, *Television and American Culture.*
4. McCarthy, "Ads Pepper Reality Shows with Product Placements."
5. Williams et al., "Product Placement Effectiveness: Revisited and Renewed."
6. Ibid.
7. "Appendix 5: Guidelines for BBC Commercial Services on Editorial Integrity and Independence from External Interests"; Morris, "How European Media Companies Are Dealing with Product Placement."

8. Mazzeo et al., "Effects of a Reality TV Cosmetic Surgery Makeover Program on Eating Disordered Attitudes and Behaviors"; Sears and Godderis, "Roar Like a Tiger on TV?"; Shufeldt and Gale, "Under the (Glue) Gun."
9. Fogel and Krausz, "Watching Reality Television Beauty Shows Is Associated with Tanning Lamp Use and Outdoor Tanning among College Students."
10. Crockett, Pruzinsky, and Persing, "He Influence of Plastic Surgery 'reality TV' on Cosmetic Surgery Patient Expectations and Decision Making."
11. Domoff et al., "The Effects of Reality Television on Weight Bias."
12. Cooke-Jackson and Hansen, "Appalachian Culture and Reality TV"; Squires, "Race and Reality TV"; Wang, "A Shot at Half-Exposure."
13. Kearney and Levine, "Media Influences on Social Outcomes."
14. Ibid.
15. McKinney, "A Lifestyle Perspective on Infertility and Pregnancy Outcome."
16. Kearney and Levine, "Media Influences on Social Outcomes."
17. Martins and Jensen, "The Relationship Between 'Teen Mom' Reality Programming and Teenagers' Beliefs About Teen Parenthood."
18. Ibid.
19. Dolgen, "Why I Created MTV's '16 and Pregnant.'"
20. The second season of *16 and Pregnant* was 19 episodes long, divided into two subsections. Only the first subsection was studied due to its availability and packaging on Amazon.com.
21. "Rates of Any and Exclusive Breastfeeding by Socio-Demographics Among Children Born in 2011 (Percentage ± Half 95% Confidence Interval)."
22. Ibid.
23. Kowalski, "Kailyn Lowry Breastfeeding: 'Teen Mom 2' Star Nurses Baby Lincoln, Mocks Gisele - Hollywood Life."
24. Mittell, *Television and American Culture.*
25. "The Social-Ecological Model: A Framework for Prevention."
26. Taveras et al., "Opinions and Practices of Clinicians Associated With Continuation of Exclusive Breastfeeding."
27. Schanler, O'Connor, and Lawrence, "Pediatricians' Practices and Attitudes Regarding Breastfeeding Promotion."
28. Wolf, "What Feminists Can Do for Breastfeeding and What Breastfeeding Can Do for Feminists."
29. Faircloth, "A Weak Formula for Legislation: How Loopholes in the Law Are Putting Babies at Risk."
30. Sender, *The Makeover: Reality Television and Reflexive Audiences.*
31. Ibid.
32. Brown and Peuchaud, "Media and Breastfeeding: Friend or Foe?"

CHAPTER 8

"The New Boob Tube?": Education, Entertainment, and Viewers' Perceptions of Breastfeeding on Social Media

In May 2014, Karlesha Thurman posted a picture of herself breastfeeding at graduation to the *Facebook* group "Black Women Do Breastfeed." Within hours, the photo went viral, as thousands of people commented on the image. While the *Facebook* group applauded her success and breastfeeding, feedback on *Twitter* was painfully negative—enough that Thurman deleted the photo, tweeting, "I can't take anymore tonight, thanks to all who have had nothing but positive things to say about my photo breastfeeding at graduation."[1] Only a few months later, another graduating senior, Jacci Sharkey, posted a similar photo of herself breastfeeding in her commencement gown. Over 200,000 people "liked" it on *Facebook*, with 6000 "shares."[2] News stories praised Sharkey for her accomplishments and commitment to both motherhood and education.[3] Again, note that comments are quoted as they were originally written and posted, including spelling, capitalization, and grammatical errors.

While both women deserved to be praised for their academic and motherhood achievements, this was clearly not what happened, even though few differences existed between them. Both were young mothers wearing commencement gowns as they breastfed their babies. However, Thurman is African American and nursed her baby at the graduation ceremony. Sharkey is Caucasian and breastfed in her posed graduation photo. These two cases, in which Thurman was publicly ridiculed and Sharkey praised for feeding their babies illustrated how public response and media's treatment of race can deeply impact messages about breastfeeding. Furthermore, the public response to both women also reinforced racial

K.A. Foss, *Breastfeeding and Media*,
DOI 10.1007/978-3-319-56442-5_8

disparities in breastfeeding rates, contradicting the title of the *Facebook* group to which Thurman celebrated her accomplishments ("Black Women Do Breastfeed"). Such negativity was disheartening, not just to Thurman, but also for nursing mothers and for breastfeeding in general.

The public responses to these *Facebook* images also demonstrated the prominent role of social media in shaping and informing perceptions about breastfeeding. Indeed, social media has become influential in everyday life. A Pew Research report noted that 71% of adult Internet users visit social media sites, with *Facebook* as the most popular.[4] Ninety percent of Internet users age 18–29 participate in social media.[5] Moreover, young adults are more likely to receive their news from Internet sources over television or print.[6] Young adults are far more likely to receive messages online than to read books, watch television, or go to the movies.

The Internet is increasingly becoming a source of advice and support. A Pew Research Center study on parents' use of social media reported that 59% had discovered information related to parenting on social media.[7] Mothers were more likely than fathers to use social media for parenting-related support and to ask parenting questions.[8] In an ethnographic study of African American mothers, Asiodu and colleagues found that participants routinely used popular social media websites and applications for pregnancy and parenting information, yet could not identify breastfeeding information from the parenting sites.[9] The researchers conclude that this gap demonstrates the need for more breastfeeding presence in social media, particularly on sites targeting African American mothers.[10] Online information can help mothers succeed at breastfeeding. Zhang, Carlton, and Fein determined a positive correlation between mothers who gleaned breastfeeding information from websites and their rates of initiation and duration.[11] Unfortunately, formula corporations regularly advertise on popular social media and other sites, undermining these messages. Abrahams identified formula marketing across *Facebook*, *Youtube*, *Twitter*, and other sites, along with hidden formula sponsorship of reviews on parenting blogs and other financial partnerships that could be perceived as violations of the International Code of Marketing of Breastmilk Substitutes.[12] Women with higher exposure to formula advertising in print and online were less likely to initiate breastfeeding and weaned sooner than those with lower rates of exposure.[13] Similarly, Huang and colleagues' analysis of the Infant Feeding Practices Study II found that over half of formula-feeding mothers had gotten their information about formula from prenatal Internet sources.[14]

For breastfeeding information, mainstream parenting websites, like *BabyCenter.com* and *The Bump*, offer some advice and support. However, these sites are sponsored so breastfeeding messages may appear next to formula advertising sidebars. That said, communities on these sites can offer camaraderie, encouragement, and immediate responses to breastfeeding concerns and questions. Gray studied discussion boards on breastfeeding, finding that posts were typically seeking information about an array of related topics.[15] These sites were also useful for providing social and emotional support in what she called "a natural setting."[16] The drawback, of course, is that anyone can respond, meaning the advice may be unhelpful or inaccurate. Breastfeeding-focused sites, notably the website of LLL, *Kellymom.com* and *Breastfeeding Inc.* (Dr. Jack Newman's site) provide more accurate information, resources, and videos to answer questions and help women overcome obstacles, like latching issues, remedies for mastitis or thrush, safe medication while nursing, and other issues. Support groups and blogs also exist for formula-feeding mothers.

Breastfeeding blogs and social media sites that celebrate breastfeeding also draw many viewers. In the virtual space of *Facebook*, *Twitter*, and others, people post, share, and discuss articles on breastfeeding benefits, stories of shamed public breastfeeding, and other relevant topics. For example, a man used *Facebook* to publicly criticize a mother breastfeeding her son in a restaurant, including a photo he took of her without her consent.[17] She responded online, questioning his behavior and defending her legal right to feed her child. The breastfeeding mother's *Facebook* reply went viral—receiving over a million "likes" in support of her response.[18] This post and its response demonstrate how social media can be used to draw attention to breastfeeding injustice and to empower women who have had negative experiences of nursing in public. These sites and groups are also used to initiate local activism, spreading news of latch-ons, in which nursing mothers breastfeed at a specific time and place to promote breastfeeding, as well as planning nurse-ins at local retailers that criticized breastfeeding mothers.

Social media sites are also used for informal milk sharing. For example, on one local private *Facebook* group, members frequently offer or request breastmilk. A member might say, "I have 10 extra bags of milk. Who can use it?" Posters then respond and set up the exchange. Similarly, members ask for breastmilk, sometimes on behalf of friends or family, with "My friend has a low supply and is having difficulty keeping up with her preemie. Does anyone have extra milk?" People then meet up to casually exchange the bags of breastmilk. As will be discussed in the next chapter, this informal swap bypasses formal milk donation banks and regulation on human milk sharing. As Geraghty, Heier, and Rasmussen outlined, outside of social media, other blogs and online outlets also serve to match donors with milk recipients.[19] These exchanges are not without risks, though, as donors are not screened and the milk is unpasteurized.[20] Still, informal milk sharing exemplifies the unique opportunities with social media to link those passionate about breastfeeding to each other.

Searching for "Breastfeeding" on *Youtube*

Building on existing research, the following section looks at the most popular breastfeeding videos on *Youtube*, along with viewers' comments. What may be surprising is the abundance of breastfeeding media content online that is not intended for breastfeeding mothers and their partners, but the general public. Breastfeeding regularly appears in news stories on mainstream sites, with extensive reader feedback. For example, Len-Rios, Bhandari, and Medvedeva examined reader comments for two online newspapers' stories questioning the evidence behind the federal government's breastfeeding recommendations.[21] They found that most comments focused more on personal experience than scientific evidence as support for their position on the issue.[22] The number and type of comments for this study illustrates the public's interest in breastfeeding controversies, even among people without children, as well as the uncensored nature of such feedback.

The video-sharing site *Youtube* brings together many of these different perspectives in its videos and viewer responses. *Youtube* videos are usually short, making them easy to watch more than once or to share on social media sites. Anyone can post videos, provided they follow the *Youtube*'s guidelines forbidding videos that violate copyright and/or are sexually explicit, violent, hateful, threatening, or harmful.[23] Users can "flag" videos that they believe violate these policies, which may be then pulled by *Youtube* employees.[24] Within these guidelines, regular people can post almost anything and quickly, without the delays of corporate gatekeepers. Anyone can post, therefore the material ranges from amateur home movies, news clips, fictional pieces, to promos from organizations. There is also financial incentive to creating popular clips. Those with heavily watched videos may receive requests from advertisers to place commercials before their videos and profit from them. And with the "views" identified and opportunity for participant responses, this site openly shows how many people are watching the videos and provide an idea of reactions to the videos—at least for the most vocal viewers.

Public health advocates have recognized the value of *Youtube* in reaching and persuading audiences. The site has been used to teach health information to college students and has been perceived as a useful tool for health educators.[25] Breastfeeding advocates have also begun to use this site to educate and persuade. The "DYI Breastfeeding" channel on *Youtube* offers short videos on a range of topics, including latching and positions, Supplemental Nursing Systems, overactive let-downs, breastfeeding multiples, and pumping advice. A more entertainment-focused (but also informative) approach is with the music video "Teach Me How to Breastfeed," posted in 2013 by "UrbanMatriarch."[26] This music video features advice in the lyrics, like the healthy color of breastfed babies' output, while incorporating positive images of women of multiple ethnicities breastfeeding their babies. WIC and other organizations also use *Youtube* to disseminate their breastfeeding promotion videos.

Most videos addressing breastfeeding on *Youtube* are not part of formal campaigns or advertising.[27] Rather, uploaded videos tend to be stories about breastfeeding. Furthermore, even those that convey health messages do not typically address latching. In an analysis of 175 *Youtube* videos on the health statements in breastfeeding videos from 2011, De Carvalho and colleagues noted that only 18% addressed proper latching.[28] While this content analysis provides a solid overview of the type of health messages, it was outside the scope of the study to explore how *Youtube* viewers interpreted and responded to these videos. Such an approach can help explain public reactions to breastfeeding videos and provide an indication as to (at least the most outspoken) responses to different types of breastfeeding videos.

"Breastfeeding" was entered in the *Youtube* keyword search—mimicking the path that people seeking breastfeeding videos might take. The top 10 videos by relevance and the top 10 videos by popularity were analyzed with the assumption that the videos appearing on the first page of search results would be most likely to be watched by people doing similar searches. Videos were analyzed for their content, noting the overall messages, tone, visuals of breastfeeding (covered or uncovered), title, and description. It was noted whether or not the videos were home movies or part of a breastfeeding campaign and if the videos were intended to be instructional or persuasive. For videos with 50 comments or less, all comments were analyzed. With those over 50, the first page of viewer comments were examined to gauge reaction to the videos. All viewer comments have been preserved in their original form, including spelling and grammatical errors.

The 10 Ten Videos by Relevance and View Count

Searching "breastfeeding" in *Youtube* prompts results by relevance. All of the top 10 "Breastfeeding" videos are home movies, and range in length from under 2 min to over 12 min. They range in length from less than 2 min to over 12 min. At the time of this analysis, the number of views ranges from 12,315 to nearly four million. Three of the top 10 videos are of the same woman from her Vlog "Mama Cabbage." Breastfeeding is clearly shown, with no cover, in all of the videos.

Most of the videos are not intended to be instructional. Rather, they feature regular women breastfeeding in their everyday lives. In the "Mama Cabbage" videos, the mother nurses her son (5 months old to around 18 months old across the three videos), as her older children run around, play music, and watch television. The "Mama Cabbage" video "Breastfeeding Entertainment" shows a mom sitting on the couch when her toddler cries. She casually pulls her breast out of her tank top and he nurses standing up. Meanwhile, she talks to the camera about how to make spaghetti noodles out of zucchini—a video that has received more than a million views. In "Breastfeeding a Toddler," a mom lies on the bed as she nurses her child. He unlatches and they sing a song, then breastfeeds some more. Likewise, "This kid is ADDICTED to breastfeeding" shows a mother nursing her 1 year-old on a couch.

Two of the videos are clearly meant to be educational. In "Breastfeeding and Breast Hygiene," a Caucasian woman sits down outside and begins nursing her baby boy (8–10 months old) and says, "Hello. Today's topic is breastfeeding and breast hygiene."She addresses myths about breastfeeding and then states, "It is your responsibility to take care of your girls while you're breastfeeding." The mother advises breastfeeding women to care for their breasts by wearing a sleeping bra, applying aloe and vitamin E, and exercising regularly, along with other tips. She concludes her video with "I hope you learned a little something," cautioning nursing mothers to be vigilant" and "act like a wet nurse" to protect their milk supplies. Throughout the video, she breastfeeds her baby. The other instructional video is "Breastfeeding Hand Expression," as a woman demonstrates how to manually express milk, using hand massage to stimulate the flow. This video does not include a baby. It should be noted that both "educational" videos are home movies of regular women providing advice. They are not affiliated with a breastfeeding organization, nor do they appear to have professional lactation training or certification.

Despite the title, "Breastfeeding Tutorial: How to Tandem Breastfeed" provides little advice about how to tandem breastfeed (nursing more than one child). While the mother demonstrates with her two children, her dialogue is more focused on how difficult it is to nurse both children at the same time. This is the only video to address tandem nursing. Even for this mother, she states, "They don't get to do it very often," suggesting that they are typically nursed individually. Overall, the tone is positive, with the children smiling and nursing and talking to their mother. At one point, she asks her daughter why she likes to nurse. Her daughter replies enthusiastically, "Because it makes me happy!" In addition to this video, three others feature the extended nursing of toddlers and older children. The scenes are peaceful and playful as the mothers chat with their nurslings and sing songs. In "Breastfeeding a Toddler," the mother playfully asks, "What are boobies for?" Her son cheerfully announces, "For milk and for drinking!" Then they cuddle and nurse. All of these videos of nursing older children are positive, calming, and sweet, with content mothers and children.

Only one video discusses weaning. In "Pregnant and Breastfeeding a 4 year old! How to wean your toddler," the same mother from the tandem nursing video addresses breastfeeding her 4-year, arguing that, against some people's beliefs that her children are too attached, her daughter is very independent and has begun to self-wean. The mother explains that her daughter's "body is automatically, naturally" having her wean. She adds, "This is exactly how I wanted it to be. I wanted it to be nature's way that she would completely self-wean." Her daughter briefly nurses during the video, as the mother reassures other extended breastfeeders, "You don't need to worry… your child will self-wean." This video is more defensive than the others and features the 4 year-old nursing.

A mother expressed ambivalence about breastfeeding in only one of the top videos. The title and caption established the mother's angst regarding her daughter's breastfeeding: "This kid is ADDICTED to

Breastfeeding," with text underneath the video stating, "1 yr old Zoe cant give up boob milk! weaning this toddler wont be easy!! SEXUAL PERVERTED OR RUDE COMMENTS WILL BE DELETED AND USER BLOCKED." In this short video, the mom says to her daughter, "So, can you explain to us your obsession?" as the tot climbs on her mother's lap and nurses. The video jumps to the next shot, in which the mother's breast is covered and the child is crying, then giggles, uncovers the breast and latches on. Her mom asks, "So when are you going to give up the boobie?" then talks in a baby voice (replying for her daughter), "I don't know. Never." She continues this "dialogue" as her daughter breastfeeds, cautioning, "You know you can't be on the boob and going to college." Then they both laugh and the mom mentions her daughter needing "rehab." While this video is playful and includes a happy, nursing child, the title, caption, and dialogue counter this image, suggesting a more negative undertone, especially given the girl's age (1 year-old).

The top 10 videos by "view count" were also analyzed. Six of the top 10 are home movies, featuring regular women breastfeeding and/or talking about breastfeeding. One video is professionally done: an instructional movie on latching produced by *Fit Pregnancy* magazine. The other two videos that are commercially-made are clearly intended for a general audience.

Only three of the top videos are educational. The top-rated video "Breastfeeding Video—Breastfeeding Tips on Scheduling" from 2009 is a 2-min piece in which a woman advises women to feed on demand, not schedule feedings, and explains how milk provides more than nutrition. She holds her baby during the video, but does not breastfeed. This video has received more than 66 million views. The *Fit Pregnancy* video, "How to Breastfeed" begins with the introduction of a board-certified lactation consultant. She talks about good breastfeeding positions and latching as the camera shows women breastfeeding properly. The final educational video is "Breast-feeding Cradle Hold," which, according to the caption, is an excerpt from a 1980s breastfeeding video. This clip features an African American mother in a hospital bed learning how to breastfeed from another woman (whose role is not defined), who goes over positioning and how to latch. As the baby starts to nurse, the camera shows the new father smiling. This inclusion of the father is unique and an important addition since other videos do not show fathers, despite their critical role in breastfeeding success.

As with the videos filtered by "relevance," home movies with no intended educational message are also extremely popular. Five videos—all with more than 10 million views—are home movies that show regular women breastfeeding. "Breastfeeding Method—The beauty of life" shows a montage of breastfeeding women and then one mother (presumably the creator of the video) talking about breastfeeding. It ends with a title slide that reads, "As I have said before I mean no harm by this video. I am a new mother and I am excited about this new skill that I am learning." Three of the videos feature toddlers, not babies nursing. "Mama Cabbage" has one of the most highly-viewed videos, entitled, "Breastfeeding a Toddler in the Nature." She nurses her toddler as she playfully asks, "Are you my little goat?" The camera focuses on the nursing toddler, not the mother. In "Breastfeeding Toddlers," a 26-s video, a woman's voice asks, "Are you going to nurse now?" A toddler answers, "Yeah!" and then latches on. This video has been watched more than 13 million times. The video "Breastfeeding Ari (3.5 years old) in the park," shows a mother nursing her toddler. They chat in a different language as the child breastfeeds. As with the "relevant" videos, these breastfeeding videos of older children are positive, relaxed, and happy overall.

A search for popular breastfeeding videos also results in videos that are clearly not targeting expectant and new parents. A clip from the television show *Family Guy*, labeled "Family Guy—Breastfeeding," is the fourth highest viewed video on breastfeeding, with over 20 million hits. In this cartoon, the father, Peter, holds his baby, Stewie. Peter lifts up his shirt and latches Stewie on his nipple. Stewie suckles for a moment. Then he unlatches, looking puzzled, and pulls a hair out of his mouth. Stewie opens his eyes and discovers that it is his dad, not his mother. He begins to gag and shiver from disgust and the clip ends. As discussed in Chap. 6, this is not the only episode of *Family Guy* that depicts breastfeeding. Yet, it is the clip of a breastfeeding Peter, not Lois (the baby's mother), that received millions of views.

Finally, an online news commentary show, *FTD Epic News Commentary*, also ranked in the top 10 with the title, "Woman Breastfeeds TV Host Live on Air." Throughout this commentary, the video from the breastfeeding scene is muted, as the *FTD* host describes the situation. He begins the story with "If human breast milk was sold in the stores, would you buy it, yes or no? . . The first story we're talking about today deals with some naked-type news." An image of a woman breastfeeding a calf appears on the screen as the host says, "Ladies, breastfeeding cows are a thing of the past because a Dutch TV host, Paul D. Liu just breastfed live on his own show." We see a clip of a man leaning over an audience member and latching on to her breast. The *FTD* host reacts to the video, declaring, "Man, TV just really sucks these days. Aha, the pun!" He then explains that the guests on the show had been discussing milk donation when "One of the ladies offered Paul a drink of her breastmilk that she pumped into a bottle. He's like 'No, no, no. I want to drink it from the source.'" The clip of the nursing TV man is replayed. The *FTD* host states, "Now people in the Netherlands got so pissed… But what I want to know is whether or not people are calling it so disgusting for this big ole' man just randomly sucking (cue video again) on this lady's breast for the milk to come out on national television or for the fact that he drank human milk." He then concludes with "I'm sure Paul will be milking the publicity for as long as he can." Following this story, the *FTD* host gives a review of a new videogame system and then discusses a story about a beautiful woman who is unemployed due to her looks. These additional topics are telling of the target audience of the breastfeeding story and explain how and why the story was framed.

Overall, these search results are surprising. The *DIY Breastfeeding Channel* appears at the top of the relevant search results. However, most of the remaining videos are amateur home movies, including the ones that aim to be educational. This absence suggests that breastfeeding advocates and organizations need to create appealing videos that people want to watch and share with their social networks, like the "Teach Me How to Breastfeed." More professionally done videos would increase the legitimate resources for breastfeeding information and create more of an online presence for breastfeeding promotion. Nearly all of the videos convey positive messages about breastfeeding, with pleasant images of numerous mothers nursing their babies without a cover and at various ages. The videos appear to be somewhat racially diverse, with different women nursing. Most of the home movies appear to be filmed by the mothers themselves. The view count of these home movies is remarkable. Why do millions of people care to watch unfamiliar women breastfeeding, particularly the short clips with no information?

Another pattern of the top videos is the absence of fathers. True, some of them may have been filming the videos, but we seldom hear their voices. In fact, fathers only appear in two videos: the smiling dad in the 1980s "Cradle Hold" video and the animated Peter Griffin, in *Family Guy*—hardly a positive role model for supportive fathers. Even though the top videos are largely home movies that are unscripted and generally unplanned, overall, they reflect a bigger problem—fathers tend to be left out of breastfeeding media, despite their significant roles in breastfeeding success.

The "entertainment" videos of *Family Guy* and the *FTD* news commentary could be potentially both an advantage and a drawback for breastfeeding promotion. To create a breastfeeding-friendly environment, we need media for the general public that addresses and shows breastfeeding. At the same time, these specific videos were humorous and critical in tone, with Stewie gagging at his father and the TV host ridiculing the breastfeeding man. Media messages that can attract and straddle audiences without demeaning breastfeeding itself would be a more progressive step.

Finally, it should be noted that nine of the 20 videos were preceded by commercials advertising home and personal hygiene products, food, and upcoming motion pictures. Such marketing is usually added after a video becomes popular, demonstrating the recognition of the high viewership of these videos. Since the video creators do not get to select the product (just receive revenue for the sponsorship), it is very possible that these breastfeeding videos could be sponsored by formula companies, meaning that people looking for breastfeeding advice could be exposed to more formula advertising. Indeed, sponsored videos for Enfamil and other formula companies actually appear above the search results of the breastfeeding videos.

Viewer Feedback to Breastfeeding on *YouTube*

How did viewers respond to these videos? Three videos had the comments disabled. "How to Breastfeed" (by *Fit Pregnancy*) yielded the most comments, with 1092. Recurring positive themes included praise for the videos, sharing of personal experience, and support for breastfeeding in general. Negative comments ridiculed the mothers or their breastfeeding, sexualized the breastfeeding experience, and criticized breastfeeding itself. People also posted irrelevant remarks to the topics in the videos.

Many videos, especially those that showed babies breastfeeding, only received positive comments, commending the mother for breastfeeding and complimenting her baby. Comments for the "Mama Cabbage" home movies, for example, are overwhelmingly positive. For her video, "Breastfeeding Entertainment," viewers responded with "Natalie this is a beautiful video"

(Anjel Hall, May 2015, "Breastfeeding Entertainment"), "beautiful family" (Chevon G., July 2015, "Breastfeeding Entertainment"), and other affirmative remarks. Similarly, comments for "Breastfeeding Dilemma" are also upbeat, most of which describe the cuteness of the child in the video. As part of praising the videos, viewers shared their own experiences with breastfeeding. To "Mama Cabbage," a poster named "Anjel Hall" wrote, "My little guy is 9 months and I have just had to stop breastfeeding him as I got really ill and had no other choice than to take medication that wasn't safe to be passed on through my milk... instead I feel so upset that I cannot continue, I wanted to feed him way into toddlerhood as you did with Joey" (Anjel Hall, May 2015, "Breastfeeding Entertainment"). These shared experiences suggest a parasocial bond with the videos' creators and may explain why people are drawn to home movies of people they do not know.

People also posted positive comments in the midst of feedback that was predominately negative. Videos with tandem and/or extended breastfeeding received largely negative feedback; thus praise, within this context, defends the nursing mothers. "Breastfeeding Tutorial: How to Tandem Breastfeed," "Pregnant and Breastfeeding a 4 year old! How to wean your toddler!" (both home movies labeled "A KoalaBearBabyXX Production"), as well as other videos of older children nursing were met with heavy criticism, focusing on the ages of the breastfed children. Viewers declared, "They do not need breast milk! Jesus women let it go!" (Booyelkawinnie, 2014, "Breastfeeding Tutorial: How to Tandem Breastfeed-3.5 yr & 2 yr Toddlers!") and "i think she's too old for that... just saying" (Tatiana Bento, Jan. 2015, "Pregnant and Breastfeeding a 4 year old! How to wean your toddler!"). Some posters directed their messages to the mothers themselves, with "I'm sorry if I sound rude to you ma'am but your son looks to old old for breast feeding. Please dont take it the wrong way" (Tyler Pagan, July 2015, "Breastfeeding a Toddler"). Likewise, "faith Duvivier" stated, "Personally I feel that people should at least stop breast feeding at the most two because you need let your daughter grow and not be too attached to you" (faith Duvivier, May 2015, "Pregnant and Breastfeeding a 4 year old! How to wean your toddler!"). Again, note that comments are quoted as they were originally written and posted, including spelling, capitalization, and grammatical errors.

Many of the comments that supported breastfeeding in general were part of the feedback for the extended videos. In other words, viewers posted positive statements about breastfeeding as responses to condemnation of breastfeeding in other posts. In the midst of ridicule for the tandem nursing video, “Jose Luis” praised the mother, stating “Breastfeeding is so important for children, please keep doing it!” (Jose Luis, Jan. 2015, “Breastfeeding Tutorial: How to Tandem Breastfeed-3.5 yr & 2 yr Toddlers!”). Another viewer wrote, “I don’t think there’s anything wrong with it. Heck it’s what God gave us breast for so we can feed our babies. It’s not like she’s 12 lol people can be so dense and like you said children do ween themselves naturally” (Not2008Me, Jan. 2015, “Pregnant and Breastfeeding a 4 year old! How to wean your toddler!”). Viewers incorporated their personal experiences into defending the extended breastfeeders. “Madam Vonkook” explained, “My daughter lots her suckle around 4 years old so they eventually will ween naturally as you said. My daughter is now 22 and a beautiful wholesome independent young woman” (Madam Vonkook, Dec. 2014, “Pregnant and Breastfeeding a 4 year old! How to wean your toddler!”). Other posters shared similar stories of breastfeeding older children and praised the women in the videos.

In addition to criticizing extended breastfeeding, other negative feedback sexualized breastfeeding. Viewers joked about feeling aroused by the videos, with “This is now my fetish” (187onaPigeon, July 2015, “Breastfeeding Tutorial: How to Tandem Breastfeed-3.5 yr & 2 yr Toddlers!”), “I’d be a very happy baby, if I had that much breast milk” (JamesReadythe5th, July 2015, “Pregnant and Breastfeeding a 4 year old! How to wean your toddler!”) and “I’ve never been so jealous of a 2 year old” (Rob W, July 2015, “Breastfeeding a Toddler”).

Feedback for the videos also blossomed into discussion and debates. Viewers expressed concerns and asked questions about breastfeeding in the feedback section, which were then answered by the video creators or other people. This interactive space was also used for fierce debates about breastfeeding, sparked by the critical remarks about breastfeeding in general, extended nursing, and the sexualization of breasts. With some of these conversations, the video creators participated. For example, in response to the declaration that the tandem nursing mother should “let it go!” (Booyelkawinnie, 2014, “Breastfeeding Tutorial: How to Tandem Breastfeed-3.5 yr & 2 yr Toddlers!”), the video’s creator replied, “They may not NEED Breastmilk (my eldest 2 kids survived perfectly fine without it for more than a few months) but, it’s sooooo good for them, full of nutrients and antibodies that protect them from any virus that my own body has fought off (continues on)" ("KoalaBreastfeedingBaby Angie," July 2014, "Breastfeeding Tutorial: How to Tandem Breastfeed-3.5 yr & 2 yr Toddlers!"). This type of exchange frequently occurred in the heavily criticized videos. Other posters also contributed to debates. Viewers ardently refuted the notion of the sexualization of breastfeeding. After a viewer stated, "Does breastfeeding a child his age beneficial? It kinda seems like he wants the breast and not so much the milk" (Robert Baratheon, May 2015, "Breastfeeding a Toddler"), 55 posts from different people followed, largely criticizing "Robert Baratheon" for proposing this idea. Other popular debates included the credentials of the women in the breastfeeding videos, the motives behind posting the videos, and benefits of extended breastfeeding.

Overall, the viewer patterns exemplify the narrow definition of what is considered "normal" and acceptable in society, with praise for breastfeeding babies and criticism for breastfeeding older children. These interactive discussions allow for viewers to ask questions and seek advice, video creators to respond to questions and concerns, and provide instantaneous feedback on the viewing experience. This set-up also enables debate and discussion about topics relating to breastfeeding, allowing posters to counter criticism. At the same time, the overwhelmingly negative comments are suggestive of the lack of gatekeeping and anonymous nature of these boards. The critical words of many of these posts are discouraging and unsupportive, giving the impression that a mother may be heavily scrutinized if she breastfeeds in front of others.

Conclusion: Using *Youtube* as a Breastfeeding Tool?

These findings reflect existing research on online coverage of breastfeeding and viewer responses. As De Carvalho and colleagues noted from their content analysis of breastfeeding on *Youtube*, most videos are narratives about breastfeeding, not instructive or educational.[29] No videos address Supplemental Nursing Systems, treatment for clogged ducts, mastitis or thrush, or other concerns of breastfeeding mothers. Furthermore, as Len-Rios, Bhandari, and Medvedeva found in their study of reader feedback for online news, posters here often used personal experience and emotion, rather than scientific evidence, to support their positions—for and against breastfeeding.[30] Expectant and new parents searching for "breastfeeding" on this site would likely view these videos, largely home movies with unverified advice on nursing. The diversity of these women, their authenticity, and the uncovered images of latching children could be encouraging to mothers early in their breastfeeding journeys. And yet, the backlash from the vocal public in the comments may threaten confidence and make new mothers feel unsupported and fear criticism when nursing in public spaces.

Why do so many viewers tune into see Mama Cabbage talk about zucchini squash while breastfeeding? Answering this question would help breastfeeding advocates design videos to educate and encourage breastfeeding. To implement change, breastfeeding organizations need to produce eye-catching, informative videos that are accurate and engaging so that people would willingly watch and share them. Such videos should include mothers of color, older babies, other challenges beyond latching and the first few days. Advocates could also create humorous videos designed for those who are not expecting or have children. Similar to the *Family Guy* clips, funny pro-breastfeeding videos that draw a childless audience could positively influence overarching cultural attitudes about breastfeeding. For both groups, polished, catchy videos could then be used as viral marketing tools, as a challenge or alternative to popular formula commercials that are widely distributed. In addition, people should speak out against sponsored formula ads on breastfeeding searches. And, to protect against harmful and disparaging remarks in the feedback area, comments should either be disabled or monitored so that negative feedback is removed. Given the pervasiveness of formula marketing online, it is imperative that breastfeeding promoted better utilized online tools like *Youtube*.

Notes

1. Velez, "Here's What Happened When A Mom Posted A Photo Of Herself Breastfeeding At Graduation."
2. Bologna, "Internet Cheers For Photo Of Mom Breastfeeding At Graduation."
3. Ibid.
4. Duggan et al., "Social Media Update 2014."
5. Street et al., "Social Networking Fact Sheet."
6. Street et al., "Internet Now Main Source of News for Young Adults."
7. Duggan et al., "Parents and Social Media."
8. Ibid.

9. Asiodu et al., "Breastfeeding and Use of Social Media Among First-Time African American Mothers."
10. Ibid.
11. Zhang, Carlton, and Fein, "The Association of Prenatal Media Marketing Exposure Recall with Breastfeeding Intentions, Initiation, and Duration."
12. Abrahams, "Milk and Social Media Online Communities and the International Code of Marketing of Breast-Milk Substitutes."
13. See note 11.
14. Huang et al., "Association of Health Profession and Direct-to-Consumer Marketing with Infant Formula Choice and Switching."
15. Gray, "Feeding On the Web."
16. Ibid.
17. "Woman Is Publicly Shamed For Breastfeeding In Public. Then She Posts This On Facebook."
18. Ibid.
19. Geraghty et al., "Buying Human Milk via the Internet."
20. Ibid.
21. Len-Ríos, Bhandari, and Medvedeva, "Deliberation of the Scientific Evidence for Breastfeeding Online Comments as Social Representations."
22. Ibid.
23. "Community Guidelines—*Youtube*."
24. Ibid.
25. Burke and Snyder, "*Youtube*"; Burke, Snyder, and Rager, "An Assessment of Faculty Usage of *Youtube* as a Teaching Resource."
26. "▶ Teach Me How To Breast Feed [MUSIC VIDEO]—*Youtube*."
27. de Carvalho et al., "Analysis of *Youtube* Videos on Breastfeeding."
28. Ibid.
29. Ibid.
30. Len-Ríos, Bhandari, and Medvedeva, "Deliberation of the Scientific Evidence for Breastfeeding Online Comments as Social Representations."

CHAPTER 9

Marginalized Milk: "Extreme" Nursing, Milk Exchange, and Erotic Breastfeeding

> Attractive, professional white male is seeking a woman who is willing to be a wet nurse. Very discreet. Just a fantasy that I would like to fulfill. ("Adult Wet Nurse Needed," May 9, 2015)

This *Craigslist* posting in Fairbanks, Alaska is not unique. Advertisements for willing female partners and erotic breastfeeding pornography are rampant online, through sites like *Lactation Fantasy*, *LactatingDreams.com*, and *FetishLactate*. This behavior that most would consider outside the norm has entered mainstream media through reality shows that include a *Strange Sex* episode on "extreme breastfeeding." Yet, there has been little uproar to these fetishes compared to the backlash that women have received for nursing in public, in uniform, or at commencement, breastfeeding older children, or the criticism surrounding human milk sharing. While breastfeeding advocates would consider erotic breastfeeding as a separate domain from nursing children, its media coverage has been similar to the discourse of other breastfeeding and human milk stories considered outside the norm. This chapter explores breastfeeding and breastmilk uses and behaviors that have been perpetuated as "spectacle" by mainstream media, looking at how this "othering" polarizes people and undermines public acceptance of breastfeeding. Specifically, this chapter addresses media frenzies over extended breastfeeding, peer-to-peer milk sharing, and alternative uses to breastmilk, in comparison to the lack of public scrutiny for adult wet nursing and erotic breastfeeding.

K.A. Foss, *Breastfeeding and Media*,
DOI 10.1007/978-3-319-56442-5_9

As in other chapters, quotations from online postings are stated verbatim, including spelling and grammatical errors.

Extended as Extreme?

The American Academy of Pediatrics (AAP) encourages women to breastfeed until at least a year.[1] The World Health Organization (WHO) recommends exclusive breastfeeding for 6 months and then nursing until at least 2 years.[2] The breastfeeding goal for *Healthy People 2020* is to have 81.9% initiation, 60.6% at 6 months, and 34.1% at a year.[3] Despite the known benefits of extended breastfeeding, media images typically do not show children nursing past the infancy stage. When women are portrayed breastfeeding older children, the response is immediate, abundant, and overwhelmingly negative. Newspapers, blogs, and online communities have criticized women who have publicly nursed toddlers and older children. In outlets ranging from *Forbes* magazine to parenting blogs, writers distinguish between appropriate ages for breastfeeding and what they consider "too old." Media and public response to extended breastfeeding in the *Extraordinary Breastfeeding* documentary, a 2012 *Time* magazine cover, and the fantasy television program *Game of Thrones* illustrate the fierce public negativity toward this natural practice.

Extraordinary Breastfeeding

In 2006, a British documentary, *Extraordinary Breastfeeding*, was released, covering the stories of women who nursed older children.[4] The headline of *The Telegraph* article about extended breastfeeding-mother Veronica Robinson stated, "There comes a point when breast is not best."[5] In the body of the article, writer Alison Palmer directly criticizes Robinson's choice, with "I love to see a woman breastfeeding her baby whenever and wherever, just as God intended. But the operative word is 'baby.' Surely I'm not wrong to feel slightly repulsed by a woman being suckled by a child who can walk, talk and, in some cases, tie her own shoelaces?"[6] She followed her remarks with a quote from a parenting psychologist who agrees with her repulsion.[7] This response reflected the vocal public's reaction to this story. An excerpt of this film, labeled "Breastfeeding at 8," was posted on *Youtube*, and by 2013 received over 42.5 million views and nearly 86,000 comments.[8] Most of the posts were negative, including "This is not normal," "Even without someone telling me this is wrong, when I see something like it, it gives me a weird, creepy feeling, and that's how I know it's not normal." Viewers expressed their repulsion, with numerous comments like "This is gross." One poster questioned the mental state of the mother, declaring, "She should be arrested for sexual abuse." Others remarked at how the breastfeeding mothers continue for their pleasure, not their babies, ignoring the numerous emotional and health benefits of extended breastfeeding.

"Are You Mom Enough?" the *Time* Magazine Cover

On May 21, 2012, the cover of *Time* magazine featured a strong, confident woman standing up, facing the camera, as her 3 year-old stood next to her on a chair breastfeeding, accompanied by the title, "Are You Mom Enough?" The cover referred to an article about the Attachment Parenting philosophy. Yet media focused exclusively on the cover image and its caption. A few positive stories praised *Time* and the mother. On *The BabySleep Site*, writer Nicole Johnson encouraged other moms to be not offended, but, "inspired" by the cover, praising the mother for her confidence.[9] Johnson then declared that the *Time* cover is "only 'shocking' because our culture does not support extended breastfeeding, but in other cultures, this would not have had the same shock value, if any at all."[10] However, the overall response was undoubtedly negative. Backlash ensued, with individual readers and other media outlets extensively criticizing the photo. *YahooNews!*'s coverage of the story received more than 17,000 viewer comments, questioning the mother's psychological state, *Time* magazine's decision to print the photo, and the practice of extended breastfeeding overall. *Forbes'* magazine responded with the headline "*Time* Magazine Asks 'Are You Mom Enough?' Every Mom Should Be Offended."[11] Its author, Sabrina Parsons, argued that the accompanying article was anti-Feminist in its implication that working moms could not follow Attachment Parenting (of which extended breastfeeding is a key part).[12]

Some media went so far as to suggest that the mother was somehow sexually deviant for nursing her child. *Fox News* writer Keith Ablow argued, "The truth is that what *Time* magazine may have unwittingly captured and been party to was a grotesque form of psychological abuse."[13] Reader feedback suggested similar responses. Numerous bloggers also responded to the cover. A *Huffington Post* story on the cover resulted in more than 4000 messages, again, mostly negative, with statements such as, "When you look at best practices—sticking your boob in a preschool age child is not developmentally appropriate-EVER!" and "Breast feeding until 5yrs old is NOT normal. Kids must be weaned at a reasonable age, 2 at the latest." While some readers wrote in favor of extended breastfeeding, they were quickly bombarded with negative feedback. For example, one reader remarked, "People are so upset over this, but will drink hormone and drug laden milk from another species, get a clue people, your worldview is upside down!" Another reader responded, "Yeah, call me silly and strange, but I don't want to drink my mother's breast milk," ending the conversation.

This cover problematized several of the ideologies about motherhood and breastfeeding. First, the title "Are You Mom Enough?" perpetuated the "intensive mothering" of contemporary "new momism" described by Douglas and Michaels.[14] Paired with the image of thin, fit, blonde mother and her angelic, air-brushed son, this cover elevates a type of "perfect" mothering that no woman could actually achieve, even with extended breastfeeding. Moreover, by using "Mom enough," this message suggests that women who do not nurse through toddlerhood are somehow inferior mothers, contrasted with the "good mother" ideology present in other media.[15] Second, the positioning of the mother and child standing together as he nurses, both facing the camera, paints a false picture of most extended breastfeeding experiences, which are typically more about the relationship of mother and child than the "in-your-face" Lactivism that the cover suggests. Backlash to this cover then, likely occurred because of its demonization of other feeding choices in as much as societal objection and discomfort with public breastfeeding. A better approach to changing cultural norms and perceptions would be for *Time* to showcase an array of breastfeeding women and experiences, with less ideologically-loaded captions that celebrate breastfeeding, as opposed to insulting those who do not.

Powerful Breastfeeding in *The Game of Thrones*

As addressed earlier, extended breastfeeding in fictional television has also been conveyed as "extreme." This othering has been reinforced and perpetuated by online discussion of fictional content. The 2011 *Game of Thrones* episode "The Wolf and the Lion" included a scene in which a woman clearly breastfeeds a child around 6 years-old. While this episode also contained images of simulated intercourse with full nudity and battle scenes with graphic violence, media backlash only addressed the breastfeeding scene. Blogger Jessica Carlson for *ImperfectParent* declared that the breastfeeding scene "has sent the Internets all a flutter."[16] Critics associated the mother's breastfeeding as an extension of her insanity in other ways. Andrew Dansbury, a blogger for the *Houston Chronicle* stated, "Cut to Lysa, Cat's sister, acting *craaaazy*. Tyrion undersold the crazy. How crazy? Well, she's breastfeeding her kid, who is a few years past baby teeth. He too is touched" (Dansbury, 2011). A *Youtube* clip of the child breastfeeding (with restricted access for those 18 and over) received nearly one million views and 478 comments, most of which were negative remarks about the "deviance" of the image, like "This scene was disturbing" (Fcuk1118, March 2015) and "oh what an awkward scene to film" (toughangel17). Many posts were sexual in nature, with "Now I wanna suck on a teat" (wiisalute, May 2015). Viewers also speculated on the mother's intentions, stating, "Let's face it Lysa got off her son sucking her tits. She got desperate for affection over the years with no true romantic relationship with Petyr" (Ketorulz, June 2015). In response to these comments, other viewers stated that the breast was a prosthetic, stating, "it's a fake tit. Calm yourselves" (Gage Tinsley, April 2015) and "Those are fake boobs! Dislikers didn't know that" (Amazing Deepak, June 2015). Again, in a show filled with other images and behaviors that are typically considered deviant, it is interesting that media and viewers honed in on this scene, demonstrating just how much people consider breastfeeding an older child to be a spectacle. The malevolent tone of the online posts convey scrutiny over Lysa's breastfeeding an older child, not just shock or fascination.

Analyzing Media and Public Response

These examples and others illustrate how extended breastfeeding has been defined by media. This analysis also reflects other scholars' examination of such discourse. For example, Norwood and Turner found that discussion boards of the *Time* magazine cover perpetuated heterosexuality and narrow definitions of "normal" breastfeeding.[17] Several themes emerge from media coverage of these three cases. First, what most people overlooked is that it was media producers that created the spectacle. The media messages here did not come from regular women making home movies. Rather, filmmakers chose to make a documentary about Veronica Robinson, selected what to film, how to edit the footage, how to package it, and decided to call the film *Extraordinary Breastfeeding*. Likewise, we have to remember that Jamie Lynn Grumet did not approach *Time* with her photo and order them to place it on the cover with "Are You Mom Enough?" Rather, the production team for *Time* magazine decided to run a story on Attachment Parenting and then hired Jamie Lynn Grumet and her son as models for the cover. In the photo shoot, the photographer and assistants chose the clothing, lighting, and then set up her pose, with her son standing on a chair (as she probably does not usually breastfeed him perched in this position). Editors selected this photo, touched it up, and placed it as the cover photo, then added the caption. Finally, *Game of Thrones* is a fictional show. Every element of the breastfeeding scene was planned as part of the overarching character development and storylines for the television program. My point here is that media set up the spectacle in such a way as to invite backlash. The title of the documentary, the bold and provocative positioning of Grumet on the cover, the articulate dialogue of the child breastfeeding from Lysa on the throne—all of it was created to incite backlash and frenzy, feeding off of the already existing negative public attitudes toward breastfeeding, especially beyond the newborn stage.

It is problematic in itself that nursing older children has been demonized. Negative speculations of the effects are unfounded. No evidence exists to support long-term harmful consequences of breastfeeding into the primary years, including some kind of sexual aberration. Rather, lengthy nursing has been shown to be beneficial, particularly in places that lack clean water and adequate food supplies.[18] Suggestions that children will breastfeed "forever" are also false as self-weaning is inevitable. In fact, in cultures in which extended nursing is normal, most children naturally self-wean between 3 and 6 years old.[19] Finally, the accusations of sexual perversion attached to extended breastfeeding also takes away from the breastfeeding relationship and suggests that nursing should not be pleasurable, delegitimizing the emotional and physical reasons for extended nursing.

Unfortunately, normalized depictions of extended nursing are missing from news, entertainment, and social media. We see a dichotomy of representations: positive images of breastfeeding infants or the highly-ridiculed extreme of nursing older toddlers or elementary school children offered as spectacle. This in itself is also detrimental to the promotion of breastfeeding duration. Few news and entertainment media offer portrayals of women nursing older babies and toddlers, suggesting that the "norm" is nursing infants and that breastmilk beyond that point will be publicly scrutinized. How can breastfeeding duration goals for age 6 months, 1 year, 2 years, and more be met if people are not accustomed to seeing children breastfed for that long? In addition, the militant nature of the extreme extended breastfeeding may seem threatening to expectant and new parents, conveying that to nurse longer than infancy is to make a political statement—to head-on combat society's definition of what is normal. In reality, for most women, nursing older babies into toddlerhood and beyond is just a natural progression as their children grow. Media's treatment of extended nursing: as always extreme and received with heavy public criticism may discourage women from breastfeeding past the early baby stages. Mothers may also feel uncomfortable nursing in public for fear of this scrutiny. Studies have shown that women who are at ease breastfeeding in public have longer duration rates.[20]

Breastmilk—not just from the Tap

Media has also treated milk donation, sales, and sharing as controversial. While most people no longer formally hire wet nurses, the well-established benefits of breastmilk have prompted corporations, non-profits, and individuals to desire its acquisition. Currently, no federal laws address or prohibit the share of human milk, even though the United States Food and Drug Administration discourages obtaining another mother's milk directly.[21] This section examines media messages of different means of acquiring breastmilk: through milk banks, informal milk sharing and selling milk online. The formal practice of distributing human milk dates back to 1910, with the creation of the first American milk bank in Boston.[22] Milk bank donation and distribution rates have fluctuated since that time, with a steady increase in the 2000s.[23] Currently, the United States has non-profit milk banks in many areas of the country, which distribute human milk to hospitals for babies who are premature and/or have serious medical complications.[24] In the past few years, more for-profit companies that accept human milk and transform it into milk fortifiers have emerged. Notably, Prolacta Bioscience accepts human milk, which is then "pasteurized and formulated into nutritional products exclusively for in hospital use, not for individual purchase."[25]

Milk banks focus on providing milk and milk fortifiers to hospitals to help medically fragile babies. Breastmilk is life-saving for low birth weight babies. Infants born early are susceptible to Necrotizing Enterocolitis, a devastating gastrointestinal disease that can lead to surgical intervention or even death.[26] Human milk dramatically reduces the risk of premature babies developing this disease, compared to babies who receive formula or even a mixture of human milk and bovine milk-based products.[27] Long-term, premature babies fed breastmilk also fare better overall, scoring higher in measures of cognitive, psychomotor, and behavioral measures.[28] Unfortunately, mothers of premature babies also tend to have more difficulty with milk supply and lower breastfeeding success overall.[29] Milk banks address this gap between the mothers' ability to provide milk and the number of babies who need it by delivering pasteurized human milk to hospitals where it can be fed in the Neonatal Intensive Care Unit. That said, milk banks do not exist in every state or even region, nor can they supply enough milk for all the babies who need it.[30] Furthermore, the delivery of human milk to those in need depends on health professionals as the intermediary, which can be problematic if they do not recognize the need or are unaware of the donor milk process.[31]

In addition to these medicalized outlets, informal milk sharing and the selling of breastmilk enables access to human milk beyond the hospital and/or for those who do not meet the milk bank criteria. *Facebook* alone has 170 milk sharing sites from 50 countries, with global and local virtual spaces for milk exchanges.[32] On the *Facebook* sites "Eats on Feets" and "Human Milk 4 Human Babies," people post requests for breastmilk, usually paired with an explanation of their needs. For example, one mother posted on a local "Eats on Feets" group, "We just unexpectedly adopted a preemie baby, now 7 weeks old. She is not doing well on formula. I nursed all of my children and am trying to relactate, but not getting anything really yet. Please let me know if you can help me." Several mothers replied, offering to help with donated milk. These exchanges are built on trust, without regulation or intervention from gatekeepers.

Aunchalee Palmquist explained how peer-to-peer milk sharing represents a demedicalization of breastmilk that is not controlled by science, but based on relationships and altruism.[33] Karleen Gribble surveyed donors and recipients on milk sharing sites, finding that this connection is one reason some women prefer to give their milk through these sites, rather than donate to milk banks.[34] Other women chose milk sharing sites because they believed the milk banks were too restrictive, found the screening process too difficult, or philosophically preferred informal milk sharing.[35] Those who had received donor milk appreciated the relationship aspect, enjoying learning more about the women who had donated.[36] Palmquist and Doehler also surveyed participants in milk sharing sites to determine the demographics and reasons for participation in these groups.[37] On average, donors were more educated and had higher incomes than recipients, although both groups had above-average household incomes.[38] Moreover, donors were more likely to have had vaginal deliveries, healthy babies, and breastfeeding support from their partners, families, and pediatricians, compared to recipients (who did not have adequate milk for their babies).[39]

Among breastfeeding advocates, milk banks and peer-to-peer milk sharing are fitting solutions to parents who want the benefits of breastmilk, but are unable to provide it themselves, either because of breastfeeding troubles, or because of adoption, surrogacy, or other situations that place children with others than the biological mother.[40] It is also a helpful response for mothers who feel guilty or ashamed if they cannot breastfeed. Steele, Martin, and Foell discussed how it is unreasonable and impractical for people to tout the benefits of breastmilk without providing safe alternatives to nursing at the breast, like milk sharing.[41]

People also buy and sell human milk online. Websites like *Onlythebreast.com* provide an outlet for both financial exchanges and donating milk. The site has channels for milk produced by women with specific diets, ages of the nursling, quantity, and other characteristics. People also find donor milk, hire wet nurses, or purchase milk for themselves (not just babies). On this site, mothers typically advertise their breastmilk (much like products on *Craigslist*), using catchy descriptions to hopefully attract buyers, emphasizing what they perceive as desirable qualities. Many of the ad titles emphasize health and diet. Advertisements posted on July 26, 2015 included the titles "EXTRA HIGH QUALITY BREASTMILK FROM HEALTHY FIT MOM," "HEALTHY MOM WITH HEALTHY BABY WITH EXTRA HIGH QUALITY MILK," and "SUPER HEALTHY, CLEAN EATING, DRUG AND ALCOHOL FREE" (emphasis in the original ads). Milk quantity is also promoted as an asset, with "1500 oz ready to go! Milk from an active healthy mom less then 3 months old!" and "Overproducing mom over 4000 oz—milk bank donor." Here, the "milk donor" status implies a reassurance of health. Intelligence and education are also played up in the ads, like "Well-educated mother of Healthy 10 Mo."

Once a potential buyer clicks on an ad, a sometimes lengthy description is provided in an attempt to make the sale. Milk sellers stress their fitness levels, diet, and lifestyle (including vitamin intake), the health and size of their nurslings, and their adherence to careful storage and freezing of the milk. "The "Well-educated mother of Healthy 10 Mo.," for example, has the following ad:

> I have over 500 oz of frozen breastmilk available, less than 2 months old. I currently produce twice my daughter's need. She is 10 months old and very healthy! She has been in daycare since she was 3 months old and has only had minor colds. She did not get the flu or hand, foot, mouth while it was going around at the daycare. Thank goodness for strong immune systems due to breastmilk.
>
> I am a very healthy 33 y/o mother of 2. I eat very healthy and take prenatal vitamins with DHA. I have been certified by a milk bank. I have recently moved and do not want to go through the lengthy wait to get recertified (2 + months) and am running out of room in my freezer. I have donated to over 3,000 oz to milk banks and local mothers. I do no smoke, take drugs, have any diseases, etc. I will have approx. 500 oz each month available for purchase.

These ads are very business-like in tone and appeal to buyers using breastfeeding benefits. Aside from having excess, the milk sellers do not mention their reasons for selling milk or the effect that the additional income will have on their lives. While donor milk posts use emotion and altruism, milk sellers use numbers, references to milk bank screening, and their own nurslings as selling points for the milk quality, even though there is no actual scientific measurement or assessment of the milk itself.

However, the *Onlythebreast.com* page "Men Buying Breast Milk" is a different story. Much like pleas for donor milk on *Facebook*, most of these ads (posted from potential buyers) explain why they would like to purchase human milk. The male buyers emphasize that the milk is not for sexual use and give bodybuilding, overall health, and other justifications for drinking human milk. offering explanations like "i'm not some creep buying it for a fetish, I want to start a diet with breastmilk for fitness." Similarly, another buyer wrote "I am clean and respectful… Looking for a local mom. freshest milk possible, I am looking for the health benefits." "Healthy Professional male looking for a supplier of fresh BM. I am willing to travel locally and to compensate. I am into Bodybuilding and very health conscious." On this site, it is clear that male buyers are on the outskirts, in the minority, and may have difficulty finding sellers. In fact, mothers can specify whether or not they are even willing to sell to men, which may explain the shift in language from the sellers (using pseudo-science) to the buyers (who offer explanation). Once the seller and buyer come to an agreement, they arrange for payment and either shipping or local meet-ups. Before consumption, the site offers instructions on how to pasteurize the milk at home and encourages people to do so.

What does milk selling convey about breastfeeding and human milk? It is not surprising that milk sharing and donation rests on the same trust and altruism that supported the co-nursing that was common before bottles and artificial food. Mothers would nurse others' babies as needed in the community.[42] For milk sellers, these ads are reminiscent of newspaper classifieds of the 1700s and 1800s, using many of the persuasive strategies of that time (i.e., describing the wet nurse and playing up the health of her baby). However, what has changed is the focus on specific diets and lifestyles, as well as the absence of using race, religion, and socio-economic class as selling points—such discriminatory language is prohibited by the site.

In our commercially-driven society, we can also ponder the value assigned to breastmilk on these sites. Sellers set the price of the milk, which can range from less than $1 an ounce in the discount lot to $4.99 an ounce and up for the milk of mothers following dairy-free, vegan, or other special diets. Given that babies, on average, consume about 19–30 oz a day, at these prices, the cheap rates would still cost $570–$4000 a month.[43] Obviously, this is cost-prohibitive for most families, hence the popularity and need for milk sharing. At the same time, this commoditization of breastmilk—at such a high price—demonstrates it value. Penny Van Esterik discussed the rise of breastmilk substitutes as status symbols, first in industrialized countries and then in developing nations, because of their cost, the restricted number of products, the separation of manufacturing from the consumer, and the product marketing.[44] These factors help associate a product with a higher social class. Using this characteristic, milk selling commoditizes breastmilk into a status symbol with its expensive price, limited availability, and distance from producer to consumer.[45] However, this association is only likely to increase perceptions of value and breastmilk if milk sales were to enter mainstream culture. As the next section discusses, human milk exchanges rarely enter into public discourse except in stories about their risks.

Media Coverage of Human Milk Distribution

As with milk banks, media discourse of milk sharing has been rather limited. Most notably, was popular news coverage of a 2013 *Pediatrics* publication about the contamination of human milk for sale.[46] In the article, entitled, "Microbial contamination of human milk," Keim and colleagues described how they anonymously purchased and then tested 101 samples of human milk for contamination, finding that 74% contained higher bacteria counts of *Staphylococcus* than milk bank samples, as well as other bacteria.[47] Numerous news websites covered the story, using facts from the study and quotations from Keim. *Fox News* used the headline "Dangerous bacteria found in breast milk sold on Internet," repeated Keim and colleagues' findings, and then declared, "The research published in medical literature cites several cases of infants getting sick from strangers' milk"—without citation or reference to specific incidents.[48] This story had no comment section so reader response could not be gauged.

The *New York Times* (*NYT*) published a similar story, entitled, "Breast Milk Donated or Sold Online Is Often Tainted, Study Says." This headline was accompanied by a photo of a woman bottle-feeding her son, above a caption that explained that she used donor milk with no major problems.[49] The article paralleled other stories using the *Pediatrics* study, acknowledging breastfeeding benefits, milk sharing and selling, and the risks. However, this article deviated from the others in the photo of the milk donor recipient and another picture of a hand pouring milk from a breastmilk storage bag. This story also incorporated the positive testimony of the donor recipient.

NYT readers gave extensive feedback on the topic, leaving 418 comments. Most posters argued that parents should avoid risks of human milk contamination by using formula. "PL" wrote, "Why would anyone ever buy an unregulated liquid from an unknown source online to give to a baby? I am all for breast-feeding and did it for almost 2 years, but there is safe and nutritious formula for those times that you cannot. The small benefit that is gained from breast milk is certainly outweighed by the very real dangers of bacterial contamination." Other readers shared similar reactions. "Dan Stackhouse" stated, "Basically the rough equivalent of ordering milk online is buying it from someone selling jars of it out of a duffel bag, at a sidewalk cafe. If people really want to take chances like that with their newborns, I suppose that's evolution in action for ya, but I'd think FDA-approved formula would be a better way to go." Some people perceived the story as a response to breastfeeding promotion: "lots of stars" argued, "Proof positive that the current societal obsession with breastfeeding has gone way too far. Some people actually think that breastmilk from a total stranger is safer and better for their baby than formula!? However well-intentioned the donors and the buyers surely are, this practice is unsanitary, dangerous, and just disgusting." "Nicoline Smits" shared the previous poster's beliefs with "Am I the only one around here who thinks the "breast is best" maffia has gone a little overboard recently? Yes, breastmilk may have all sorts of benefits, but if you cannot breast feed, for whatever reason, formula is a perfectly acceptable alternative. There is no need to drive yourself crazy and unnecessarily expose your child to bacterial infections."

At the same time, other readers questioned the validity and implications of the results.

"Disco" pointed out, "The big missing piece of this article is whether any children have been sickened. There may indeed be quality issues here, but are there really any safety issues?" Likewise, "gm" questioned, "Why didn't this article research if any infants were sickened by donated breast milk?" Readers also criticized the story for not suggesting improvements to human milk distribution or offer solutions for safer milk sharing. "Ann" clearly stated, "It seems to me that the answer to this whole question is to have screened, safely-treated breast milk more widely available at an affordable price" as did the poster "LVL," with "Help improve the safety of breast milk donations—don't scrap the system." Finally, "physician in NYC" summed up the pro-breastfeeding reactions, stating:

> I agree with other commenters that a big missing piece of this article is whether any children have been sickened by bacterial contamination issues. Breast milk has advantages over formula, but only from a healthy source, and when handled sanitarily. The article should also have included protocols for safe screening and handling of milk - why just the scare mongering? Provide information to improve practices!

USA Today also ran an article on this topic, with "Buying breast milk online? It may be contaminated," providing a similar overview of the study, listing the bacteria count and risks. The story concluded with a quotation from Keim stating that her study results may not apply in some milk sharing connections. All of the 25 comments were negative. "Jon Gibson," responded, "the title caused me to heave. . . what a revolting idea." "S. Fred Taylor Jr." asked, "Who is stupid enough to do this anyway." And "Andrew Goetz:" "Sorry, but that's just wrong to use some strange womans breast milk... if you can't produce enough then why would you risk your childs health on some strangers breast milk when formula is proven safe and plenty of benefits." Other comments expressed similar opinions.

Two years later, *Pediatrics* published a second study, in which Keim and colleagues revealed that 10 of 102 human milk samples purchased online contained evidence of cow's milk, suggesting that it had been added unscrupulously.[50] The online news stories had similar angles and responses to the 2013 study, preaching the "dangers" of giving milk from another mother to a baby. A *CBS News* headline read, "Breast milk sold online often contaminated by cow's milk," then argued that because of the emphasis on breastfeeding's benefits, "some mothers have turned to the Internet to buy breast milk, thinking it will be better for their newborn than formula. But new research indicates that breast milk bought online isn't always pure."[51] The author then described the findings from Keim's study and discussed the risks of purchasing milk online.[52] Only three people commented on the story, all on its "absurdity," as "LogicalMagic" said, "This is the most ridiculous thing I've ever heard of." *NPR* published the research as "Breast Milk Sold Online Contaminated with Cow's Milk," explaining milk sales, its risks, including dilution with cow's milk (from the *Pediatrics* study) and a description of milk banks and their drawbacks.[53] As with the other news stories on milk selling, posters questioned "risking" their babies' health, instead of using formula. However, unlike the other news outlets, a debate ensued about the risks of formula, as "zen zen" replied to the negative comments with, "Breastmilk is far superior to anything made in a lab with high fructose corn syrup and other additives that are not expressly produced for the needs of the baby. It's all part of the microbiom. Formula is not safe for all babies." This post spurred a lengthy argument that focused on the drawbacks and health of formula.

This debate highlighted a point that breastfeeding advocates have made about the risk language used against direct human milk exchange. Vogel, as well as Gribble and Hausman, emphasized that naysayers toward human milk sharing overlook the risks of not breastfeeding, including the established risk of bacterial and chemical contamination, documented evidence of unsanitary conditions in formula preparation, and the long-term risks of disease and developmental issues.[54] Carroll described how donor milk used in neonatal intensive care units has been distinguished by doctors and the medical profession as "safe," from the unregulated online exchange to convince parents of its necessity.[55] That said, no documented cases of babies becoming ill from contaminated breastmilk have been publicized. In addition to higher mortality rates of formula-fed babies overall, in 2008, tainted formula caused the deaths of six babies in China, with over 300,000 ill babies.[56] Yet, the mere speculation of risk for milk sharing and selling prompts most people to regard it as unsafe.

Furthermore, none of the news stories mentioned academic responses to the 2013 *Pediatrics* article. In a published electronic reply, Stuebe, Gribble, and Palmquist refuted many of the conclusions made by Keim and colleagues, arguing that their set-up for milk acquisition (purchasing milk anonymously without screening the donors and then having it shipped to a rented mailbox) is not reflective of most milk exchanges.[57] These scholars also pointed out that milk selling is not the same as milk sharing. This response added much-needed context to the study and could have established ground for discussing safe milk exchanges in the news stories.

Overall, the distribution and consumption of breastmilk has been largely invisible in media, especially considering its prevalence. Apart from a few brief periods of spectacle focusing on contamination, human milk exchange has been on the periphery, eschewing public scrutiny. At the same time, more attention could help families without a successful lactating mother access breastmilk through milk sharing or purchasing sites. Other debates that occasionally appear in media are the for-profit milk banks and whether or not the milk donors should profit from their milk. On the one hand, they are producing and distributing a desired commodity, which Prolacta Bioscience and other corporations turn into profit as milk fortifiers. At the same time, paying mothers may detract from the altruism that motivates them to donate. Concerns about milk selling have included the possibility of diluting or putting additives into the milk as supported by Keim and colleagues' studies in *Pediatrics*. As argued, though, the benefits likely outweigh the risks.

In recent years, breastmilk has been used for purposes beyond the nourishment of babies and young children. An episode of the television medical drama *House, M.D.* included a storyline in which an adult cancer patient asked Dr. House for breastmilk. This fictional narrative addressed an emerging trend. With the recognition of breastmilk's benefits, more than just children now desire and consume breastmilk. As the *Onlythebreast.com* ads illustrate, human milk is becoming a popular supplement for bodybuilders and other fitness buffs. The possibility of helping those with cancer and other disease may also prompt more attention to human milk usage beyond childhood.

Media discourse of milk sharing and alternative uses for breastmilk have varied. Fear of disease and other biological transmissions ground one objection to consuming breastmilk outside of the mother-child relationship. As with milk from other animals, laboratory sterilization and processing can eliminate this risk. However, an increase in monitoring and regulation could shut down informal , making breastmilk expensive and difficult to acquire in a timely manner, which is obviously crucial for feeding babies. Who should profit? Would further commodification of breastmilk infuse value into breastfeeding or make human milk inaccessible to most of the population? Currently, though, milk exchange and alternative uses for human milk are largely unheard of by the general public.

Behind Closed Doors: Erotic Breastfeeding

With the emphasis on scientific evidence in breastfeeding promotion and its overall medicalization, the experience of breastfeeding has often been overlooked. In her book *Fresh Milk: The Secret Life of Breasts*, Fiona Giles outlined the division between "the clinical management of breast milk" and the experience of breastfeeding as "a relational bodily process that engages with food, babies, and sex within a plenitude model of curiosity, irreverence, and pleasure."[58] She argued that sexuality outside of the narrow heteronormative definitions is overlooked and marginalized, including the reality that breastfeeding can be sensual.[59] Moreover, pleasure in breastfeeding and maternal sexuality has been considered inappropriate or taboo, possibly threatening intimacy between partners.[60] This absence of recognizing pleasure is evident in several ways. Health care providers tend to avoid postpartum discussions of breastfeeding and sexuality, even with the hormonal and physical changes that make the topic medically relevant (i.e., reassuring mothers that arousal during breastfeeding is normal).[61] Pleasure in breastfeeding is also missing from promotional campaigns, with the belief that it would undermine the messages, a misguided perception that again divorces emotion from benefits.[62] Prenatal and parenting books exemplify the "othering" of breastfeeding's sensuality, as it is ignored, denied, or marginalized. Except for a few rare examples, popular culture has not associated sexuality with breastfeeding—at least not in an empowering way.[63]

Women's pleasure from breastfeeding should be considered distinct from the sexual objectification of the breastfeeding woman by men enjoying the sexualization of breastfeeding as voyeurs, illustrated by the lustful *Youtube* comments of a mother nursing her baby or the "Breast Feeding Juggies" of *The Man Show*. More serious demonstrations of pleasure in breastfeeding has also been limited to male enjoyment in media coverage, and depictions of male arousal to lactation pornography or the consumption of human milk acquired online or from a lactating mother, as well as men's erotic experience of suckling partners' breasts. As with other fetishes, most people have been unaware of this practice, as stories of these activities are almost unheard of in public discourse.

Erotic breastfeeding (primarily for men's pleasure) entered the mainstream in 2012 when The Learning Channel (TLC) featured it as part of the reality program *Strange Sex*. The episode "Adult Breastfeeding and Revirginization," begins with a voice-over stating, "A woman's breasts are objects of both desire and nourishment, but for some, breastmilk isn't just for babies," as a man, Jeff, pours milk into a cereal bowl. Jeff tells the camera, "The best way to drink breastmilk is straight from the source." He then explains how he becomes aroused by breastfeeding from his wife, which has helped with his erectile dysfunction. A title slide appears, with "Jeff has been feeding on Michelle's breastmilk for the past year and a half." After that, Michelle expresses how she did not think she would care for him nursing, "but when Jeff started feeding from me, it was very erotic." An "expert" then mentions some possible benefits, but also said that the fetish could become problematic when the woman stopped lactating. In the episode, we see Jeff nursing from Michelle, covered up, without the latch shown.

This episode sparked online debate about the function and sexuality of breastfeeding on the "Weird News" page of the *Huffington Post* and in the comments portion of its *Youtube* clip.[64] Compared to the reaction to the "extreme" extended breastfeeding, media coverage and readers were surprisingly indifferent to a man "treating" his erectile dysfunction by drinking his wife's breastmilk. Despite the program title *Strange Sex*, most media outlets either ignored the show or appeared neutral on the topic, as exemplified by the *Huffington Post* title "Breastfeeding Man: Jeff says drinking wife Michelle's breastmilk helped his erectile dysfunction."[65] Many of the 395 comments suggested that Jeff's behavior was "normal," with remarks like, "Sucking on a woman's breasts gives a man an erection?! I had no idea!" and "Wow. Boobs in my face would cure ED for me too. LOL." Another reader wrote, "Just when I think I've heard it all. I guess as long as no one is hurt and both are willing, whatever floats their boat." Other readers agreed, applauding them for identifying a fetish that worked for them.

By placing erotic breastfeeding in a program entitled *Strange Sex*, producers defined the practice as deviant, as a spectacle. The viewer response, though, suggests that it is far less scrutinized than other marginalized breastfeeding acts. Possibly, the lack of reaction is because of Jeff (the man) is the main person deriving pleasure from this act, thus preserving the "Madonna and Child" image of the mostly asexual mother.[66] Michelle's experience is not at the center. It is not her needs or desires that are met, but her husband's. This media framing (and the public cheers for Jeff) conveyed that the mother's sexual desires are less important than the man's. In other words, had Michelle spoke about her pleasure and her yearnings, the public apathy likely would have turned to rampant accusations of perversion, much like what was (mis) directed at the "extreme" extended breastfeeders. It is about his pleasure, his desires, as reinforced by a patriarchal public that celebrates male sexuality, but degrades female sexuality. This contradiction relates back to Giles' work that calls for a rediscovery of female pleasure and sexuality, including breastfeeding, without shame.[67]

Conclusion: Breastfeeding as Spectacle

What do media presentations of "othered" breastfeeding practices tell us about what is considered "normal" and "deviant?" Why has there been a stronger public reaction to stories of nursing older children than erotic breastfeeding or alternative uses to human milk or breastfeeding? Conventional beliefs about private versus public space may help explain this difference. In a Feminist analysis of breastfeeding and celebrities, Spring-Serenity Duvall discussed how these online media stories unnervingly bridge the public and private.[68] Likewise, media representations of the *Extraordinary Breastfeeding* documentary, *Time* magazine cover, and *Game of Thrones* episode brought the "extreme" breastfeeding into the public sphere. In other words, acts that some people perceive as private were made public, possibly inviting criticism. If nothing else, the negative reactions may have stemmed from conservative Victorian notions of covering one's body—something that is not an issue with the exchange of human milk, in which negative reactions are to the substance, not the body. However, the "private" into the "public" space hardly explained the lack of response to Jeff, the erotic breastfeeder.

We could also analyze the discourse disparities in a Feminist framework. The "extreme" extended breastfeeding media depictions featured strong women, confident in their breastfeeding and positions of power: Victoria speaks to the camera about her decision to breastfeed her children until they self-wean. Jamie Grummet, the *Time* magazine mom, stands while breastfeeding, facing the camera, with the confrontational headline "Are You Mom Enough?" In *Game of Thrones*, the breastfeeding mother, Lysa, sits elevated on a throne as she speaks down to her sister and her entourage of soldiers. The scene ends with Lysa ordering the prisoner, Tyrion Lannister (a main character), to another part of the castle. For these three women, breastfeeding is framed as an extension of their powerful identities.

On the contrary, Jeff, not his lactating wife, Michelle, controls the narrative in the reality show *Strange Sex*. He explains the history behind his desire to suckle at his wife's breasts. And while Michelle seems to be a willing participant, Jeff, as the patriarch of the family, appears to make the decision. It is his erectile dysfunction that must be cured. It is his fantasy to nurse. He is the one who keeps her lactating. The lack of response to Jeff, the "erotic breastfeeder," may have been due to the maternal disempowerment of his wife, that it was his desire, his fetish, his fantasy—an extension of the "normal" man's attraction to breasts. In a society that has celebrated male sexual needs and desires over female comfort, perhaps it is this male control that deters criticism. Here, erotic breastfeeding merely supports a hegemonic structure in which women give their bodies to their male partners. Erotic breastfeeding is presented as exotic breastfeeding, much like other fetishes that occasionally and superficially appear in popular culture. Like the rape narratives in *Fifty Shades of Grey* masked as fetishes, erotic breastfeeding is dismissed as personal choice, while extended breastfeeding is publicly flogged for its "sexual perversion."

Aside from its gendered implications, *Strange Sex* and other mainstreamed discussions of erotic breastfeeding may also be problematic in further sexualizing the breast. For centuries, some women have chosen not to breastfeed to "save" their breasts for male partners and have been denied their own sexuality.[69] The overall point here is not to demonize erotic breastfeeding. Rather, I am pointing out that the unequal public response to the media's treatment of acts that contradict what has been considered "the breastfeeding norm" indicates larger problems that help explain less than ideal breastfeeding success rates. More attention to female pleasure and the experience of breastfeeding would help celebrate and empower the nursing mother.

Media discourse on human milk exchange fits into these discussion by exemplifying the medicalization and separation of breastmilk from the maternal producers. As Palmquist and Giles argued, the medical model distances scientific frameworks of breastfeeding from cultural and shared experience.[70] More media stories on human milk donation and sharing, which returns trust and emotion back to breastfeeding, would help broaden how we perceive the benefits of breastfeeding. Moreover, such stories would help to counter the human milk as "pollutant" or "biohazard" messages that dominate news about donated and sold milk.[71]

What do "extreme" extended breastfeeding, erotic breastfeeding, and and alternative uses for breastmilk have in common? All are presented in media as vastly different than conventional breastfeeding, of societal definitions of "normal." These definitions of "normal" constantly change, as exemplified by fluctuating breastfeeding attitudes and rates over the last 150 years. Therefore, new media portrayals of breastfeeding offer opportunities to enact change, expanding and redefining normal. Increasing depictions of breastfeeding 6 month-olds, 1 year-olds, 2 year-olds, and up would help people grow accustomed to nursing older children. At the same time, milk sharing and alternative uses for breastmilk would create public awareness of the importance of breastmilk and its health benefits. It is only with messages that challenge and counter narrow definitions of acceptable breastfeeding and breastmilk that we can change the cultural climate.

Notes

1. Breastfeeding, "Breastfeeding and the Use of Human Milk."
2. "WHO | Breastfeeding."
3. "Maternal, Infant, and Child Health| Healthy People 2020."
4. Buchanan, *Extraordinary Breastfeeding.*
5. Palmer, "There Comes a Point When Breast Is Not Best."
6. Ibid.
7. Ibid.
8. This specific video has been removed. However, another posting of the clip remains on *Youtube.*
9. Johnson, ""Are You Mom Enough?"
10. Ibid.
11. Parsons, "Time Magazine Asks 'Are You Mom Enough?' Every Mom Should Be Offended."
12. Ibid.
13. Ablow, "Time Magazine Cover – Forget the Breast, What about the Boy?"
14. Douglas and Michaels, *The Mommy Myth: The Idealization of Motherhood and How It Has Undermined Women.*
15. Hausman, "Feminism and Breastfeeding"; Callaghan and Lazard, "'Please Don't Put the Whole Dang Thing out There!'."
16. Carlson, "Game of Thrones."
17. Norwood and Turner, "The Breast Is (Always) for Sex."
18. Mandel et al., "Fat and Energy Contents of Expressed Human Breast Milk in Prolonged Lactation"; Onyango, Receveur, and Esrey, "The Contribution of Breast Milk to Toddler Diets in Western Kenya."
19. Dettwyler, "A Time to Wean: The Hominid Blueprint for the Natural Age of Weaning in Modern Human Populations."
20. Stuebe and Bonuck, "What Predicts Intent to Breastfeed Exclusively?"
21. Commissioner, "Pediatrics - Use of Donor Human Milk."
22. Jones, "History of North American Donor Milk Banking."
23. Updegrove, "Nonprofit Human Milk Banking in the United States."
24. Ibid.
25. "FAQs - Prolacta Bioscience."
26. Schnabl et al., "Necrotizing Enterocolitis."
27. McGuire and Anthony, "Donor Human Milk versus Formula for Preventing Necrotising Enterocolitis in Preterm Infants"; Sullivan et al., "An Exclusively Human Milk-Based Diet Is Associated with a Lower Rate of Necrotizing Enterocolitis than a Diet of Human Milk and Bovine Milk-Based Products"; Sisk et al., "Early Human Milk Feeding Is Associated with a Lower Risk of Necrotizing Enterocolitis in Very

Low Birth Weight Infants"; Meinzen-Derr et al., "Role of Human Milk in Extremely Low Birth Weight Infants|[rsquo]| Risk of Necrotizing Enterocolitis or Death."

28. Vohr et al., "Beneficial Effects of Breast Milk in the Neonatal Intensive Care Unit on the Developmental Outcome of Extremely Low Birth Weight Infants at 18 Months of Age."
29. Bishara et al., "Volume of Foremilk, Hindmilk, and Total Milk Produced by Mothers of Very Preterm Infants Born at Less Than 28 Weeks of Gestation"; Smith et al., "Initiation of Breastfeeding Among Mothers of Very Low Birth Weight Infants."
30. Updegrove, "Nonprofit Human Milk Banking in the United States."
31. Ibid.
32. Gribble, "Peer-to-Peer Milk Donors' and Recipients' Experiences and Perceptions of Donor Milk Banks."
33. Palmquist, "Demedicalizing Breastmilk."
34. Gribble, "Peer-to-Peer Milk Donors' and Recipients' Experiences and Perceptions of Donor Milk Banks."
35. Ibid.
36. Ibid.
37. Palmquist and Doehler, "Contextualizing Online Human Milk Sharing."
38. Ibid.
39. Ibid.
40. Palmquist, "Demedicalizing Breastmilk."
41. Steele, Martyn, and Foell, "Risks of the Unregulated Market in Human Breast Milk."
42. Fildes, *Breasts, Bottles and Babies—a History of Infant Feeding.*; Golden, *A Social History of Wet Nursing in America.*
43. Bonyata, "KellyMom.com : How Much Expressed Milk Will My Baby Need?"
44. Van Esterik, *Beyond the Breast-Bottle Controversy.*
45. Ibid.
46. Keim et al., "Microbial Contamination of Human Milk Purchased via the Internet."
47. Ibid.
48. "Dangerous Bacteria Found in Breast Milk Sold on Internet| Fox News."
49. Bakalar, "Breast Milk Donated or Sold Online Is Often Tainted, Study Says."
50. Keim et al., "Cow's Milk Contamination of Human Milk Purchased via the Internet."
51. Firger, 2015, and Pm, "Breast Milk Sold Online Often Contaminated by Cow's Milk."
52. Ibid.

53. Doucleff, "Breast Milk Sold Online Contaminated With Cow's Milk."
54. Vogel, "Milk Sharing"; Gribble and Hausman, "Milk Sharing and Formula Feeding."
55. Carroll, "Body Dirt or Liquid Gold?"
56. Huang, "The 2008 Milk Scandal Revisited."
57. Stuebe, Gribble, and Palmquist, "Differences between Online Milk Sales and Peer-to-Peer Milk sharing. (E-Letter Reply to Keim et Al., Microbial Contamination of Human Milk Purchased via the Internet)."
58. Giles, "Reinstating Pleasure in Reality: Promoting Breastfeeding through Ars Erotica," p. 216.
59. Giles, "'Relational, and Strange.'"
60. Bartlett, "Maternal Sexuality and Breastfeeding."
61. "Sexuality & Breastfeeding."
62. Giles, "Reinstating Pleasure in Reality: Promoting Breastfeeding through Ars Erotica."
63. Ibid.
64. Hanson, "Breastfeeding Man: Jeff Says Drinking Wife Michelle's Milk Helped His Erectile Dysfunction Symptoms."
65. Ibid.
66. Giles, "Reinstating Pleasure in Reality: Promoting Breastfeeding through Ars Erotica."
67. Ibid.
68. Duvall, "Not 'Simply the Breast' Media Discourses of Celebrity, Breastfeeding, and Normalcy."
69. Fildes, *Breasts, Bottles and Babies - a History of Infant Feeding.*
70. Palmquist, "Demedicalizing Breastmilk"; Giles, "Reinstating Pleasure in Reality: Promoting Breastfeeding through Ars Erotica."
71. Palmquist, "Demedicalizing Breastmilk"; Vogel, "Milk Sharing"; Hausman, *Viral Mothers.*

CHAPTER 10

Concluding Thoughts: Media's Role in Improving Breastfeeding Success

It is now common knowledge that breastfeeding is best for babies. While some naysayers occasionally question the extent of these advantages, most people, including college students and others that do not have children, agree on breastfeeding's superiority.[1] At this point, the problem is that most people are uncomfortable with breastfeeding and that we have numerous social, cultural, and institutional barriers to successful breastfeeding.[2] Media strongly contribute to society's discomfort, the normalization of bottle-feeding, narrow definitions of breastfeeding mothers, scrutiny over public nursing, angry responses to breastfeeding photos and videos, and fictional tales of breastfeeding used in criminally-deviant ways. These messages are then situated within an environment rich with well-funded and strategized formula marketing that is so engaging that people willingly distribute its products to their friends and family.

This book is not about the breast vs. bottle dichotomy/"controversy," but about media's dominant role in emphasizing individual choice, individual behavior, and individual responsibility for breastfeeding success and failure, while persistently undermining breastfeeding by creating a culture that is far more conducive to formula-feeding. We have legislation that protects a mother's right to breastfeed *anywhere* she wishes. However, news, entertainment, and social media convey to the public that she will likely be publicly shamed for her behavior.

A study of media's coverage and representations from the mid-1800s until contemporary times reveals that many of the issues with perceptions of breastfeeding today stem from the nineteenth century. First, media

K.A. Foss, *Breastfeeding and Media*,
DOI 10.1007/978-3-319-56442-5_10

has repeatedly conveyed the (false) message that breastfeeding will fail. Starting with artificial food ads of the 1880s, this discourse introduces myths of "insufficient milk," threatening mothers' confidence in breastfeeding success. This approach, while profitable for the formula companies, injects doubt into the burgeoning breastfeeding relationship. Since self-efficacy is the best predictor of success, these messages can damage confidence beyond repair, particularly for certain groups of women already at-risk.[3]

A consistent theme is that people are generally uncomfortable with breastfeeding. Before bottle-feeding became common in the 1800s, this was obviously not the case. Babies were breastfed, period. And prior to industrialization, women also had more familiarity with childbirth and breastfeeding through their relationships with family and community members.[4] The popularity of bottle-feeding not only meant that fewer women breastfed but that society itself was less exposed to breastfeeding.[5] Children did not grow up watching their mothers, aunts, and family friends nurse. Breastfeeding became a less common sight in public spaces as it was replaced by bottle-feeding. Media reinforced this invisibility, so rarely showing breastfeeding in film and television that one could have questioned it as a means of feeding a baby. Until contemporary times, babies on the big and small screens have been almost exclusively bottle-fed, likely due to self-censorship of the industry and perceived public reaction. Even in parenting magazines and childrearing books, photos and drawings of bottle-feeding have historically far outweighed the natural way of feeding babies. It is not surprising then that people are uncomfortable with breastfeeding since most have not seen it. The public's discomfort with breastfeeding extends to breastmilk. Instead of equating human milk to the dairy products of other animals, popular culture representations have largely associated breastmilk with other bodily fluids. For example, Al Bundy of *Married with Children* compares public breastfeeding to public urination. With such messages, it is no wonder most people gasp at the idea of sharing milk.

A continued disparity exists among different groups of women. Cultural beliefs stemming from painful collective histories, as well as attitudes toward health professionals and perceptions of infant nourishment, continue to hinder breastfeeding rates.[6] Differences among groups of women tend to be overlooked in media. Assumptions about ethnicity, age, and other factors are not addressed, including ways in which interventions could help increase overall breastfeeding rates. Furthermore, news and entertainment media perpetuate blame, particularly for African

American women, criticize them for nursing in public, and generally refrain from offering positive representations of women of color breastfeeding.[7]

Competing Discourses

Through this study of 200 years of media, competing discourses emerge, many of which have detracted from successful breastfeeding promotion. Magazine articles and ads, medical journals, pregnancy promotional materials, new baby books for parents and children, reality programs, fictional television, *Youtube* videos, and online responses to breastfeeding "as spectacle" were analyzed to ascertain media's messages about breastfeeding, infant feeding, and related topics and products. While the technology has evolved, marketing strategies, the role of medical "experts" in infant feeding, and other barriers to breastfeeding continue to create divisions among groups of people that impede breastfeeding promotion and success.

Breastfeeding as Health Prevention or Cultural Experience

Much of the mainstream media coverage (and the first chapter of this book) touts the wealth of scientific evidence that breastfeeding improve short- and long-term health for both mother and child. Aside from a few vocal critics, the benefits in reducing risks and overall better health are what sell breastfeeding to health policy makers, care providers, and the general public. This knowledge is well-established, difficult to refute, and reflects the American focus on quantifiable evidence reminiscent of the rise of logic and reason with industrialization. The focus on benefits is important and has been effective in raising general awareness of breastfeeding. However, as scholars have pointed out, the medical aspects are only part of understanding breastfeeding and its success. In some ways, we can compare breastfeeding to healthy eating. The public has been taught to consume vegetables and fruit more than bacon and fast food. That said, the rampant obesity in the United States suggests that there is a gap between knowing the benefits of healthy eating and adopting a healthy lifestyle. Eating can be social, emotional, and cultural and is linked to socio-economic status, geography, religion, access to healthy food, and knowledge of how to prepare the food. Like breastfeeding, it is also hard to maintain a healthy diet if you are surrounded by people eating junk food. Effective campaigns at changing behavior offer specific, achieveable modifications—for example, the "1% or Less" community education effort raised awareness of the importance of drinking low-fat milk instead of whole or 2%.[8] A follow-up survey indicated that 38.2% of respondents had switched from high- to low-fat milk and maintained the switch for 6 months.[9] Obviously, breastfeeding promotion is more complex than purchasing different milk. And yet, the importance of understanding a community's barrier to change, paired with specific goals (i.e. more lactation support) could help with effective breastfeeding promotion, especially if women's feelings and experiences are considered in the message design.

To only discuss the impact of the physiological process of lactation removes the very intimate and emotional experience of the the mother and child. It divorces the product from its relationship. While some women may be prompted to breastfeed for the benefits, it is not the only reason to breastfeed and to keep breastfeeding. Charlotte Faircloth conducted an ethnographic study with LLL groups in the United Kingdom, which included interviews on the breastfeeding experience. She explained how many women decided to nurse because that was the decision that felt "right."[10] Just as importantly, emotion is a factor in early weaning. Mozingo and colleagues interviewed mothers who stopped breastfeeding within two weeks and found that their experiences significantly influenced their desire to wean.[11] Instead of focusing on physical obstacles, mothers reported feeling tired, frustrated, uncomfortable, and inadequate with breastfeeding—that their experiences did not match their expectations of what nursing would be like.[12] They expressed feelings of relief, as well as shame and guilt at "failing."[13] Likewise, Hauck and Irurita also found a disconnect between mothers' expectations of breastfeeding and their (often disappointing) experiences.[14] These studies serve not only as a reminder that breastfeeding is about the whole mother and her feelings, not just her breasts, but also holds clinical implications. The researchers stress the importance of health care providers who are sensitive to mothers' emotions about breastfeeding and acknowledge and address them in a positive way.[15]

The scientific and the cultural frameworks of breastfeeding can and do overlap. Breastfeeding support is not just about physical instruction on latching and positioning, or prescriptions for treating mastitis. As Aimee Eden discussed, lactation consultants straddle both the medical and the cultural approaches to breastfeeding, offering physiological and emotional support.[16] A mother's perceptions of support influence her confidence and overall breastfeeding success.[17] LLL groups and peer-to-peer support help to guide and reassure new mothers.[18] Palmquist demonstrated the connection experienced by those involved in milk sharing, noting how these relationships help to demedicalize breastfeeding.[19] This approach has and can certainly apply to support for breastfeeding mothers. In addition to encouraging mothers, highlighting the cultural framework of breastfeeding also acknowledges and celebrates other emotional aspects, including enjoyment and pain, pleasure and discomfort.[20] More media discourse that encompasses mothers' various feelings and array of experiences could help prepare women for the range of sensations experienced in breastfeeding, helping to create realistic expectations and reassure them that their experiences are normal, not shameful.

Breastfeeding as Feminist?

Tension exists between discourses that promote breastfeeding as Feminist and those that claim that breastfeeding tethers babies to their mothers and therefore strips away agency. In "What Can Feminists Do for Breastfeeding?," Jacqueline Wolf outlined the various ways in which improving conditions for breastfeeding would also heighten public awareness, improving policies and legislation that benefit women's rights overall, including maternity leaves and reproductive rights.[21] Van Esterik argued that to encourage breastfeeding is to encourage women to seize control of their breasts and their bodies, empowering women to be independent and to have faith in their bodies.[22] Paralleling these words, Paige Hall Smith has pointed out that promoting breastfeeding values women's bodies, helping to bridge the private and public spheres.[23] Furthermore, Smith argued, the barriers that have impeded breastfeeding derive from overall obstacles to women's equality—the sexualization and objectification of women, the domination of men over women, and the deeply entrenched sexual division of labor, where private sphere work (i.e. caring for the home) is unpaid and perceived as inferior.[24] Breastfeeding promotion, then, should consider the overall implications for gender equality, without, as Smith stated, "defining women's essence by their bodily abilities."[25] Blum offered a similar argument, integrating breastfeeding into discourse on gender inequality and the construction of motherhood.[26] Both scholars concur that careful strategies, including the incorporation of pleasure and experience, can promote breastfeeding without objectifying breasts.[27]

As opposed to Wolf, Smith, Hausman, Blum and others that regard breastfeeding and Feminism as being inextricably connected, some Feminists argue that breastfeeding runs counter to gender equality. Notably, Joan Wolf, in *Is Breast Best? Taking on the Breastfeeding Experts and the New High Stakes of Motherhood* (2010) declared that breastfeeding, as part of "the total motherhood," is disempowering by encouraging mothers to place their children's need to breastfeed above their own needs, and creating guilt and shame for bottle-feeding women.[28] Amy Koerber argued that the rhetorical strategies of overusing "science-based messages" to promote breastfeeding was often problematic, especially from a Feminist standpoint.[29] Hausman analyzed the rhetoric of both Feminist breastfeeding advocates and Feminists who do not perceive breastfeeding as Feminist, discovering distinct associations between position and perception of infant feeding in culture. Pro-bottle-feeding scholars present the world as more breastfeeding-friendly, yet Feminist breastfeeding advocates see the dominance of bottles in public discourse, with numerous obstacles to success.[30] Yet, Feminists on both sides have agreed that it is problematic to promote breastfeeding within socio-cultural contexts that impede breastfeeding.[31] Bottle-feeding Feminists argue for less attention to breastfeeding and more on freedom to choose the mode of infant feeding.[32] Feminist breastfeeding advocates, on the other hand, push for shifting the socio-cultural context to make it more conducive to breastfeeding.[33] We see this tension played out in different ways in media texts, with messages that establish a false dichotomy of the "good breastfeeder" and "bad bottle-feeder" or the breastfeeder as "Supermom" in the *Time* magazine cover, and fictional Lactivists on television who use breastfeeding as political statements. On the contrary, some parenting books present breastfeeding as isolating, binding a mother to her home and her baby—a message also conveyed by television's criticism of the public breastfeeder, the lonely teen mom in her short breastfeeding stint, or the backlash to "extreme" breastfeeders. Even the more positive messages about breastfeeding are troubling, as they shift focus (and guilt) to individual mothers, ignoring a system that sets up women to fail.

Discourses of the *Mommy Wars*

As the Similac "Mother 'Hood" ad capitalizes on, breastfeeding (or at least media's coverage of it) can polarize women, attaching it to an identity of "superior" motherhood.[34] Much of the opposition to the *Time* magazine cover involved the title of "Are You Mom Enough?" paired with the image of the breastfeeding child. These messages are perpetuated throughout media channels, at least for mothers whose breastfeeding relationships fall within societal definitions of "normal." For example, viewers react positively to *Youtube* videos of breastfeeding small babies, praising the mothers for their success. Such media examples reinforce a battle between those who breastfeed and those who do not, associating not breastfeeding with failure and inferior mothering. Breastfeeding is intertwined with conceptualizations and identities of motherhood.[25] Joan Wolf used this implication of blame as justification to stop breastfeeding promotion. However, I hold that this argument reflects a misplaced assessment of the issue and the solution.

Indeed, mothers have reported feelings of guilt and shame for not breastfeeding.[36] Marianne Neifert contended that pressure and guilt placed on women to breastfeed can result in babies' failure to thrive and other tragedies from breastfeeding.[37] Stories of undernourished babies due to breastfeeding pressure have been common in media, playing up rare cases in which children starved.[38] Hausman has discussed these frames of tragedy, stating that they implicate blame, particularly for women of color.[39] These fears of inducing guilt have been used as one argument against risk messages in breastfeeding promotion.[40] Most promotion, in fact, does not use risk messages.[41] And yet, as we have seen, media have no issues with disseminating exaggerated stories about breastfeeding risks. One tragedy, the Walrond case, was distorted into a broad generalization that breastfeeding could starve your baby, which completely ignored the damaging health effects of not breastfeeding. In addition, Hausman and Gribble have laid out how media rarely touch upon risks, and then tragedies, of not breastfeeding.[42] To simply blame mothers for not breastfeeding unfairly ignores the numerous people and factors that come together to make breastfeeding work. Labbok outlined how responsibility for successful breastfeeding rests on others beyond the mother, demonstrating how health professionals and the health care system need to set up mothers to meet their nursing goals.[43] In addition, policymakers, employers, media producers, and numerous other people play a role in an individual woman's success.[44]

With all of these factors in mind, it is possible to bridge the fierce division of the *Mommy Wars.* First, more diversified media messages and representations of breastfeeding women will help broaden the image of the noble breastfeeding woman to encompass a variety of lifestyles, personalities, and situations. More images of military moms breastfeeding in uniform, women in same-sex couples, more women of color and teenage mothers breastfeeding will expand and transform what has been upheld as the breastfeeding mother—a process that will also help women of different groups feel that they can breastfeed. Second, creating a cultural climate conducive to breastfeeding will not only improve success, but also shift blame for not breastfeeding away from mothers. We should not shy away from risk-messages, but incorporate and acknowledge barriers in the socio-cultural context. Finally, as a society, we should not encourage media that promote the *Mommy Wars.* Stop sharing and "liking" videos that parody or celebrate this division and look for media support of partnerships.

What's Overlooked in Media?

Most of this book has focused on what is talked about and portrayed in media messages about breastfeeding. Little attention has been given to what is missing or nearly invisible. As stated, the type of women breastfeeding has been limited in these constructions. While rates are higher for certain groups (older, more educated, higher income, average weight, Caucasian or Hispanic, etc.), that does not mean that no one is breastfeeding outside of these social intersections. We need more visibility of breastfeeding mothers across these groups—teen mothers, women of different ethnicities, working women, various body types, people who are LGBTQ, and the abundant ways in which these characteristics intersect. [45] Stories with a diversity of breastfeeding mothers need to appear in news and entertainment media, in reality television, online, and in parenting and children's books so that role models exist, not just for expectant parents, but for society in general.

We also need more images and stories of breastfeeding older children and in public spaces, without backlash and criticism. The more that people see breastfeeding mothers, the more they will accept breastfeeding and be comfortable with it. This is the first step in creating a breastfeeding-friendly environment. Media lack stories addressing the breastfeeding of adopted children, surrogates expressing milk, relactation, positive stories about human milk donation and selling, and the use of Supplemental Nursing Systems. Again, more attention to these overlooked issues will not only help mothers, but broaden the public's definition of what nursing is and should look like.

We have established the benefits of breastfeeding to the extent to which college students know of its superiority.[46] What we need now is more discourse on breastfeeding experiences, including the array of emotion and feelings, so that mothers and fathers can set realistic expectations and we can celebrate pleasure in breastfeeding.[47] More information on how to overcome obstacles and difficult situations is needed in mainstream media, including fictional and reality TV, parenting books and news stories so that mothers can meet their breastfeeding goals. Advice on specific challenges is essential, such as increasing milk supply, thrush, mastitis, sleepy or fussy babies, awkward positioning and painful latches, as well as encouragement on emotional issues (i.e., postpartum depression, feelings of inadequacy and doubt, or other concerns).

The many people that can help with breastfeeding have been largely ignored, including the important role of partners, but also lactation consultants, IBCLCs, peer support counselors, and breastfeeding educators. These breastfeeding experts and helpers can significantly improve success, especially for women at-risk for not breastfeeding.[48] In addition, more information about doulas would also improve success. In a study of Medicaid recipients and breastfeeding rates, women who had doulas (who were ethnically diverse, reflecting the population) had a 97% initiation rate, compared to 80% for women birthing without doulas.[49] Of the African American women with doula care, 92.7% initiated breastfeeding, while only 70.3% mothers without doula support started breastfeeding.[50] More attention to this network of support would help mothers and their partners become aware of the possible resources available to them.

Finally, media tend to reinforce division, not unification. More messages are required to bring people together about breastfeeding: men and women; fathers to fathers; breast, bottle, and mixed feeders; working and stay-at-home mothers; academics and practitioners; physicians, nurses, and those in lactation support and other groups, to work together to help create a breastfeeding-friendly environment.

How can we create a more breastfeeding-friendly society and what are media's roles in this shift? Labbok, Hall Smith, Wolf, Hausman, and other scholars have prescribed ways to improve breastfeeding in society.[51] Media play a significant role in this success. At the policy level, the implementation of formula regulation that adheres to the tenets of the International Code of Breastmilk Substitutes would call attention to the ways in which formula marketing undermines breastfeeding success, especially with contemporary technology.[52] Specifically, laws are needed that prohibit direct-to-consumer marketing of formula, meaning no more television and Internet commercials. While some may argue that this regulation is not possible in the free-market society of the United States, we can point to the voluntarily cessation of direct-to-consumer marketing that was upheld from the 1920s until the late 1980s.[53]

At the institutional level, health professionals could refuse to distribute formula samples or coupons to their patients. As Howard, Howard, and Weitzman discussed, this distribution is a mark of endorsement.[54] The increase of Baby-Friendly hospitals would also help create an environment more conducive to breastfeeding. Furthermore, recognition of points of weakness within Baby-Friendly identification and compliance would also help breastfeeding.[55] Media stories that praise hospitals with this distinction would heighten its prestige and could be used to help draw potential patients. Furthermore, media within hospitals could communicate the importance of the Baby-Friendly practices to health care providers who question the adoption of these practices and offer additional training on breastfeeding.[56]

Media creators themselves could also be more proactive in promoting breastfeeding. Much like the writers of *The Big Bang Theory*, *The Office*, and *Bones*, television producers could integrate pro-breastfeeding storylines and refuse formula product placement. These actions could be particularly important in reality television, especially with teen programming. Online, website managers could better serve as gatekeepers to reduce formula marketing, labeling formula sponsorship of content or refusing to run formula ads, especially on breastfeeding websites. Those that maintain websites could also flag or remove anti-breastfeeding messages.

Communities should create spaces to support breastfeeding. Local media could recognize retail stores, other places of employment, and public venues that are supportive of breastfeeding. Linked to this community level is the general public. Consumers can make a commitment to boycott viral videos that promote formula, refuse to click on formula marketing, and protest when sneaky sponsorship is used without disclosure. And of course, people can support each other, by encouraging expectant parents to take breastfeeding classes, supporting breastfeeding in public and bringing discussion about breastfeeding into the public sphere. Just as important, we need to acknowledge that breastfeeding success is a societal responsibility, not an individual choice.[57] These measures will help create a breastfeeding-friendly culture in which every mother feels supported and that every person can feel confident that children are truly receiving the best.

Notes

1. Kavanagh et al., "Breastfeeding Knowledge, Attitudes, Prior Exposure, and Intent among Undergraduate Students"; Foss and Blake, "'It's Natural and Healthy, But I Don't Want To See It': The Impact of Entertainment Television on Breastfeeding Attitudes."
2. Foss and Blake, "'It's Natural and Healthy, But I Don't Want To See It': The Impact of Entertainment Television on Breastfeeding Attitudes"; Spear, "College Students' Experiences and Attitudes Regarding Middle and High School–Based Breastfeeding Education"; Kavanagh et al., "Breastfeeding Knowledge, Attitudes, Prior Exposure, and Intent among Undergraduate Students."
3. de Jager et al., "The Role of Psychosocial Factors in Exclusive Breastfeeding to Six Months Postpartum"; Meedya, Fahy, and Kable, "Factors That Positively Influence Breastfeeding Duration to 6 Months"; Kools et al., "The Motivational Determinants of Breast-Feeding: Predictors for the Continuation of Breast-Feeding."
4. Wolf, *Don't Kill Your Baby: Public Health and the Decline of Breastfeeding in the 19th and 20th Centuries.*
5. Ibid.
6. Blum, *At the Breast*; Horodynski, Calcatera, and Carpenter, "Infant Feeding Practices"; Johnson et al., "Enhancing Breastfeeding Rates among African American Women."
7. Hausman, *Mother's Milk.*
8. Reger et al., "1% or Less."
9. Ibid.
10. Faircloth, "'It Feels Right in My Heart.'"
11. Mozingo et al., "It Wasn't Working."
12. Ibid.
13. Ibid.
14. Hauck and Irurita, "Incompatible Expectations."

15. Mozingo et al., "It Wasn't Working."
16. Eden, "New Professions and Old Practice: Lactation Consulting and the Medicalization of Breastfeeding."
17. Mannion et al., "Maternal Perceptions of Partner Support during Breastfeeding"; Schmied et al., "Women's Perceptions and Experiences of Breastfeeding Support."
18. Rossman, "Breastfeeding Peer Counselors in the United States"; Chapman et al., "Effectiveness of Breastfeeding Peer Counseling in a Low-Income, Predominantly Latina Population"; Faircloth, "'It Feels Right in My Heart.'"
19. Palmquist, "Demedicalizing Breastmilk."
20. Giles, "Reinstating Pleasure in Reality: Promoting Breastfeeding through Ars Erotica."
21. Wolf, "What Feminists Can Do for Breastfeeding and What Breastfeeding Can Do for Feminists."
22. Van Esterik, *Beyond the Breast-Bottle Controversy.*
23. Smith, "Breastfeeding Promotion through Gender Equality."
24. Ibid.
25. Ibid, p. 34.
26. Blum, "Mothers, Babies, and Breastfeeding in Late Capitalist America."
27. Smith, "Breastfeeding Promotion through Gender Equality"; Blum, "Mothers, Babies, and Breastfeeding in Late Capitalist America."
28. Wolf, *Is Breast Best?*
29. Koerber, *Breast or Bottle?: Contemporary Controversies in Infant-Feeding Policy and Practice.*
30. Hausman, "Breastfeeding, Rhetoric, and the Politics of Feminism."
31. Ibid.
32. Ibid.; Wolf, *Is Breast Best?*
33. Hausman, "Breastfeeding, Rhetoric, and the Politics of Feminism."
34. Similac, "The Mother 'Hood Official Video."
35. Knaak, "Contextualising Risk, Constructing Choice."
36. Taylor and Wallace, "Feminist Breastfeeding Promotion and the Problem of Guilt"; Labbok, "Exploration of Guilt Among Mothers Who Do Not Breastfeed."
37. Neifert, "Prevention of Breastfeeding Tragedies."
38. Hausman, *Mother's Milk.*
39. Ibid.
40. Wolf, "Is Breast Really Best?"
41. Stuebe, "The Risks of Not Breastfeeding for Mothers and Infants."
42. Gribble and Hausman, "Milk Sharing and Formula Feeding."
43. Labbok, "Exploration of Guilt Among Mothers Who Do Not Breastfeed."
44. Ibid.

45. Jones et al., "Factors Associated With Exclusive Breastfeeding in the United States"; Wojcicki, "Maternal Prepregnancy Body Mass Index and Initiation and Duration of Breastfeeding"; Forste, Weiss, and Lippincott, "The Decision to Breastfeed in the United States"; Hauff, Leonard, and Rasmussen, "Associations of Maternal Obesity and Psychosocial Factors with Breastfeeding Intention, Initiation, and Duration."
46. Marrone, Vogeltanz-Holm, and Holm, "Attitudes, Knowledge, and Intentions Related to Breastfeeding Among University Undergraduate Women and Men"; Foss and Blake, "'It's Natural and Healthy, But I Don't Want To See It': The Impact of Entertainment Television on Breastfeeding Attitudes."
47. Giles, "Reinstating Pleasure in Reality: Promoting Breastfeeding through Ars Erotica"; Hauck and Irurita, "Incompatible Expectations."
48. Chapman et al., "Effectiveness of Breastfeeding Peer Counseling in a Low-Income, Predominantly Latina Population"; Rossman, "Breastfeeding Peer Counselors in the United States"; Semenic et al., "Barriers, Facilitators, and Recommendations Related to Implementing the Baby-Friendly Initiative (BFI)."
49. Kozhimannil et al., "Doula Care Supports Near-Universal Breastfeeding Initiation among Diverse, Low-Income Women."
50. Ibid.
51. Labbok, "Breastfeeding in Public Health"; Smith, "Breastfeeding Promotion through Gender Equality"; Wolf, "What Feminists Can Do for Breastfeeding and What Breastfeeding Can Do for Feminists"; Gribble and Hausman, "Milk Sharing and Formula Feeding"; Hausman, "Breastfeeding, Rhetoric, and the Politics of Feminism."
52. Abrahams, "Milk and Social Media Online Communities and the International Code of Marketing of Breast-Milk Substitutes."
53. Greer and Apple, "Physicians, Formula Companies, and Advertising."
54. Howard, Howard, and Weitzman, "THE PHYSICIAN AS ADVERTISER."
55. Nickel et al., "The Extent That Noncompliance with the Ten Steps to Successful Breastfeeding Influences Breastfeeding Duration."
56. Koenig, "Breastfeeding Education for Healthier Babies. Baby-Friendly Designation Improves Infant, Mother and Community Health."
57. Labbok, "Exploration of Guilt Among Mothers Who Do Not Breastfeed."

References

▸ Teach Me How To Breast Feed [MUSIC VIDEO] - YouTube. https://www.youtube.com/watch?v=SZ3QO-7h4YA. Accessed 29 July 2015.

6 Ways to Fat-Proof Your Child. *Parents*. 2004.

2004.06.04: Public Service Campaign to Promote Breastfeeding Awareness Launched. http://archive.hhs.gov/news/press/2004pres/20040604.html. Accessed 29 July 2015.

A Wet Nurse. *Weekly Museum*, March 21, 1795.

A Wet Nurse. *The Time Piece; and Literary Companion*, August 25, 1797.

A Wet Nurse. *The Intellectual Regale or Ladies' Tea Tray*, November 25, 1815.

Aaronson, Lauren S., Carol Macnee Mural, and Susan K. Pfoutz. 1988. Seeking Information: Where Do Pregnant Women Go? *Health Education & Behavior* 15 (3): 335–345. doi:10.1177/109019818801500307.

Ablow, Keith. 2012. Time Magazine Cover—Forget the Breast, What about the Boy? | Fox News. Text.Article. *FoxNews.com*, May 11, 2012. http://www.foxnews.com/opinion/2012/05/11/time-magazine-cover-forget-breast-what-about-boy.html.

About JAMA. *The JAMA Network*, 2016. http://jama.jamanetwork.com/public/About.aspx.

About NEJM Past and Present. *The New England Journal of Medicine*, 2016. http://www.nejm.org/page/about-nejm/history-and-mission.

Abrahams, Sheryl W. 2012. Milk and Social Media Online Communities and the International Code of Marketing of Breast-Milk Substitutes. *Journal of Human Lactation* 28 (3): 400–406. doi:10.1177/0890334412447080.

Al-Sahab, Ban, Andrea Lanes, Mark Feldman, and Hala Tamim. 2010. Prevalence and Predictors of 6-Month Exclusive Breastfeeding among Canadian Women: A National Survey. *BMC Pediatrics* 10 (1): 20. doi:10.1186/1471-2431-10-20.

K.A. Foss, *Breastfeeding and Media*,
DOI 10.1007/978-3-319-56442-5

Amazon.com. 2015. On Becoming Baby Wise: Giving Your Infant the GIFT of Nighttime Sleep: (Amazon Entry). http://www.amazon.com/Becoming-Baby-Wise-Giving-Nighttime/dp/1932740139/ref=sr_1_1?ie=UTF8&qid=1438218819&sr=8-1&keywords=On+Becoming+Babywise.

Ample Supply of Bottles, Nipples. *Parents*, 1943.

Anglo-Swiss Milk Food. *The Ladies' Home Journal and Practical Housekeeper*, 1884.

Anstey, Erica H., Carol MacGowan, and Jessica A. Allen. 2016. Five-Year Progress Update on the Surgeon General's Call to Action to Support Breastfeeding, 2011. *Journal of Women's Health*, August 1, 2016. doi:10.1089/jwh.2016.5990.

Appendix 5: Guidelines for BBC Commercial Services on Editorial Integrity and Independence from External Interests. *BBC.com*, 2016. http://www.bbc.co.uk/editorialguidelines/guidelines/appendix5/product-placement.

Apple, Rima D. 1987. *Mothers and Medicine: A Social History of Infant Feeding*. Madison, WI: University of Wisconsin Press. https://books.google.com/books/about/Mothers_and_Medicine.html?id=GNpSsJSkobEC.

Apple, Rima D. 1995. Constructing Mothers: Scientific Motherhood in the Nineteenth and Twentieth Centuries. *Social History of Medicine* 8 (2): 161–178. doi:10.1093/shm/8.2.161.

Apple, Rima D. 2006. *Perfect Motherhood*. New Brunswick, NJ: Rutgers University Press. https://books.google.com/books/about/Perfect_Motherhood.html?id-=73PMY8itf3cC.

Arora, Samir, Cheryl McJunkin, Julie Wehrer, and Phyllis Kuhn. 2000. Major Factors Influencing Breastfeeding Rates: Mother's Perception of Father's Attitude and Milk Supply. *Pediatrics* 106 (5): e67–e67.

Article 2. *The Ladies' Home Journal and Practical Housekeeper*, August 1885.

ASH/OPHS. The Surgeon General's Call to Action to Support Breastfeeding. http://www.surgeongeneral.gov/library/calls/breastfeeding/index.html. Accessed 28 July 2015.

Asiodu, Ifeyinwa V., Catherine M. Waters, Dawn E. Dailey, Kathryn A. Lee, and Audrey Lyndon. 2015. Breastfeeding and Use of Social Media Among First-Time African American Mothers. *Journal of Obstetric, Gynecologic, & Neonatal Nursing* 44 (2): 268–278. doi:10.1111/1552-6909.12552.

Avery, Melissa, Laura Duckett, Joan Dodgson, Kay Savik, and Susan J. Henly. n.d. Factors Associated with Very Early Weaning Among Primiparas Intending to Breastfeed. *Maternal and Child Health Journal* 2 (3): 167–179. doi:10.1023/A:1021879227044.

Baby-Friendly Hospital Initiative. 2012. *Baby-Friendly USA*. https://www.babyfriendlyusa.org/about-us/baby-friendly-hospital-initiative.

Bakalar, Nicholas. 2013. Breast Milk Donated or Sold Online Is Often Tainted, Study Says. *The New York Times*, October 21. http://www.nytimes.com/2013/10/21/health/breast-milk-donated-or-sold-online-is-often-tainted-study-says.html.

Barona-Vilar, Carmen, Vincenta Escribá-Agüir, and Raquel Ferrero-Gandía. 2009. A Qualitative Approach to Social Support and Breast-Feeding Decisions. *Midwifery* 25 (2): 187–194. doi:10.1016/j.midw.2007.01.013.

Bartick, Melissa, and Arnold Reinhold. 2010. The Burden of Suboptimal Breastfeeding in the United States: A Pediatric Cost Analysis. *Pediatrics* 125 (5): e1048–1056. doi:10.1542/peds.2009-1616.

Bartlett, Alison. 2007. Maternal Sexuality and Breastfeeding. *Sex Education*, January 23. doi:10.1080/1468181420000301894.

Baumslag, Naomi, and Dia L. Michels. 1995. *Milk, Money, and Madness: The Culture and Politics of Breastfeeding*. New York: Praeger Pub Text.

Beard, Meg. 2014. 'Bfed' Texting Program and 'Breastfeeding: A Smart Choice' Class: Using Cell Phones to Reach Gen Y Mothers. *Clinical Lactation* 5 (4): 123–127.

Becker, Marshall H., Lois A. Maiman, John P. Kirscht, Don P. Haefner, and Robert H. Drachman. 1977. The Health Belief Model and Prediction of Dietary Compliance: A Field Experiment. *Journal of Health and Social Behavior* 18 (4): 348–366. doi:10.2307/2955344.

Belamarich, Peter F., Risa E. Bochner, and Andrew D. Racine. 2016. A Critical Review of the Marketing Claims of Infant Formula Products in the United States. *Clinical Pediatrics* 55 (5): 437–442. doi:10.1177/0009922815589913.

Bentley, Margaret E., Deborah L. Dee, and Joan L. Jensen. 2003. Breastfeeding among Low Income, African-American Women: Power, Beliefs and Decision Making. *The Journal of Nutrition* 133 (1): 305S–309S.

Berger, Peter L., and Thomas Luckmann. 1967. *The Social Construction of Reality: A Treatise in the Sociology of Knowledge*. New York: Anchor.

Bernath, Maja. 1960. A Bottle for Baby with Love. *Parents*, May 1960.

Bernstein, Nina. 1999a. Mother Charged With Starving Baby Tells of Frantic Effort to Save Him. *New York Times*, May 1999.

Bernstein, Nina. 1999b. Mother Convicted in Infant's Starvation Death Gets 5 Years' Probation. *New York Times*, September 9, 1999. http://www.nytimes.com/1999/09/09/nyregion/mother-convicted-in-infant-s-starvation-death-gets-5-years-probation.html?ref=topics.

Bernstein, Nina. 1999c. Trial Begins for Mother in Breast-Fed Infant's Starvation Death. *New York Times*, April 28, 1999. http://www.nytimes.com/1999/04/28/nyregion/trial-begins-for-mother-in-breast-fed-infant-s-starvation-death.html?ref=topics.

Beyerlein, Andreas, and Rüdiger von Kries. 2011. Breastfeeding and Body Composition in Children: Will There Ever Be Conclusive Empirical Evidence for a Protective Effect against Overweight? *The American Journal of Clinical Nutrition* 94 (6): 1772S–1775S. doi:10.3945/ajcn.110.000547.

Bishara, Rosine, Michael S. Dunn, Susan E. Merko, and Pauline Darling. 2009. Volume of Foremilk, Hindmilk, and Total Milk Produced by Mothers of Very

Preterm Infants Born at Less Than 28 Weeks of Gestation. *Journal of Human Lactation* 25 (3): 272–279. doi:10.1177/0890334409334606.

Blair, Peter S., Jon Heron, and Peter J. Fleming. 2010. Relationship Between Bed Sharing and Breastfeeding: Longitudinal. *Population-Based Analysis. Pediatrics* 126 (5): e1119–1126. doi:10.1542/peds.2010-1277.

Blum, Linda M. 1993. Mothers, Babies, and Breastfeeding in Late Capitalist America: The Shifting Contexts of Feminist Theory. *Feminist Studies* 19 (2): 291–311.

Blum, Linda M. 1999. *At the Breast*. Boston, MA: Beacon Press.

Bologna, Caroline. 2015. A Playful Reminder That Judging Other Parents Is Wrong. *Huffington Post*, January 22, 2015. http://www.huffingtonpost.com/2015/01/22/mommy-wars-similac-video_n_6517242.html.

Bologna, Chelsea. 2014. Internet Cheers For Photo Of Mom Breastfeeding At Graduation. *The Huffington Post*, November 5, 2014. http://www.huffingtonpost.com/2014/11/05/breastfeeding-graduation-photo_n_6108164.html.

Bolton, Tracie A., Tan Chow, Patricia A. Benton, and Beth H. Olson. 2009. Characteristics Associated With Longer Breastfeeding Duration: An Analysis of a Peer Counseling Support Program. *Journal of Human Lactation* 25 (1): 18–27. doi:10.1177/0890334408325985.

Bonyata, Kelly. 2015. KellyMom.com: How Much Expressed Milk Will My Baby Need? *Kellymom.com*. http://kellymom.com/bf/pumpingmoms/pumping/milkcalc/#howmuch.

Bottle-Feeding Guilt. *Parents*, 2002.

Bracken, Beth. 2012. *Henry Helps with the Baby*. Mankato, MN: Picture Window Books.

Bramson, Leslie, Jerry W. Lee, Elizabeth Moore, Susanne Montgomery, Christine Neish, Khaled Bahjri, and Carolyn Lopez Melcher. 2010. Effect of Early Skin-to-Skin Mother–Infant Contact During the First 3 Hours Following Birth on Exclusive Breastfeeding During the Maternity Hospital Stay. *Journal of Human Lactation*, January 28, 2010. doi:10.1177/0890334409355779.

Breast Milk for Infants. *The New York Times*, May 30, 1867.

Breastfeeding Benefits | HealthCare.gov. https://www.healthcare.gov/coverage/breast-feeding-benefits/. Accessed 29 July 2015.

Breastfeeding Boom. *Parents*, May.

Breastfeeding Report Card–United States, 2010. Centers for Disease Control & Prevention, August 2010. http://www.cdc.gov/breastfeeding/pdf/BreastfeedingReportCard2010.pdf.

Breastfeeding Report Card: United States, 2014 - 2014breastfeedingreportcard.pdf. http://www.cdc.gov/breastfeeding/pdf/2014breastfeedingreportcard.pdf. Accessed 28 July 2015.

Breastfeeding State Laws. http://www.ncsl.org/research/health/breastfeeding-state-laws.aspx. Accessed 28 July 2015.

Brimdyr, Kajsa. 2002. Lactation Management: A Community of Practice. In *Reclaiming Breastfeeding for the United States*, ed. Karin Cadwell, 51–65. Mississauga: Jones and Bartlett Publishers.

Brodie, Mollyann, Ursula Foehr, Vicky Rideout, Neal Baer, Carolyn Miller, Rebecca Flournoy, and Drew Altman. 2001. Communicating Health Information Through The Entertainment Media. *Health Affairs* 20 (1): 192–199. doi:10.1377/hlthaff.20.1.192.

Brodribb, Wendy. 2011. Barriers to Translating Evidence-Based Breastfeeding Information into Practice. *Acta Paediatrica* 100 (4): 486–490. doi:10.1111/j.1651-2227.2010.02108.x.

Brott, Armin A., and Jennifer Ash. 2015. *The Expectant Father: The Ultimate Guide for Dads-to-Be*, 4th ed. New York: Abbeville Press.

Brown, Jane D., and Sheila Rose Peuchaud. 2008. Media and Breastfeeding: Friend or Foe? *International Breastfeeding Journal* 3 (15). http://www.biomedcentral.com/content/pdf/1746-4358-3-15.pdf.

Buchanan, Katie. 2006. *Extraordinary Breastfeeding*. Documentary.

Burke, S., Shonna Snyder, and Robin C. Rager. n.d. An Assessment of Faculty Usage of YouTube as a Teaching Resource. *The Internet Journal of Allied Health Sciences and Practice* 7 (1): 1–8.

Burke, Sloane C., and Shonna L. Snyder. 2008. YouTube: An Innovative Learning Resource for College Health Education Courses. *International Electronic Journal of Health Education* 11: 39–46.

Bylaska-Davies, Paula. 2015. Exploring the Effect of Mass Media on Perceptions of Infant Feeding. *Health Care for Women International*, January 22. http://www.tandfonline.com/doi/abs/10.1080/07399332.2015.1005304.

Cadwell, Karin. 2002. *Reclaiming Breastfeeding For The United States: Protection, Promotion And Support*, 1st ed. Boston: Jones & Bartlett Learning.

Callaghan, Jane E. M., and Lisa Lazard. 2012. 'Please Don't Put the Whole Dang Thing out There!': A Discursive Analysis of Internet Discussions around Infant Feeding. *Psychology & Health*, June 8, 2012. http://www.tandfonline.com/doi/abs/10.1080/08870446.2011.634294.

Cancel Bear. 2009. MTV's Season Finale of '16 & Pregnant' Hits Series High 2.1 Million Total Viewers Thursday - Ratings. *TVbytheNumbers.Zap2it.com*, July 20, 2009. http://tvbythenumbers.zap2it.com/2009/07/20/mtvs-season-finale-of-16-pregnant-hits-series-high-2-1-million-total-viewers-thursday/23134/.

Capucilli, Alyssa Satin. 2014. *Hannah Is a Big Sister*. Barron's Educational Series, Inc.

Carlson, Jessica. 2015. Game of Thrones: Extending Extended Breastfeeding and beyond. *Imperfect Parent*. http://www.imperfectparent.com/blog/2011/05/16/game-of-thrones-extending-extended-breastfeeding-and-beyond/. Accessed 29 July 2015.

Carnation Milk. This Gold Age for Babies. *Parents*, 1938.

Carnrick's Soluble Food. *The Ladies' Home Journal and Practical Housekeeper*, October 1887.

Carnrick's Soluble Food. *The Ladies' Home Journal and Practical Housekeeper*, March 1888.

Carroll, Katherine. 2014. Body Dirt or Liquid Gold? How the 'safety' of Donated Breastmilk Is Constructed for Use in Neonatal Intensive Care. *Social Studies of Science* 44 (3): 466–485. doi:10.1177/0306312714521705.

Carvalho, Jaidnara Alves de, Polyanna Keitte Fernandes Gurgel, Kálya Yasmine Nunes de Lima, Cilene Nunes Dantas, Cláudia Cristiane Filgueira Martins, and Francis Solange Vieira Tourinho. 2013. Analysis of YouTube Videos on Breastfeeding: Relevance and Benefit. *Journal of Nursing UFPE on Line [JNUOL/doi:* 10.5205/01012007*]* 7 (3): 1016–1022. doi:10.5205/3530.

Caulfield, Ernest. 1938. How Baby Care Has Changed. *Parents*, January 1938.

Chantry, Caroline J., Kathryn G. Dewey, Janet M. Peerson, Erin A. Wagner, and Laurie A. Nommsen-Rivers. 2014. In-Hospital Formula Use Increases Early Breastfeeding Cessation Among First-Time Mothers Intending to Exclusively Breastfeed. *The Journal of Pediatrics* 164 (6): 1339–1345.e5. doi:10.1016/j.jpeds.2013.12.035.

Chapman, Donna J., Grace Damio, Sara Young, and Rafael Pérez-Escamilla. 2004. Effectiveness of Breastfeeding Peer Counseling in a Low-Income, Predominantly Latina Population: A Randomized Controlled Trial. *Archives of Pediatrics & Adolescent Medicine* 158 (9): 897–902. doi:10.1001/archpedi.158.9.897.

Chen, Peggy G., Lara W. Johnson, and Marjorie S. Rosenthal. 2012. Sources of Education about Breastfeeding and Breast Pump Use: What Effect Do They Have on Breastfeeding Duration? An Analysis of the Infant Feeding Practices Survey II. *Maternal and Child Health Journal* 16 (7): 1421–1430.

Chetley, Andrew. 1986. *The Politics of Baby Foods: Successfully Challenges to International Marketing Strategies*. New York: Palgrave Macmillan.

Chezem, JoCarol, Carol Friesen, and Joan Boettcher. 2003. Breastfeeding Knowledge, Breastfeeding Confidence, and Infant Feeding Plans: Effects on Actual Feeding Practices. *Journal of Obstetric, Gynecologic, and Neonatal Nursing: JOGNN/NAACOG* 32 (1): 40–47.

Civardi, Anne. 2005. *Usborne First Experiences The New Baby*, ed. Michelle Bates. Tulsa, OK: Usborne Pub Ltd.

Cole, Joanna. 2010. *I'm a Big Brother*, Revised edition. New York: HarperFestival.

Collins, R.E. 1992. Fathering by Touch. *Parents*, 1992.

Community Guidelines - YouTube. https://www.youtube.com/yt/policyandsafety/communityguidelines.html. Accessed 29 July 2015.

Conrad, Peter. 2008. *The Medicalization of Society: On the Transformation of Human Conditions into Treatable Disorders*. Baltimore: JHU Press.

Cook, Amanda Barnes. 2015. Breastfeeding, Feminism, and Political Theory. The University of North Carolina at Chapel Hill. http://gradworks.umi.com/37/03/3703748.html.

Cooke-Jackson, Angela, and Elizabeth K. Hansen. 2008. Appalachian Culture and Reality TV: The Ethical Dilemma of Stereotyping Others. *Journal of Mass Media Ethics*, August 5, 2008. doi:10.1080/08900520802221946.

Coolidge, Emelyn Lincoln. 1902. The Care of the Baby in Summer. *The Ladies' Home Journal.*

Coolidge, Emelyn Lincoln. 1903. What to Do for a Baby Month By Month. *The Ladies' Home Journal.*

Coolidge, Emelyn Lincoln. 1904a. Mother's Calendar: Four Breast-Fed Babies Who Did Not Thrive, and How. *The Ladies' Home Journal.*

Coolidge, Emelyn Lincoln. 1904b. Mother's Calendar: The Care of Premature and Backward Children. *The Ladies' Home Journal.*

Coolidge, Emelyn Lincoln. 1904c. The Young Mother's Calendar: The Baby's Mouth and Teeth. *The Ladies' Home Journal.*

Coolidge, Emelyn Lincoln. 1904d. The Young Mother's Calendar: What to Do for Summer Complaint. *The Ladies' Home Journal.*

Coolidge, Emelyn Lincoln. 1904e. The Young Mother's Calendar: : Why Four Babies Could Not Sleep. *The Ladies' Home Journal.*

Coolidge, Emelyn Lincoln. 1905a. The Young Mother and Her Child. *The Ladies' Home Journal.*

Coolidge, Emelyn Lincoln. 1905b. The Young Mother and Her Child: The Proper Management of Breast-Fed Infants. *The Ladies' Home Journal.*

Coolidge, Emelyn Lincoln. 1906a. The Young Mothers' Home Club: An Ounce of Prevention Is Better Than a Pound of Cure. *The Ladies' Home Journal.*

Coolidge, Emelyn Lincoln. 1906b. The Young Mothers' Home Club: The Prevention of Rheumatism in Children. *The Ladies' Home Journal.*

Coolidge, Emelyn Lincoln. 1906c. The Young Mothers' Summer Club. *The Ladies' Home Journal.*

Coolidge, Emelyn Lincoln. 1909. *The Mothers' Manual: A Month By Month Guide for Young Mothers.* New York: A.S. Barnes & Company.

Corbin, H. 1944. How to Prepare the Baby's Formula. *Parents*, 1944.

Country Implementation of the International Code of Marketing of Breast-Milk Substitutes: Status Report 2011. Geneva: World Health Organization, 2011. http://apps.who.int/iris/bitstream/10665/85621/1/9789241505987_eng.pdf.

Crockett, Richard J., Thomas Pruzinsky, and John A. Persing. 2007. He Influence of Plastic Surgery 'reality TV' on Cosmetic Surgery Patient Expectations and Decision Making. *Plastic and Reconstructive Surgery* 120 (1): 316–324.

Cromi, Antonella, Maurizio Serati, Ilario Candeloro, Stefano Uccella, Sara Scandroglio, Massimo Agosti, and Fabio Ghezzi. 2015. Assisted Reproductive Technology and Breastfeeding Outcomes: A Case-Control Study. *Fertility and Sterility* 103 (1): 89–94. doi:10.1016/j.fertnstert.2014.10.009.

Cumming, Robert G., and Robin J. Klineberg. 1993. Breastfeeding and Other Reproductive Factors and the Risk of Hip Fractures in Elderly Women. *International Journal of Epidemiology* 22 (4): 684–691. doi:10.1093/ije/22.4.684.

Damon-Moore, Helen. 1994. *Magazines for the Millions: Gender and Commerce in the Ladies' Home Journal and the Saturday Evening Post, 1880–1910.* Albany: State University of New York Press.

Dangerous Bacteria Found in Breast Milk Sold on Internet| Fox News. http://www.foxnews.com/health/2013/10/21/bacteria-found-in-breast-milk-sold-on-internet/. Accessed 29 July 2015.

Davidson Health Nipple. *The Ladies' Home Journal*, 1897.

Davin, Solange. 2004. Healthy Viewing: The Reception of Medical Narratives. In *Health and the Media*, ed. Clive Seale, 143–159. Malden, MA: Blackwell Publishing.

Davis, Susan Kinney, Jaynelle F. Stichler, and Debra M. Poeltler. 2012. Increasing Exclusive Breastfeeding Rates in the Well-Baby Population. *Nursing for Women's Health* 16 (6): 460–470.

Dettwyler, Katherine A. 1995. A Time to Wean: The Hominid Blueprint for the Natural Age of Weaning in Modern Human Populations. In *Breastfeeding: Biocultural Perspectives*, ed. Patricia Stuart-Macadam and Katherine A. Dettwyler, 39–73. Hawthorne, NY: Aldine de Gruyter. https://books.google.com/books/about/Breastfeeding.html?id=uEylIbDr5RgC.

DiGirolamo, Ann M., Laurence M. Grummer-Strawn, and Sara B. Fein. 2003. Do Perceived Attitudes of Physicians and Hospital Staff Affect Breastfeeding Decisions? *Birth* 30 (2): 94–100. doi:10.1046/j.1523-536X.2003.00227.x.

Dixon, Travis L. 2007. Black Criminals and White Officers: The Effects of Racially Misrepresenting Law Breakers and Law Defenders on Television News. *Media Psychology* 10 (2): 270–291. doi:10.1080/15213260701375660.

Dobson, Mary. 2008. *Disease: The Extraordinary Stories Behind History's Deadliest Killers.* London: Quercus Books.

Dolgen, Lauren. 2011. Why I Created MTV's '16 and Pregnant.' *CNN*, May 5, 2011. http://www.cnn.com/2011/SHOWBIZ/TV/05/04/teen.mom.dolgen/index.html.

Domoff, Sarah E., Nova G. Hinman, Afton M. Koball, Amy Storfer-Isser, Victoria L. Carhart, Kyoung D. Baik, and Robert A. Carels. 2012. The Effects of Reality Television on Weight Bias: An Examination of The Biggest Loser. *Obesity* 20 (5): 993–998. doi:10.1038/oby.2011.378.

Dong, Qingwen, and Arthur Phillip Murrillo. 2007. The Impact of Television Viewing on Young Adults' Stereotypes Towards Hispanic Americans. *Human Communication* 10 (1): 33–44.

Doucleff, Michaeleen. 2015. Breast Milk Sold Online Contaminated With Cow's Milk. *NPR.org*, April 7, 2015. http://www.npr.org/sections/health-shots/2015/04/07/397369416/breast-milk-sold-online-contaminated-with-cows-milk.

Douglas, Susan J., and Meredith W. Michaels. 2004. *The Mommy Myth: The Idealization of Motherhood and How It Has Undermined Women*. New York: Free Press.

Dublin, J.W. 2004. Boost You Baby's IQ. *Parents*, 2004.

Duggan, Maeve, Am, a Lenhart, Cliff Lampe, and Nicole B. Ellison. 2015. Parents and Social Media. *Pew Research Center: Internet, Science & Tech*. http://www.pewinternet.org/2015/07/16/parents-and-social-media/. Accessed 29 July 2015.

Duggan, Maeve, Nicole B. Ellison, Cliff Lampe, Am, a Lenhart, and Mary Madden. 2015. Social Media Update 2014. *Pew Research Center: Internet, Science & Tech*. http://www.pewinternet.org/2015/01/09/social-media-update-2014/. Accessed 29 July 2015.

Duijts, Liesbeth, Vincent W.V. Jaddoe, Albert Hofman, and Henriëtte A. Moll. 2010. Prolonged and Exclusive Breastfeeding Reduces the Risk of Infectious Diseases in Infancy. *Pediatrics* 126 (1): e18–25. doi:10.1542/peds.2008-3256.

Dungy, Claibourne I., Jay Christensen-Szalanski, Mary Losch, and Daniel Russell. 1992. Effect of Discharge Samples on Duration of Breast-Feeding. *Pediatrics* 90 (2): 233–237.

Duvall, Spring-Serenity. 2015. Not 'Simply the Breast' Media Discourses of Celebrity, Breastfeeding, and Normalcy. *Feminist Media Studies* 15 (2): 324–340.

Eden, Aimee R. n.d. New Professions and Old Practice: Lactation Consulting and the Medicalization of Breastfeeding. In *Beyond Health, Beyond Choice: Breastfeeding Constraints and Realities*, ed. Paige Hall Smith, Bernice L. Hausman, and Miriam Labbok, 98–109. New Brunswick, NJ: Rutgers University Press,

Ehrenreich, Barbara, and Deirdre English. 1978. *For Her Own Good: 150 Years of the Experts' Advice to Women*. New York: Anchor Boods.

Employment Characteristics of Families Summary. http://www.bls.gov/news.release/famee.nr0.htm. Accessed 30 July 2015.

Enger, S.M., R.K. Ross, B. Henderson, and L. Bernstein. 1997. Breastfeeding History, Pregnancy Experience and Risk of Breast Cancer. *British Journal of Cancer* 76 (1): 118–123.

Eskay's Albumenized Food. It's Worth Crying for. *The Ladies' Home Journal*, 1898.

Evans, Sara. 'Is Breast Best?' Q & A. *Parents*, 1988.

Ezzo, Gary, and Robert Bucknam. 2012. *On Becoming Baby Wise: Giving Your Infant the GIFT of Nighttime Sleep*, Rev Upd edition. Mount Pleasant, SC: Parent-Wise Solutions.

Faircloth, Charlotte. 2007. A Weak Formula for Legislation: How Loopholes in the Law Are Putting Babies at Risk. NICEF UK/National Childbirth Trust/ Save the Children UK. http://www.savethechildren.org.uk/sites/default/ files/docs/babymilk_legislation_1.pdf.

Faircloth, Charlotte. 2011. 'It Feels Right in My Heart': Affective Accountability in Narratives of Attachment. *The Sociological Review* 59 (2): 283–302. doi:10.1111/j.1467-954X.2011.02004.x.

FAQs - Prolacta Bioscience. *Prolacta Bioscience*, 2015. http://www.prolacta.com/faqs.

Fein, Sara B., Bidisha Mandal, and Brian E. Roe. 2008. Success of Strategies for Combining Employment and Breastfeeding. *Pediatrics* 122 (2): S56–62. doi:10.1542/peds.2008-1315g.

Feldman-Winter, Lori. 2013. Evidence-Based Interventions to Support Breastfeeding. *Pediatric Clinics of North America* 60 (1): 169–187.

Feldman-Winter, Lori, Lauren Barone, Barry Milcarek, Krystal Hunter, Joan Meek, Jane Morton, Tara Williams, Audrey Naylor, and Ruth A. Lawrence. 2010. Residency Curriculum Improves Breastfeeding Care. *Pediatrics* 126 (2): 289–297. doi:10.1542/peds.2009-3250.

Fentiman, Linda Christine. 2009. Marketing Mothers' Milk: The Commodification of Breastfeeding and the New Markets for Breast Milk and Infant Formula. doi:10.2139/ssrn.1370425.

Ferber, Richard. 2006. *Solve Your Child's Sleep Problems: New, Revised, and Expanded Edition*, Rev Exp edition. New York: Touchstone.

Fildes, Valerie. 1986. *Breasts, Bottles and Babies—A History of Infant Feeding*. Edinburgh: Edinburgh University Press. http://www.cabdirect.org/ abstracts/19880428999.html;jsessionid=C18DA1D2B9571BC1F2D0F6FE 954B568D.

Find Facilities. *Baby-Friendly USA*, September 23, 2016. http://www.baby-friendlyusa.org/find-facilities.

Firger, Jessica. 2015, and 12:50 Pm. Breast Milk Sold Online Often Contaminated by Cow's Milk. *CBS News*, April 6, 2015. http://www.cbsnews.com/news/breast-milk-sold-online-often-contaminated-by-cows-milk/.

Fogel, Joshua, and Faye Krausz. 2013. Watching Reality Television Beauty Shows Is Associated with Tanning Lamp Use and Outdoor Tanning among

College Students. *Journal of the American Academy of Dermatology* 68 (5): 784–789. doi:10.1016/j.jaad.2012.09.055.

Folb, Kate Langrall. 2000. 'Don't Touch That Dial!': TV as a–What!?–Positive Influence. *SIECUS Report* 28 (5): 16–18.

Fomon, Samuel J. 2001. Infant Feeding in the 20th Century: Formula and Beikost. *The Journal of Nutrition* 131 (2): 409S–420S.

Forde, Kathy Roberts, and Katherine A. Foss. 2012. 'The Facts—The Color!—The Facts': The Idea of a Report in American Print Culture. *Book History* 15 (1): 123–151. doi:10.1353/bh.2012.0003.

Forste, Renata, Jessica Weiss, and Emily Lippincott. 2001. The Decision to Breastfeed in the United States: Does Race Matter? *Pediatrics* 108 (2): 291–296. doi:10.1542/peds.108.2.291.

Foss, Katherine A. 2010. Perpetuating 'Scientific Motherhood': Infant Feeding Discourse in Parents Magazine, 1930–2007. *Women & Health*, May 27, 2010. http://www.tandfonline.com/doi/abs/10.1080/03630242.2010.480905.

Foss, Katherine A. 2014. *Television and Health Responsibility in an Age of Individualism*. Lanham, Maryland: Lexington Books.

Foss, Katherine A., and Ken Blake. 'It's Natural and Healthy, But I Don't Want To See It': The Impact of Entertainment Television on Breastfeeding Attitudes. Montreal, Canada, 2014.

Foss, Katherine A., and Brian G. Southwell. 2006. Infant Feeding and the Media: The Relationship between Parents' Magazine Content and Breastfeeding, 1972–2000. *International Breastfeeding Journal* 1 (10): 1–9.

Fox, Bonnie J. 1990. Selling the Mechanized Household: 70 Years of Ads in *Ladies' Home Journal*. *Gender & Society* 4 (1): 25–40. doi:10.1177/089124390004001003.

Franiuk, Renae, Jennifer L. Seefelt, Sandy L. Cepress, and Joseph A. Vandello. 2008. Prevalence and Effects of Rape Myths in Print Journalism The Kobe Bryant Case. *Violence Against Women* 14 (3): 287–309. doi:10.1177/1077801207313971.

Freed, Gary L., J. Kennard Fraley, and Richard J. Schanler. 1992. Attitudes of Expectant Fathers Regarding Breast-Feeding. *Pediatrics* 90 (2): 224–227.

Freed, Gary L., Sarah J. Clark, James Sorenson, Jacob A. Lohr, Robert Cefalo, and Peter Curtis. 1995. National Assessment of Physicians' Breast-Feeding Knowledge, Attitudes, Training, and Experience. *JAMA* 273 (6): 472–476. doi:10.1001/jama.1995.03520300046035.

Frerichs, Leah, Julie L. Andsager, Shelly Campo, Mary Aquilino, and Carolyn Stewart Dyer. 2006. Framing Breastfeeding and Formula-Feeding Messages in Popular US Magazines. *Women & Health* 44 (1): 95–118.

Gale, Chris, Karen M. Logan, Shalini Santhakumaran, James RC Parkinson, Matthew J. Hyde, and Neena Modi. 2012. Effect of Breastfeeding Compared with Formula Feeding on Infant Body Composition: A Systematic Review and Meta-Analysis. *The American Journal of Clinical Nutrition*, March 1, ajcn.027284. doi:10.3945/ajcn.111.027284.

GAO-06-282 Breastfeeding: Some Strategies Used to Market Infant Formula May Discourage Breastfeeding; State Contracts Should Better Protect Against Misuse of WIC Name - d06282.pdf. http://www.gao.gov/new.items/d06282.pdf. Accessed 28 July 2015.

Gartner, Lawrence M., Jane Morton, Ruth A. Lawrence, Audrey J. Naylor, Donna O'Hare, Richard J. Schanler, Arthur I. Eidelman, and American Academy of Pediatrics Section on Breastfeeding. 2005. Breastfeeding and the Use of Human Milk. *Pediatrics* 115 (2): 496–506. doi:10.1542/peds.2004-2491.

Gebrian, Bette. 2014. Bottles to Breastfeeding in Rural Haiti. *Journal of Health Care for the Poor and Underserved* 25 (4): 1514–1519. doi:10.1353/hpu.2014.0161.

Geraghty, Sheela R., Kelly A. McNamara, Chelsea E. Dillon, Joseph S. Hogan, Jesse J. Kwiek, and Sarah A. Keim. 2013. Buying Human Milk via the Internet: Just a Click Away. *Breastfeeding Medicine* 8 (6): 474–478.

Gerbner, George, and Larry Gross. 1976. Living With Television: The Violence Profile. *Journal of Communication* 26 (2): 172–194. doi:10.1111/j.1460-2466.1976.tb01397.x.

Germs and Babies. *Parents*, 2005.

Giles, Fiona. 2010. 'Relational, and Strange': A Preliminary Foray into a Project to Queer Breastfeeding. *Australian Feminist Studies*, June 9, 2010. doi:10.1080/0816464042000278981.

Giles, Fiona. 2012. Reinstating Pleasure in Reality: Promoting Breastfeeding through Ars Erotica. In *Beyond Health, Beyond Choice: Breastfeeding Constraints and Realities*, ed. Paige Hall Smith, Bernice L. Hausman, and Miriam Labbok, 215–225. New Brunswick, NJ: Rutgers University Press.

Gillman, Matthew W., Sheryl L. Rifas-Shiman, Carlos A. J.r, Catherine S. Camargo, A. Lindsay Berkey, Helaine R.H. Frazier, Alison E. Field Rockett, and Graham A. Colditz. 2001. Risk of Overweight Among Adolescents Who Were Breastfed as Infants. *JAMA* 285 (19): 2461–2467. doi:10.1001/jama.285.19.2461.

Gitlin, Todd. 1979. Prime Time Ideology: The Hegemonic Process in Television Entertainment. *Social Problems* 26 (3): 251–266. doi:10.2307/800451.

Givens, Sonja M. Brown, and Jennifer L. Monahan. 2005. Priming Mammies, Jezebels, and Other Controlling Images: An Examination of the Influence of Mediated Stereotypes on Perceptions of an African American Woman. *Media Psychology* 7 (1): 87–106. doi:10.1207/S1532785XMEP0701_5.

Glik, Deborah, Emil Berkanovic, Kathleen Stone, Leticia Ibarra, Marcy Connell Jones, Bob Rosen, Myrl Schreibman, Lisa Gordon, Laura Minassian, and

Darcy Richardes. 2010. Health Education Goes Hollywood: Working with Prime-Time and Daytime Entertainment Television for Immunization Promotion. *Journal of Health Communication*, October 29, 2010. doi:10.1080/108107398127364.

Golden, Janet. 1996. *A Social History of Wet Nursing in America*. Cambridge: Cambridge University Press. https://books.google.com/books/about/A_Social_History_of_Wet_Nursing_in_Ameri.html?id=0TgAoZnZ2jEC.

Goldreich, G. 1970. Facts and Fallacies about Cesarean Births. *Parents*, 1970.

Graham, J. 2000. A Smart Start. *Parents*, 2000.

Grantham, Susan, Lee Ahern, and Colleen Connolly-Ahern. 2011. Merck's One Less Campaign: Using Risk Message Frames to Promote the Use of Gardasil® in HPV Prevention. *Communication Research Reports* 28 (4): 318–326. doi: 10.1080/08824096.2011.616243.

Gray, Jennifer. 2013. Feeding On the Web: Online Social Support in the Breastfeeding Context. *Communication Research Reports*, January 18, 2013. http://www.tandfonline.com/doi/abs/10.1080/08824096.2012.746219.

Greer, Frank R., and Rima D. Apple. 1991. Physicians, Formula Companies, and Advertising: A Historical Perspective. *American Journal of Diseases of Children* 145 (3): 282–286. doi:10.1001/archpedi.1991.02160030050019.

Gregory, Emily F., Arlene M. Butz, Sharon R. Ghazarian, Susan M. Gross, and Sara B. Johnson. 2015. Are Unmet Breastfeeding Expectations Associated With Maternal Depressive Symptoms? *Academic Pediatrics* 15 (3): 319–325. doi:10.1016/j.acap.2014.12.003.

Gribble, Karleen D. 2013. Peer-to-Peer Milk Donors' and Recipients' Experiences and Perceptions of Donor Milk Banks. *Journal of Obstetric, Gynecologic, & Neonatal Nursing* 42 (4): 451–461. doi:10.1111/1552-6909.12220.

Gribble, Karleen D., and Bernice L. Hausman. 2012. Milk Sharing and Formula Feeding: Infant Feeding Risks in Comparative Perspective? *The Australasian Medical Journal* 5 (5): 275. doi:10.4066/AMJ.2012.1222.

Hall, Stuart, Jessica Evans, and Sean Nixon. 2013. *Representation: Cultural Representations and Signifying Practices*, 2nd ed. Los Angeles: Sage.

Hanson, Hilary. 2012. Breastfeeding Man: Jeff Says Drinking Wife Michelle's Milk Helped His Erectile Dysfunction Symptoms. *Huffington Post*, July 11, 2012. http://www.huffingtonpost.com/2012/07/11/breastfeeding-sex-erectile-dysfunction-jeff-michelle_n_1666073.html.

Harms, Richard (ed.). 2004. *Mayo Clinic Guide to a Healthy Pregnancy by Mayo Clinic (2004) Paperback*. New York: Harper Collins.

Haroon, Sarah, Jai K. Das, Rehana A. Salam, Aamer Imdad, and Zulfiqar A. Bhutta. 2013. Breastfeeding Promotion Interventions and Breastfeeding Practices: A Systematic Review. *BMC Public Health* 13 (3): S20. doi:10.1186/1471-2458-13-S3-S20.

Harris, Robie H. 2000. *Hi New Baby!*, 1st ed. Cambridge, MA: Candlewick.

Hauck, Fern R., John M.D. Thompson, Kawai O. Tanabe, Rachel Y. Moon, and Mechtild M. Vennemann. 2011. Breastfeeding and Reduced Risk of Sudden Infant Death Syndrome: A Meta-Analysis. *Pediatrics* 128 (1): 103–110. doi:10.1542/peds.2010-3000.

Hauck, Yvonne, and Vera Irurita. 2003. Incompatible Expectations: The Dilemma of Breastfeeding Mothers. *Health Care for Women International* 24 (1): 62–78. doi:10.1080/07399330390170024.

Hauff, Laura E., Stephanie A. Leonard, and Kathleen M. Rasmussen. 2014. Associations of Maternal Obesity and Psychosocial Factors with Breastfeeding Intention, Initiation, and Duration. *The American Journal of Clinical Nutrition*, March 1, 2014, ajcn.071191. doi:10.3945/ajcn.113.071191.

Hausman, Bernice L. 2003. *Mother's Milk: Breastfeeding Controversies in American Culture*. Psychology Press.

Hausman, Bernice L. 2011. *Viral Mothers: Breastfeeding in the Age of HIV/AIDS*. University of Michigan Press.

Hausman, Bernice L. 2012. Feminism and Breastfeeding. In *Beyond Choice: Breastfeeding Constraints and Realities*, ed. Beyond Health, 15–24. New Brunswick, NJ: Rutgers University Press.

Hausman, Bernice L. 2013. Breastfeeding, Rhetoric, and the Politics of Feminism. *Journal of Women, Politics & Policy*, November 8, 2013. http://www.tandfonline.com/doi/abs/10.1080/1554477X.2013.835673.

Haynes, Suzanne G. 2015. Evaluation of the National Breastfeeding Awareness Campaign. *The National Academies of Science, Engineering, Medicine*. http://iom.nationalacademies.org/~/media/Files/Activity%20Files/Nutrition/USDABreastfeeding/09_Haynes_Suzanne.pdf. Accessed 29 July 2015.

Hazell, Ada. 1888. Timely Hints About Baby. *The Ladies' Home Journal and Practical Housekeeper*, March.

Health Q & A. *Parents*, 2007.

Hesse, Bradford W., David E. Nelson, Gary L. Kreps, Robert T. Croyle, Neeraj K. Arora, Barbara K. Rimer, and Kasisomayajula Viswanath. 2005. Trust and Sources of Health Information: The Impact of the Internet and Its Implications for Health Care Providers: Findings From the First Health Information National Trends Survey. *Archives of Internal Medicine* 165 (22): 2618–2624. doi:10.1001/archinte.165.22.2618.

Hirschman, Charles, and Marilyn Butler. n.d. Trends and Differentials in Breast Feeding: An Update. *Demography* 18 (1): 39–54. doi:10.2307/2061048.

Horlick's Food. 1884. Our Baby. *The Ladies' Home Journal and Practical Housekeeper*, October.

Hornik, Robert. 2002. *Public Health Communication: Evidence for Behavior Change*. Routledge.

Horodynski, Mildred A., Mary Calcatera, and Amanda Carpenter. 2011. Infant Feeding Practices: Perceptions of Native American Mothers and Health Paraprofessionals. *Health Education Journal*, February 28, 2011 doi:10.1177/0017896911398814.

How Working Moms Can Breast-Feed. *Parents*, May 1992.

Howard, Cynthia, Fred Howard, Ruth Lawrence, Elena Andresen, Elisabeth DeBlieck, and Michael Weitzman. 2000. Office Prenatal Formula Advertising and Its Effect on Breast-Feeding patterns1. *Obstetrics & Gynecology* 95 (2): 296–303. doi:10.1016/S0029-7844(99)00555-4.

Howard, Fred, Cynthia R. Howard, and Michael Weitzman. 1993. The Physician as Advertiser: The Unintentional Discouragement of Breastfeeding. *Obstetrics & Gynecology* 81 (6): 1048–1051.

Howell, Elizabeth A., Susan Bodnar-Deren, Amy Balbierz, Michael Parides, and Nina Bickell. 2014. An Intervention to Extend Breastfeeding among Black and Latina Mothers after Delivery. *American Journal of Obstetrics and Gynecology* 210 (3): 239.e1–239.e5. doi:10.1016/j.ajog.2013.11.028.

Huang, Yanzhong. The 2008 Milk Scandal Revisited. *Forbes*. http://www.forbes.com/sites/yanzhonghuang/2014/07/16/the-2008-milk-scandal-revisited/. Accessed 29 Sept 2016.

Huang, Yi, Judith Labiner-Wolfe, Hui Huang, Conrad J. Choiniere, and Sara B. Fein. 2013. Association of Health Profession and Direct-to-Consumer Marketing with Infant Formula Choice and Switching. *Birth* 40(1) (March 1): 24–31. doi:10.1111/birt.12025.

Imdad, Aamer, Mohammad Yawar Yakoob, and Zulfiqar A. Bhutta. 2011. Effect of Breastfeeding Promotion Interventions on Breastfeeding Rates, with Special Focus on Developing Countries. *BMC Public Health* 11(Suppl 3) (April 13): S24. doi:10.1186/1471-2458-11-S3-S24.

International Code of Marketing of Breast-Milk Substitutes. Geneva: World Health Organization, 1981. http://www.who.int/nutrition/publications/code_english.pdf.

Iovine, Vicki. 2007. *The Girlfriends' Guide to Pregnancy*, 2nd ed. Pocket Books.

Jacobson, Sandra W., Lisa M. Chiodo, and Joseph L. Jacobson. 1999. Breastfeeding Effects on Intelligence Quotient in 4- and 11-Year-Old Children. *Pediatrics* 103(5) (May 1): e71–e71.

Jager de, Emily, Jaclyn Broadbent, Matthew Fuller-Tyszkiewicz, and Helen Skouteris. 2013. The Role of Psychosocial Factors in Exclusive Breastfeeding to Six Months Postpartum. *Midwifery* 29 (5): 506–518.

Janz, Nancy K., and Marshall H. Becker. 1984. The Health Belief Model: A Decade Later. *Health Education & Behavior* 11(1) (March 1): 1–47. doi:10.1177/109019818401100101.

Jarlenski, Marian P., Wendy L. Bennett, Sara N. Bleich, Colleen L. Barry, and Elizabeth A. Stuart. 2014. Effects of Breastfeeding on Postpartum Weight

Loss among U.S. Women. *Preventive Medicine* 69: 146–150. doi:10.1016/j.ypmed.2014.09.018.

Jenner, Emma. 2014. The Perils of Attachment Parenting. *The Atlantic*, August 10, 2014. http://www.theatlantic.com/health/archive/2014/08/the-perils-of-attachment-parenting/375198/.

John's Wife. 1885a. An Answer to 'Mrs. S.' *The Ladies' Home Journal and Practical Housekeeper*, July 1885.

John's Wife. 1885b. When Shall the Baby Be Weaned? *The Ladies' Home Journal and Practical Housekeeper*, May 1885.

Johnson, Angela, Rosalind Kirk, Katherine Lisa Rosenblum, and Maria Muzik. 2015. Enhancing Breastfeeding Rates among African American Women: A Systematic Review of Current Psychosocial Interventions. *Breastfeeding Medicine* 10 (1): 45–62.

Johnson, Nicole. 2012. 'Are You Mom Enough?' Time Magazine Cover Should Inspire You. *The Baby Sleep Site—Baby Sleep Help | Toddler Sleep Help.* https://www.babysleepsite.com/attachment-parenting-2/time-magazine-cover-mom-enough-should-inspire-you/.

Jones, Frances. 2003. History of North American Donor Milk Banking: One Hundred Years of Progress. *Journal of Human Lactation* 19 (3): 313–318. doi:10.1177/0890334403255857.

Jones, Jessica R., Michael D. Kogan, Gopal K. Singh, Deborah L. Dee, and Laurence M. Grummer-Strawn. 2011. Factors Associated With Exclusive Breastfeeding in the United States. *Pediatrics* 128 (6): 1117–1125. doi:10.1542/peds.2011-0841.

Jordan, Susan J., Victor Siskind, Adèle C. Green, David C. Whiteman, and Penelope M. Webb. 2009. Breastfeeding and Risk of Epithelial Ovarian Cancer. *Cancer Causes & Control* 21 (1): 109–116. doi:10.1007/s10552-009-9440-x.

Kahlor, LeeAnn, and Matthew S. Eastin. 2011. Television's Role in the Culture of Violence Toward Women: A Study of Television Viewing and the Cultivation of Rape Myth Acceptance in the United States. *Journal of Broadcasting & Electronic Media* 55 (2): 215–231. doi:10.1080/08838151.2011.566085.

Kahlor, LeeAnn, and Dan Morrison. 2007. Television Viewing and Rape Myth Acceptance among College Women. *Sex Roles* 56 (11–12): 729–739. doi:10.1007/s11199-007-9232-2.

Kaminetzky, H., and D. Meilach. 1967. When Another Baby Is on the Way. *Parents*, 1967.

Karlsrud, K., and D. Schultz. 1988. Food to Grow on. *Parents*, 1988.

Karp, Harvey. 2008. *The Happiest Baby on the Block: The New Way to Calm Crying and Help Your Newborn Baby Sleep Longer*. New York: Bantam.

Kaufman, Leslie, Swarna Deenadayalan, and Adam Karpati. 2009. Breastfeeding Ambivalence Among Low-Income African American and Puerto Rican Women in North and Central Brooklyn. *Maternal and Child Health Journal* 14 (5): 696–704. doi:10.1007/s10995-009-0499-5.

Kavanagh, Katherine F., Zixin Lou, Jennifer C. Nicklas, Mona F. Habibi, and Lee T. Murphy. 2012. Breastfeeding Knowledge, Attitudes, Prior Exposure, and Intent among Undergraduate Students. *Journal of Human Lactation* 28 (4): 556–564. doi:10.1177/0890334412446798.

Kearney, Melissa S., and Phillip B. Levine. 2014. Media Influences on Social Outcomes: The Impact of MTV's 16 and Pregnant on Teen Childbearing. National Bureau of Economic Research, January 16, 2014. http://www.nber.org/papers/w19795.

Keim, Sarah A., Joseph S. Hogan, Kelly A. McNamara, Vishnu Gudimetla, Chelsea E. Dillon, Jesse J. Kwiek, and Sheela R. Geraghty. 2013. Microbial Contamination of Human Milk Purchased via the Internet. *Pediatrics* 132 (5): e1227–e1235.

Keim, Sarah A., Manjusha M. Kulkarni, Kelly McNamara, Sheela R. Geraghty, Rachael M. Billock, Rachel Ronau, Joseph S. Hogan, and Jesse J. Kwiek. 2015. Cow's Milk Contamination of Human Milk Purchased via the Internet. *Pediatrics* 135 (5): e1157–e1162. doi:10.1542/peds.2014-3554.

Kendall-Tackett, Kathleen A. 2007. Violence Against Women and the Perinatal Period The Impact of Lifetime Violence and Abuse on Pregnancy, Postpartum, and Breastfeeding. *Trauma, Violence, & Abuse* 8 (3): 344–353. doi:10.1177/1524838007304406.

Khan, Jehangir, Linda Vesel, Rajiv Bahl, and José Carlos Martines. 2014. Timing of Breastfeeding Initiation and Exclusivity of Breastfeeding During the First Month of Life: Effects on Neonatal Mortality and Morbidity—A Systematic Review and Meta-Analysis. *Maternal and Child Health Journal* 19 (3): 468–479. doi:10.1007/s10995-014-1526-8.

Khoury, Amal J., S. Wakerul Moazzem, Chad M. Jarjoura, Cathy Carothers, and Agnes Hinton. 2005. Breast-Feeding Initiation in Low-Income Women: Role of Attitudes, Support, and Perceived Control. *Women's Health Issues* 15 (2): 64–72. doi:10.1016/j.whi.2004.09.003.

Kim, Pilyoung, Ruth Feldman, Linda C. Mayes, Virginia Eicher, Nancy Thompson, James F. Leckman, and James E. Swain. 2011. Breastfeeding, Brain Activation to Own Infant Cry, and Maternal Sensitivity. *Journal of Child Psychology and Psychiatry* 52 (8): 907–915. doi:10.1111/j.1469-7610.2011.02406.x.

Kim, Younghae. 1998. The Effects of a Breastfeeding Campaign on Adolescent Korean Women. *Pediatric Nursing* 24 (3): 235–240.

King Silver Nipple. 1899. Don't Risk the Baby's Health. *The Ladies' Home Journal*.

Knaak, Stephanie J. 2010. Contextualising Risk, Constructing Choice: Breastfeeding and Good Mothering in Risk Society. *Health, Risk & Society*, July 5. doi:10.1080/13698571003789666.

Koenig, Harris F. 2014. Breastfeeding Education for Healthier Babies. Baby-Friendly Designation Improves Infant, Mother and Community Health. *Healthcare Executive* 29 (4): 46–48.

Koerber, Amy. 2005. 'You Just Don't See Enough Normal' Critical Perspectives on Infant-Feeding Discourse and Practice. *Journal of Business and Technical Communication* 19 (3): 304–327. doi:10.1177/1050651905275635.

Koerber, Amy. 2006. Rhetorical Agency, Resistance, and the Disciplinary Rhetorics of Breastfeeding. *Technical Communication Quarterly* 15 (1): 87–101. doi:10.1207/s15427625tcq1501_7.

Koerber, Amy. 2013. *Breast or Bottle?: Contemporary Controversies in Infant-Feeding Policy and Practice*. Columbia, SC: University of South Carolina Press.

Kools, Els J., Carel Thijs, Arnold D.M. Kester, and Hein de Vries. n.d. The Motivational Determinants of Breast-Feeding: Predictors for the Continuation of Breast-Feeding. *Preventive Medicine* 43 (5): 394–401.

Kornides, Melanie, and Panagiota Kitsantas. 2013. Evaluation of Breastfeeding Promotion, Support, and Knowledge of Benefits on Breastfeeding Outcomes. *Journal of Child Health Care*, February 25, 2013. 1367493512461460. doi: 10.1177/1367493512461460.

Kowalski, Kristine Hope. 2013. Kailyn Lowry Breastfeeding: 'Teen Mom 2' Star Nurses Baby Lincoln, Mocks Gisele—Hollywood Life. *Hollywood Life*, December 12, 2013. http://hollywoodlife.com/2013/12/12/kailyn-lowry-breastfeeding-pic-baby-lincoln-mocking-gisele-bundchen/.

Kozhimannil, Katy B., Laura B. Attanasio, Rachel R. Hardeman, and Michelle O'Brien. 2013. Doula Care Supports Near-Universal Breastfeeding Initiation among Diverse, Low-Income Women. *Journal of Midwifery & Women's Health* 58 (4): 378–382. doi:10.1111/jmwh.12065.

Kramer, Michael S. 2011. Breastfeeding and Allergy: The Evidence. *Annals of Nutrition and Metabolism* 59 (s1): 20–26. doi:10.1159/000334148.

Krugman, R. 1973. What Does a Baby Need Most? *Parents*, 1973.

Kwok, Man Ki, C. Mary Schooling, Tai Hing Lam, and Gabriel M. Leung. 2010. Does Breastfeeding Protect against Childhood Overweight? Hong Kong's 'Children of 1997' Birth Cohort. *International Journal of Epidemiology* 39 (1): 297–305. doi:10.1093/ije/dyp274.

Labbok, Miriam H. 2001. Effects of Breastfeeding on the Mother. *Pediatric Clinics of North America*, Breastfeeding 2001, Part 1: The Evidence for Breastfeeding 48 (1): 143–158. doi:10.1016/S0031-3955(05)70290-X.

Labbok, Miriam. 2008. Exploration of Guilt Among Mothers Who Do Not Breastfeed: The Physician's Role. *Journal of Human Lactation* 24 (1): 80–84. doi:10.1177/0890334407312002.

Labbok, Miriam. 2012. Breastfeeding in Public Health. In *Beyond Health, Beyond Choice: Breastfeeding Constraints and Realities*, ed. Paige Hall Smith, Bernice L. Hausman, and Miriam Labbok, 36–50. New Brunswick, NJ: Rutgers University Press.

Lactated Food. *The Ladies' Home Journal and Practical Housekeeper*, 1886.

Lactated Food. Crying Babies. *The Ladies' Home Journal and Practical Housekeeper*, 1887a.

Lactated Food. *The Ladies' Home Journal and Practical Housekeeper*, 1887b.

Lactated Food. Baby's Life Saved. *The Ladies' Home Journal*, 1889.

Lactated Food. Proper Food for Infants. *The Ladies' Home Journal*, 1892.

Lamberti, Laura M., Christa L. Fischer, Adi Noiman Walker, Cesar Victora, and Robert E. Black. 2011. Breastfeeding and the Risk for Diarrhea Morbidity and Mortality. *BMC Public Health* 11 (Suppl 3): S15. doi:10.1186/1471-2458-11-S3-S15.

Lamberti, Laura M., Irena Zakarija-Grković, Christa L. Fischer, Evropi Theodoratou Walker, Harish Nair, Harry Campbell, and Robert E. Black. 2013. Breastfeeding for Reducing the Risk of Pneumonia Morbidity and Mortality in Children under Two: A Systematic Literature Review and Meta-Analysis. *BMC Public Health* 13 (Suppl 3): S18. doi:10.1186/1471-2458-13-S3-S18.

Lamott, Anne. 1993. And Baby Makes Two. *Parents*, May 1993.

Landolf, Diane Wright. 2009. *What a Good Big Brother!* New York: Random House Books for Young Readers.

Langreuter, Jutta. 1998. *Little Bear Is A Big Brother*. Brookfield, Conn: Millbrook Press.

Lapinski, Maria Knight, and Rajiv N. Rimal. 2005. An Explication of Social Norms. *Communication Theory* 15 (2): 127–147.

Len-Ríos, María E., Manu Bhandari, and Yulia S. Medvedeva. 2014. Deliberation of the Scientific Evidence for Breastfeeding Online Comments as Social Representations. *Science Communication* 36 (6): 778–801. doi:10.1177/1075547014556195.

Lepore, Jill. 2009. Baby Food: If Breast Is Best, Why Are Women Bottling Their Milk? *The New Yorker*, January 19, 2009. http://www.newyorker.com/magazine/2009/01/19/baby-food.

Lewallen, Lynne Porter, Margaret J. Dick, Janet Flowers, Wanda Powell, Kimberly Taylor Zickefoose, Yolanda G. Wall, and Zula M. Price. 2006. Breastfeeding Support and Early Cessation. *Journal of Obstetric, Gynecologic, & Neonatal Nursing* 35 (2): 166–172. doi:10.1111/j.1552-6909.2006.00031.x.

Li, Ruowei, Sara B. Fein, Jian Chen, and Laurence M. Grummer-Strawn. 2008. Why Mothers Stop Breastfeeding: Mothers' Self-Reported Reasons for Stopping During the First Year. *Pediatrics* 122 (Supplement 2): S69–76. doi:10.1542/peds.2008-1315i.

Li, Ruowei, Jason Hsia, Fred Fridinger, Abeda Hussain, Sandra Benton-Davis, and Laurence Grummer-Strawn. n.d. Public Beliefs about Breastfeeding Policies in Various Settings. *Journal of the American Dietetic Association* 104 (7): 1162–1168.

Lightfoot, D. 2000. Sleepless and Showing It. *Parents*, 2000.

Littman, Heidi, Sharon VanderBrug Medendorp, and Johanna Goldfarb. 1994. The Decision to Breastfeed The Importance of Fathers' Approval. *Clinical Pediatrics* 33 (4): 214–219. doi:10.1177/000992289403300405.

Liu, Bette, Louisa Jorm, and Emily Banks. 2010. Parity, Breastfeeding, and the Subsequent Risk of Maternal Type 2 Diabetes. *Diabetes Care* 33 (6): 1239–1241. doi:10.2337/dc10-0347.

Lockwood, Charles J. 2008. Foreword to the Fourth Edition. In *What to Expect When You're Expecting*, ed. Heidi Murkoff and Sharon Mazel, Fourth, xx. New York: Workman Publishing Company.

Lu, Michael C., Linda Lange, Wendy Slusser, Jean Hamilton, and Neal Halfon. 2001. Provider Encouragement of Breast-Feeding: Evidence from a National Survey. *Obstetrics & Gynecology* 97 (2): 290–295. doi:10.1016/S0029-7844(00)01116-9.

Lubbers, Marcel, Peer Schneepers, and Maurice Vergeer. 2000. Exposure to Newspapers and Attitudes toward Ethnic Minorities: A Longitudinal Analysis. *Howard Journal of Communications* 11 (2): 127–143. doi:10.1080/106461700246661.

Lupton, Samantha J., Christine L. Chiu, Sanja Lujic, Annemarie Hennessy, and Joanne M. Lind. Association between Parity and Breastfeeding with Maternal High Blood Pressure. *American Journal of Obstetrics and Gynecology* 208 (6): 454.e1–454.e7. doi:10.1016/j.ajog.2013.02.014.

Maddock, Jay, Christine Maglione, Jodi D. Barnett, Cynthia Cabot, Susan Jackson, and Bill Reger-Nash. 2007. Statewide Implementation of the 1% or Less Campaign. *Health Education & Behavior* 34 (6): 953–963. doi:10.1177/1090198106290621.

Mandel, Dror, Ronit Lubetzky, Shaul Dollberg, Shimon Barak, and Francis B. Mimouni. 2005. Fat and Energy Contents of Expressed Human Breast Milk in Prolonged Lactation. *Pediatrics* 116 (3): e432–35. doi:10.1542/peds.2005-0313.

Manjilalal, J.Februhartanty, and D.N. Basuki. 2014. Assessment of Breastfeeding Problems Experienced by Mothers in the First Six Months Postpartum: A Process of Tool Development. *Malaysian Journal of Nutrition* 20 (3): 351–365.

Mannion, Cynthia A., Amy J. Hobbs, Sheila W. McDonald, and Suzanne C. Tough. 2013. Maternal Perceptions of Partner Support during Breastfeeding. *International Breastfeeding Journal* 8 (1): 4.

Manushkin, Fran. 2014. *Big Brothers Are the Best.* Picture Window Books.

Marchand, Roland. 1985. *Advertising the American Dream: Making Way for Modernity, 1920–1940.* Berkeley, CA: University of California Press.

Marrone, Sonia, Nancy Vogeltanz-Holm, and Jeffrey Holm. 2008. Attitudes, Knowledge, and Intentions Related to Breastfeeding Among University Undergraduate Women and Men. *Journal of Human Lactation* 24 (2): 186–192. doi:10.1177/0890334408316072.

Martin R.M., Patel R., Kramer M.S. et al. 2013. Effects of Promoting Longer-Term and Exclusive Breastfeeding on Adiposity and Insulin-like Growth Factor-I at Age 11.5 Years: A Randomized Trial. *JAMA* 309 (10): 1005–1013. doi:10.1001/jama.2013.167.

Martins, Nicole, and Robin E. Jensen. 2014. The Relationship Between 'Teen Mom' Reality Programming and Teenagers' Beliefs About Teen Parenthood. *Mass Communication and Society*, November 24, 2014. http://www.tandfonline.com/doi/abs/10.1080/15205436.2013.851701.

Marvel, M. Kim, Ronald M. Epstein, Kristine Flowers, and Howard B. Beckman. 1999. Soliciting the Patient's Agenda: Have We Improved? *JAMA* 281 (3): 283–287. doi:10.1001/jama.281.3.283.

Maternal, Infant, and Child Health | Healthy People 2020. 2014. *Healthypeople.gov*, 2014. http://www.healthypeople.gov/2020/topics-objectives/topic/maternal-infant-and-child-health/objectives.

Maycock, Bruce, Colin W. Binns, Satvinder Dhaliwal, Jenny Tohotoa, Yvonne Hauck, Sharyn Burns, and Peter Howat. 2013. Education and Support for Fathers Improves Breastfeeding Rates A Randomized Controlled Trial. *Journal of Human Lactation* 29 (4): 484–490. doi:10.1177/0890334413484387.

Mazzeo, Suzanne E., Sara E. Trace, Karen S. Mitchell, and Rachel Walker Gow. 2007. Effects of a Reality TV Cosmetic Surgery Makeover Program on Eating Disordered Attitudes and Behaviors. *Eating Behaviors* 8 (3): 390–397. doi:10.1016/j.eatbeh.2006.11.016.

McCall, Robert B. 1982. Starting Solids. *Parents*, September 1982.

McCarter-Spaulding, Deborah. 2007. How Does Postpartum Depression Affect Breastfeeding?: MCN: The American Journal of Maternal/Child Nursing. *MCN: The American Journal of Maternal/Child. Nursing* 32 (1): 10–17.

McCarthy, Michael. 2001. Ads Pepper Reality Shows with Product Placements. *USATODAY.com*, July 23, 2001. http://usatoday30.usatoday.com/money/advertising/2001-07-23-reality-ads.htm.

McClellan, Holly L., Anna R. Hepworth, Catherine P. Garbin, Marnie K. Rowan, Jane Deacon, Peter E. Hartmann, and Donna T. Geddes. 2012.

Nipple Pain during Breastfeeding with or without Visible Trauma. *Journal of Human Lactation* 28 (4): 511–521. doi:10.1177/0890334412444464.

McCrory, Cathal, and Richard Layte. 2012. Breastfeeding and Risk of Overweight and Obesity at Nine-Years of Age. *Social Science & Medicine* 75 (2): 323–330. doi:10.1016/j.socscimed.2012.02.048.

McDivitt, Judith A., Susan Zimicki, Hornik, and Ayman Abulaban. 1993. The Impact of the Healthcom Mass Media Campaign on Timely Initiation of Breastfeeding in Jordan on JSTOR. *Studies in Family Planning* 24 (4): 295–309.

McFadden, Alison, Frances Mason, Jean Baker, France Begin, Fiona Dykes, Laurence Grummer-Strawn, Natalie Kenney-Muir, Heather Whitford, Elizabeth Zehner, and Mary J. Renfrew. 2016. Spotlight on Infant Formula: Coordinated Global Action Needed. *The Lancet* 387 (10017): 413–415. doi:10.1016/S0140-6736(16)00103-3.

McGuire, W., and M. Y. Anthony. 2003. Donor Human Milk versus Formula for Preventing Necrotising Enterocolitis in Preterm Infants: Systematic Review. *Archives of Disease in Childhood—Fetal and Neonatal Edition* 88 (1): F11–14. doi:10.1136/fn.88.1.F11.

McKinney, Amanda. 2015. A Lifestyle Perspective on Infertility and Pregnancy Outcome. *American Journal of Lifestyle Medicine*, April 24 2015, 1559827615584020. doi:10.1177/1559827615584020.

Meedya, Shahla, Kathleen Fahy, and Ashley Kable. 2010. Factors That Positively Influence Breastfeeding Duration to 6 Months: A Literature Review. *Women and Birth* 23 (4): 135–145. doi:10.1016/j.wombi.2010.02.002.

Meinzen-Derr, J., B. Poindexter, L. Wrage, A.L. Morrow, B. Stoll, and E.F. Donovan. 2009. Role of Human Milk in Extremely Low Birth Weight Infants|[rsquo]| Risk of Necrotizing Enterocolitis or Death. *Journal of Perinatology* 29 (1): 57–62. doi:10.1038/jp.2008.117.

Mellin's Food. *The Ladies' Home Journal and Practical Housekeeper*, 1884.

Mellin's Food. *The Ladies' Home Journal and Practical Housekeeper*, 1887.

Mellin's Food, Horlick's Food, Anglo-Swiss Milk Food. *The Ladies' Home Journal and Practical Housekeeper*, 1885.

Metzger, Molly W., and Thomas W. McDade. 2010. Breastfeeding as Obesity Prevention in the United States: A Sibling Difference Model. *American Journal of Human Biology* 22 (3): 291–296. doi:10.1002/ajhb.20982.

Microsoft Word - Prenatal_visit_pattern.doc - Prenatal_visit_pattern.pdf. http://www.mc.vanderbilt.edu/dept/obgyn/LD_Policies/Prenatal_visit_pattern.pdf. Accessed 29 July 2015.

Mindich, David T. Z. 2000. *Just the Facts: How Objectivity Came to Define American Journalism*. NYU Press.

Mitchell, L. 2004. Hospital Hints. *Parents*, 2004.

Mittell, Jason. 2009. *Television and American Culture*. Oxford, UK: Oxford University Press. http://www.amazon.com/Television-American-Culture-Jason-Mittell/dp/0195306678/ref=sr_1_2?ie=UTF8&qid=1438194336&sr=8-2&keywords=jason+mittell.

Mizpah Valve Nipples. *The Ladies' Home Journal*, 1891.

Mondello, Bob. 2015. Remembering Hollywood's Hays Code, 40 Years On. *NPR.org*. http://www.npr.org/templates/story/story.php?storyId=93301189. Accessed 31 July 2015.

Montagu, A. 1964. What Babies Need Most. *Parents*, 1964.

Morice, Madge. 1884. 'Nater' vs. the Milk-Bottle Again. *The Ladies' Home Journal and Practical Housekeeper*, June 1884.

Morris, James. 2011. How European Media Companies Are Dealing with Product Placement. *Advertising Age*, June 13. http://adage.com/article/global-news/european-media-companies-dealing-product-placement/228121/.

Morrissey, Tracie Egan. 2012. Attachment Parenting: Freakish or Feminist? *Jezebel*, May 10. http://jezebel.com/5909225/attachment-parenting-freakish-or-feminist.

Mozingo, Johnie N., Mitzi W. Davis, Patricia Droppleman, and Amy Merideth. 2000 'It Wasn't Working': Women's Experiences with Short-Term Breastfeeding. *MCN: The American Journal of Maternal/Child Nursing* 25 (3): 120–126.

Mrs. M. McO. 1885. *The Ladies' Home Journal and Practical Housekeeper*, December 1885.

Muller, Mike. 1974. *The Baby Killer: A War on Want Investigation into the Promotion and Sale of Powdered Baby Milks in the Third World*. War on Want.

Mulvey. 2006. Visual Pleasure and Narrative Cinema. In *Media and Cultural Studies: Keyworks*, ed. Meenakshi Gigi Durham and Douglas M. Kellner, 342–352. Malden, MA: Blackwell.

Murfreesboro, Tennessee (TN) Profile: Population, Maps, Real Estate, Averages, Homes, Statistics, Relocation, Travel, Jobs, Hospitals, Schools, Crime, Moving, Houses, News, Sex Offenders. http://www.city-data.com/city/Murfreesboro-Tennessee.html. Accessed 29 July 2015.

Murkoff, Heidi. 2001. *What to Expect When the New Baby Comes Home*. 1st ed. New York: HarperFestival.

Murkoff, Heidi, and Sharon Mazel. 2008. *What to Expect When You're Expecting*, 4th ed. New York: Workman.

Murray, Linda J., Leah Hennen, Jim Scott, and BabyCenter Editorial Team. 2005. *The Babycenter Essential Guide to Pregnancy and Birth: Expert Advice and Real-World Wisdom from the Top Pregnancy and Parenting Resource*. Emmaus, PA: Rodale Books.

'Nater' Vs. Milk-Bottles. 1884. *The Ladies' Home Journal and Practical Housekeeper*, March 1884.

Nathanson, Laura. 2001. Doctor on Call: Kids' Health & Safety: Noted Pediatrician Laura Nathanson Tackles Your Tough Question: Switching Formulas. *Parents*, January 2001.

National Breastfeeding Campaign 'Ladies Night' TV Advert. *YouTube*. http://www.youtube.com/watch?v=WM8NLxCXlp0. Accessed 29 July 2015.

National Implementation of the International Code of Marketing of Breastmilk Substitutes* - State_of_the_Code_by_Country_April2011.pdf. http://www.unicef.org/nutrition/files/State_of_the_Code_by_Country_April2011.pdf. Accessed 29 July 2015.

Nattinger, Ann Butler, Raymond G. Hoffmann, Alicia Howell-Pelz, and James S. Goodwin. 1998. Effect of Nancy Reagan's Mastectomy on Choice of Surgery for Breast Cancer by US Women. *JAMA* 279 (10): 762–766. doi:10.1001/jama.279.10.762.

Neff, Jack. 2015. Similac Wants to End Mommy Wars Over Breastfeeding: Abbot Brand Stages Playground Battle to Help End the Shaming. *Advertising Age*, January 27, 2015. http://adage.com/article/cmo-strategy/similac-end-mommy-wars-breastfeeding/296817/.

Neifert, Marianne R. 2001. Prevention of Breastfeeding Tragedies. *Pediatric Clinics of North America* 48 (2): 273–297. doi:10.1016/S0031-3955(08)70026-9.

Nestle's Food. *The Ladies' Home Journal and Practical Housekeeper*, 1888.

Nestle's Milk Food. *The Ladies' Home Journal and Practical Housekeeper*, 1885.

Nestle's Milk Food. Ringer's Ringing Recommendation. *The Ladies' Home Journal and Practical Housekeeper*, 1887a.

Nestle's Milk Food. *The Ladies' Home Journal and Practical Housekeeper*, 1887b.

Nestle's Milk Food. About Your Baby's Teeth. *The Ladies' Home Journal and Practical Housekeeper*, 1888a.

Nestle's Milk Food. Hot Weather. *The Ladies' Home Journal and Practical Housekeeper*, 1888b.

Nestle's Milk Food. Secure Strong Hard Teeth for Baby. *The Ladies' Home Journal and Practical Housekeeper*, 1888c.

Nestle's Milk Food. "Winter Diet." *The Ladies' Home Journal and Practical Housekeeper*, 1888d.

Nestle's Milk Food. Natural Law in the Baby World. *The Ladies' Home Journal*, 1889.

Nestle's Milk Food. One Minute's Talk with Baby's Mother. *The Ladies' Home Journal*, 1890.

Nestle's Milk Food. When the Stork Has Brought the Baby. *The Ladies' Home Journal*, 1902.

Newman, Jack. 2003. Breastfeeding Your Adopted Baby or Baby Born by Surrogate/Gestational Carrier. *International Breastfeeding Centre*. http://

www.nbci.ca/index.php?option=com_content&id=11:breastfeeding-your-adopted-baby-or-baby-born-by-surrogategestational-carrier&Itemid=17.

Newton, Niles. 1967. Psychologic Aspects of Lactation. *New England Journal of Medicine* 277 (22): 1179–1188.

Nickel, Nathan Christopher, Miriam H. Labbok, Michael G. Hudgens, and Julie L. Daniels. 2012. The Extent That Noncompliance with the Ten Steps to Successful Breastfeeding Influences Breastfeeding Duration. *Journal of Human Lactation* 0890334412464695.

Nickerson, Lauren E., Abby C. Sykes, and Teresa T. Fung. 2012. Mothers' Experience of Fathers' Support for Breast-Feeding (15): 1780–1787.

Nommsen-Rivers, Laurie A., Caroline J. Chantry, Roberta J. Cohen, and Kathryn G. Dewey. 2010. Comfort with the Idea of Formula Feeding Helps Explain Ethnic Disparity in Breastfeeding Intentions Among Expectant First-Time Mothers. Research-article. *Http://Dx.doi.org/10.1089/bfm.2009.0052*, February 1, 2010. http://online.liebertpub.com/doi/abs/10.1089/bfm.2009.0052.

Northup, Temple. 2010. Is Everyone a Little Bit Racist? Exploring Cultivation Using Implicit and Explicit Measures. *Southwestern Mass Communication Journal* 26 (1): 29–41.

Norwood, Kristen, and Paaige K. Turner. 2013. The Breast Is (Always) for Sex: Breastfeeding Discourse in Response to May 21, 2012 TIME Magazine Cover. *Qualitative Research Reports in Communication*, November 5. http://www.tandfonline.com/doi/abs/10.1080/17459435.2013.835345.

Now to Kill the Baby. 1886. *The Ladies' Home Journal and Practical Housekeeper*, December 1886.

O'Brien, M.L., M. Zareai, and A.B. Fallon. 2007. Creating a Breastfeeding Culture: A Comparison of Breastfeeding Practises in Australia and Iran. *Breastfeeding Review* 15 (2): 15.

O'Connor, Jane. 2014. *Lulu and the Witch Baby: I Can Read Level 2*. Reprint edition. HarperCollins.

Oddy, Wendy H., Garth E. Kendall, Jianghong Li, Peter Jacoby, Monique Robinson, Nicholas H. de Klerk, Sven R. Silburn, Stephen R. Zubrick, Louis I. Landau, and Fiona J. Stanley. 2010. The Long-Term Effects of Breastfeeding on Child and Adolescent Mental Health: A Pregnancy Cohort Study Followed for 14 Years. *The Journal of Pediatrics* 156 (4): 568–574. doi:10.1016/j.jpeds.2009.10.020.

Oddy, Wendy H., Jianghong Li, Andrew J.O. Whitehouse, Stephen R. Zubrick, and Eva Malacova. 2011. Breastfeeding Duration and Academic Achievement at 10 Years. *Pediatrics* 127 (1): e137–145. doi:10.1542/peds.2009-3489.

Odijk, J. van, I. Kull, M.P. Borres, P. Brandtzaeg, U. Edberg, L.Å. Hanson, A. Høst, et al. 2003. Breastfeeding and Allergic Disease: A Multidisciplinary Review of the Literature (1966–2001) on the Mode of Early Feeding in

Infancy and Its Impact on Later Atopic Manifestations. *Allergy* 58 (9): 833–843. doi:10.1034/j.1398-9995.2003.00264.x.

Odland, Sarah Burke. 2010. Unassailable Motherhood, Ambivalent Domesticity: The Construction of Maternal Identity in Ladies' Home Journal in 1946. *Journal of Communication Inquiry* 34 (1): 61–84. doi: 10.1177/0196859909343762.

Odom, Erika C., Ruowei Li, Kelley S. Scanlon, Cria G. Perrine, and Laurence Grummer-Strawn. 2014. Association of Family and Health Care Provider Opinion on Infant Feeding with Mother's Breastfeeding Decision. *Journal of the Academy of Nutrition and Dietetics* 114 (8): 1203–1207.

Office of the Commissioner. 2010. Pediatrics—Use of Donor Human Milk. http://www.fda.gov/ScienceResearch/SpecialTopics/PediatricTherapeuticsResearch/ucm235203.htm.

Olds, Sally Wendkos. 1980. All About Breastfeeding, 25 Vital Questions and Answers. *Parents*, January 1980.

Onyango, Adelheid W., Olivier Receveur, and Steven A. Esrey. 2002. The Contribution of Breast Milk to Toddler Diets in Western Kenya. *Bulletin of the World Health Organization* 80 (4): 292.

Østbye, Truls, Katrina M. Krause, Geeta K. Swamy, and Cheryl A. Lovelady. 2010. Effect of Breastfeeding on Weight Retention from One Pregnancy to the next: Results from the North Carolina WIC Program. *Preventive Medicine* 51 (5): 368–372. doi:10.1016/j.ypmed.2010.07.017.

Owen, Christopher G., Richard M. Martin, Peter H. Whincup, George Davey Smith, and Derek G. Cook. 2006. Does Breastfeeding Influence Risk of Type 2 Diabetes in Later Life? A Quantitative Analysis of Published Evidence. *The American Journal of Clinical Nutrition* 84 (5): 1043–1054.

Palmer, Alison. 2006. There Comes a Point When Breast Is Not Best. *The Telegraph*, February 3, 2006. http://www.telegraph.co.uk/news/health/3336122/There-comes-a-point-when-breast-is-not-best.html.

Palmer, Brian. n.d. The Influence of Breastfeeding on the Development of the Oral Cavity: A Commentary. *Journal of Human Lactation* 14 (2): 93–98.

Palmquist, Aunchalee. 2015. Demedicalizing Breastmilk: The Discourses, Practices, and Identities of Informal Milk Sharing. *Ethnographies of Breastfeeding: Cultural Contexts and Confrontations* 23.

Palmquist, Aunchalee E.L., and Kirsten Doehler. 2014. Contextualizing Online Human Milk Sharing: Structural Factors and Lactation Disparity among Middle Income Women in the US. *Social Science & Medicine* 122: 140–147.

Pantley, Elizabeth, and William Sears. 2002. *The No-Cry Sleep Solution: Gentle Ways to Help Your Baby Sleep Through the Night*, 1st ed. Chicago: McGraw-Hill Education.

PARAAMStatement.pdf. June 30, 2014. http://www.meredith.com/mediakit/parents/print/PARAAMStatement.pdf.

Parents Guide: Breast & Bottle Feeding. *Parents*, September 1992.

Parents Magazine—Encyclopedia of Children and Childhood in History and Society. http://www.faqs.org/childhood/Me-Pa/Parents-Magazine.html. Accessed 29 July 2015.

Parry, Kathleen, Emily Taylor, Pam Hall-Dardess, Marsha Walker, and Miriam Labbok. 2013. Understanding Women's Interpretations of Infant Formula Advertising. *Birth* 40 (2): 115–124. doi:10.1111/birt.12044.

Parsons, Sabrina. 2012. Time Magazine Asks 'Are You Mom Enough?' Every Mom Should Be Offended. *Forbes*, May 12, 2012. http://www.forbes.com/sites/sabrinaparsons/2012/05/12/time-magazine-asks-are-you-mom-enough-every-mom-should-be-offended/.

Pearl, Michael, and Debi Pearl. 1994. *To Train Up a Child*. Pleasantville, TN: No Greater Joy Ministries.

Pechmann, Cornelia. 2009. A Comparison of Health Communication Models: Risk Learning Versus Stereotype Priming. *Media Psychology*, November 17. doi:10.1207/S1532785XMEP0302_04.

Pérez-Escamilla, Rafael, Josefa L. Martinez, and Sofia Segura-Pérez. 2016. Impact of the Baby-friendly Hospital Initiative on Breastfeeding and Child Health Outcomes: A Systematic Review. *Maternal & Child Nutrition* 12 (3): 402–417. doi:10.1111/mcn.12294.

Perrine, Cria, Jian Chen, and Kelley Scanlon. Early Formula Supplementation and Breastfeeding Duration (131.4). *The FASEB Journal* 28 (1 Supplement): 131.4.

Pfeiffer, John. 2013. *Dude, You're a Dad!: How to Get (All of You) Through Your Baby's First Year*. Adams Media.

Piwoz, Ellen G., and Sandra L. Huffman. 2015. The Impact of Marketing of Breast-Milk Substitutes on WHO-Recommended Breastfeeding Practices. *Food and Nutrition Bulletin*, August 27, 2015, 0379572115602174. doi: 10.1177/0379572115602174.

Pondillo, Robert. 2010. *America's First Network TV Censor: The Work of NBC's Stockton Helffrich*. Carbondale: Southern Illinois University.

Port, David, and John Ralston. 2006. *The Caveman's Pregnancy Companion: A Survival Guide for Expectant Fathers*. New York: Sterling.

Potter, Beth, Judy Sheeshka, and Ruta Valaitis. 2000. Content Analysis of Infant Feeding Messages in a Canadian Women's Magazine, 1945 to 1995. *Journal of Nutrition Education* 32 (4): 196–203. doi:10.1016/S0022-3182(00)70557-7.

Pratt, Helenor F. 1984. Breastfeeding and Eczema. *Early Human Development* 9 (3): 283–290. doi:10.1016/0378-3782(84)90039-2.

Prior, Emily, Shalini Santhakumaran, Chris Gale, Lara H. Philipps, Neena Modi, and Matthew J. Hyde. 2012. Breastfeeding after Cesarean Delivery: A Systematic Review and Meta-Analysis of World Literature. *The American*

Journal of Clinical Nutrition, May 1, 2012, ajcn.030254. doi:10.3945/ajcn.111.030254.

Pyrex. 1930. For Your Baby. *Parents*, 1930.

Quigley, Maria A., Christine Hockley, Claire Carson, Yvonne Kelly, Mary J. Renfrew, and Amanda Sacker. 2012. Breastfeeding Is Associated with Improved Child Cognitive Development: A Population-Based Cohort Study. *The Journal of Pediatrics* 160 (1): 25–32. doi:10.1016/j.jpeds.2011.06.035.

Rates of Any and Exclusive Breastfeeding by Socio-Demographics Among Children Born in 2011 (Percentage +/− Half 95% Confidence Interval). *Centers for Disease Control*. http://www.cdc.gov/breastfeeding/data/nis_data/rates-any-exclusive-bf-socio-dem-2011.htm. Accessed 29 July 2015.

Reger, B., M.G. Wootan, S. Booth-Butterfield, and H. Smith. 1998. 1% or Less: A Community-Based Nutrition Campaign. *Public Health Reports* 113 (5): 410.

Rideout, Vicky. 2008. Television As A Health Educator: A Case Study of Grey's Anatomy. Kaiser Family Foundation. https://kaiserfamilyfoundation.files.wordpress.com/2013/01/7803.pdf.

Ridge's Food for Infants and Invalids. *The Ladies' Home Journal*, 1890.

Rockwell, Lizzy. 2015. *Hello Baby!* Reprint edition. Knopf Books for Young Readers.

Rogers, Fred. 1996. *The New Baby*, Reissue ed. New York: Puffin Books.

Rollins, Nigel C., Nita Bhandari, Nemat Hajeebhoy, Susan Horton, Chessa K. Lutter, Jose C. Martines, Ellen G. Piwoz, Linda M. Richter, and Cesar G. Victora. 2016. Why Invest, and What It Will Take to Improve Breastfeeding Practices? *The Lancet* 387 (10017): 491–504. doi:10.1016/S0140-6736(15)01044-2.

Rorer, Mrs., S.T. 1898. Proper Cooking for the Nursery: New Cooking Lessons: Number Three. *The Ladies' Home Journal*.

Rorer, Mrs., S.T. 1900. The Proper Food for a Child in Summer. *The Ladies' Home Journal*.

Rosenberg, Kenneth D., Carissa A. Eastham, Laurin J. Kasehagen, and Alfredo P. Sandoval. 2008. Marketing Infant Formula Through Hospitals: The Impact of Commercial Hospital Discharge Packs on Breastfeeding. *American Journal of Public Health* 98 (2): 290. doi:10.2105/AJPH.2006.103218.

Rossman, Beverly. 2007. Breastfeeding Peer Counselors in the United States: Helping to Build a Culture and Tradition of Breastfeeding. *Journal of Midwifery & Women's Health* 52 (6): 631–637. doi:10.1016/j.jmwh.2007.05.006.

Rotch, Thomas. 1898. The General Principles Underlying All Good Methods of Infant Feeding. *Boston Medical and Surgical Journal* 129 (21): 505–506.

Rozga, Mary R., Jean M. Kerver, and Beth H. Olson. 2015. Impact of Peer Counselling Breast-Feeding Support Programme Protocols on Any and Exclusive Breast-Feeding Discontinuation in Low-Income Women. *Public Health Nutrion* 18 (3): 453–463.

Rubenstein-Gillis, Sarah. 2008. Reel Milk: Sexual? Maternal? Investigating the Portrayal of Breastfeeding in American Cinema. *Mothering*.

Ryan, Alan S., Zhou Wenjun, and Andrew Acosta. 2002. Breastfeeding Continues to Increase Into the New Millennium. *Pediatrics* 110 (6): 1103–1109.

Sanipure. 1907. Have Your Baby Thrive. *The Ladies' Home Journal*.

Saunders, Katie. 2015. *Olive Marshmallow*. New York: little bee books.

Schaaf, Rachelle Vander. 1998. New Breast-Feeding Guidelines. *Parents*, May 1998.

Schanler, Richard J., Karen G. O'Connor, and Ruth A. Lawrence. 1999. Pediatricians' Practices and Attitudes Regarding Breastfeeding Promotion. *Pediatrics* 103 (3): e35. doi:10.1542/peds.103.3.e35.

Schlossman, Steven. 1985. Perils of Popularization: The Founding of 'Parents' Magazine'. *Monographs of the Society for Research in Child Development* 50 (4/5): 65–77.

Schmied, Virginia, Sarah Beake, Athena Sheehan, Christine McCourt, and Fiona Dykes. 2011. Women's Perceptions and Experiences of Breastfeeding Support: A Metasynthesis. *Birth* 38 (1): 49–60. doi:10.1111/j.1523-536X.2010.00446.x.

Schnabl, Kareena L., John E. Van Aerde, Alan B.R. Thomson, and Michael T. Clandinin. 2008. Necrotizing Enterocolitis: A Multifactorial Disease with No Cure. *World Journal of Gastroenterology: WJG* 14 (14): 2142. doi:10.3748/wjg.14.2142.

Schudson, Michael. 1981. *Discovering the News: A Social History of American Newspapers*. New York: Basic Books.

Scott, Jane A., and Tricia Mostyn. 2003. Women's Experiences of Breastfeeding in a Bottle-Feeding Culture. *Journal of Human Lactation* 19 (3): 270–277. doi:10.1177/0890334403255225.

Scovil, Elizabeth. 1891. Feeding Very Young Babies. *The Ladies' Home Journal*.

Scovil, Elizabeth. 1890a. Words for Young Mothers. *The Ladies' Home Journal*.

Scovil, Elizabeth. 1890b. Words for Young Mothers. *The Ladies' Home Journal and Practical Housekeeper*, October 1890.

Scovil, Elizabeth Robinson. 1906. *How to Bring Up a Baby: A Hand Book for Mothers*. Cincinnati, OH: The Proctor & Gamble.

Sears, Camilla A., and Rebecca Godderis. 2010. Roar Like a Tiger on TV? *Feminist Media Studies*. http://www.tandfonline.com/doi/abs/10.1080/14680777.2010.521626.

Sears, Martha, and William Sears. 2008. *The Breastfeeding Book: Everything You Need to Know About Nursing Your Child from Birth Through Weaning.* Boston: Little Brown.

Sears, William, and Martha Sears. 2001. *The Attachment Parenting Book: A Commonsense Guide to Understanding and Nurturing Your Baby.* Boston: Little Brown.

Sears, William, Martha Sears, and Christie Watts Kelly. 2001. *What Baby Needs*, 1st ed. Boston: Little, Brown Books for Young Readers.

Section On Breastfeeding. 2012. Breastfeeding and the Use of Human Milk. *Pediatrics*, February 27, 2012. doi:10.1542/peds.2011-3552.

Security Nipple. *The Ladies' Home Journal.* 1898.

Semenic, Sonia, Janet E. Childerhose, Julie Lauzière, and Danielle Groleau. 2012. Barriers, Facilitators, and Recommendations Related to Implementing the Baby-Friendly Initiative (BFI): An Integrative Review. *Journal of Human Lactation.* doi: 10.1177/0890334412445195.

Sender, Katherine. 2012. *The Makeover: Reality Television and Reflexive Audiences.* New York: New York University Press.

Sexuality & Breastfeeding: What Do You Know? : MCN: The American Journal of Maternal/Child Nursing. *LWW.* http://journals.lww.com/mcnjournal/Fulltext/2009/07000/Sexuality___Breastfeeding__What_Do_You_Know_.6.aspx. Accessed 29 July 2015.

Shainess, N. 1968. The Fine Art of Mothering. *Parents*, 1968.

Sharf, Barbara F., and Vicki S. Freimuth. 2010. Confronting Cancer on Thirtysomething: Audience Response to Health Content on Entertainment Television. *Journal of Health Communication*, 157–172. doi:10.1080/108107396128121.

Sheeshka, Judy, Beth Potter, Emilie Norrie, Ruta Valaitis, Gerald Adams, and Leon Kuczynski. 2001. Women's Experiences Breastfeeding in Public Places. *Journal of Human Lactation* 17 (1): 31–38. doi:10.1177/089033440101700107.

Sheldon, Annette. 2005. *Big Sister Now: A Story about Me and Our New Baby*, 1st ed. Washington, D.C: Magination Press.

Shelov, Steven P. 2004. *Caring for Your Baby and Young Child: Birth to Age Five.* Bantam Books.

Shoemaker, Pamela J., and Timothy Vos. 2009. *Gatekeeping Theory.* New York: Routledge. https://books.google.com/books/about/Gatekeeping_Theory.html?id=Fn2QAgAAQBAJ.

Shu, Xiao Ou, Martha S. Linet, Michael Steinbuch, Wan Qing Wen, Jonathan D. Buckley, Joseph P. Neglia, John D. Potter, Gregory H. Reaman, and Leslie L. Robison. 1999. Breast-Feeding and Risk of Childhood Acute Leukemia. *Journal of the National Cancer Institute* 91 (20): 1765–1772. doi:10.1093/jnci/91.20.1765.

Shubber, Sami. 2011. *The WHO International Code of Marketing of Breast-Milk Substitutes: History and Analysis*, 2nd ed. London: Pinter & Martin.

Shufeldt, Madeleine, and Kendra Gale. 2007. Under the (Glue) Gun: Containing and Constructing Reality in Home Makeover TV. *Popular Communication*. doi:10.1080/15405700701608980.

Similac. 2015. The Mother 'Hood Official Video. *Youtube*. January 17, 2015. https://www.youtube.com/watch?v=Me9yrREXOj4.

Simon, N. 1984. Why Breast-Feed? *Parents*, 1984.

Sisk, P.M., C. A. Lovelady, R. G. Dillard, K. J. Gruber, and T. M. O'Shea. 2007. Early Human Milk Feeding Is Associated with a Lower Risk of Necrotizing Enterocolitis in Very Low Birth Weight Infants. *Journal of Perinatology* 27 (7): 428–433. doi:10.1038/sj.jp.7211758.

Smith, Melanie M., Maureen Durkin, Veronica J. Hinton, David Bellinger, and Louise Kuhn. 2003. Initiation of Breastfeeding Among Mothers of Very Low Birth Weight Infants. *Pediatrics* 111 (6): 1337–1342.

Smith, Paige Hall. 2012. Breastfeeding Promotion through Gender Equality. In *Beyond Health, Beyond Choice: Breastfeeding Constraints and Realities*, ed. Paige Hall Smith, Bernice L. Hausman, and Miriam Labbok, 25–35. New Brunswick, NJ: Rutgers University Press.

Smith-Gagen, Julie, Robin Hollen, Marsha Walker, Daniel M. Cook, and Wei Yang. 2014. Breastfeeding Laws and Breastfeeding Practices by Race and Ethnicity. *Women's Health Issues* 24 (1): e11–e19. doi:10.1016/j.whi.2013.11.001.

Sonnenschein-van der Voort, Agnes M.M., Vincent W.V. Jaddoe, Hein Raat, Henriëtte A. Moll, Albert Hofman, Johan C. de Jongste, and Liesbeth Duijts. 2012. Fetal and Infant Growth and Asthma Symptoms in Preschool Children. *American Journal of Respiratory and Critical Care Medicine* 185 (7): 731–737. doi:10.1164/rccm.201107-1266OC.

Soumerai, Stephen, Dennis Ross-Degnan, and Jessica Spira Kahn. 2002. The Effects of Professional and Media Warnings about the Association between Asprin Use in Children and Reye's Syndrome. In *Public Health Communication: Evidence for Behavior Change*, 265–288. Mahwah, NJ: Lawrence Erlbaum Associates.

Spear, Hila J. 2007. College Students' Experiences and Attitudes Regarding Middle and High School–Based Breastfeeding Education. *The Journal of School Nursing* 23 (5): 276–282. doi:10.1177/10598405070230050601.

Squires, Catherine. 2008. Race and Reality TV: Tryin' to Make It Real—but Real Compared to What? *Critical Studies in Media Communication*. doi: 10.1080/15295030802328038.

Stang, Jamie, Kathleen Hoss, and Mary Story. 2010. Health Statements Made in Infant Formula Advertisements in Pregnancy and Early Parenting Magazines

A Content Analysis. *ICAN: Infant, Child, & Adolescent Nutrition* 2 (1): 16–25. doi:10.1177/1941406409359806.

Starr, Paul. 1982. *The Social Transformation of American Medicine*. New York: Basic Books.

Steele, Sarah, Jeanine Martyn, and Jens Foell. 2015. Risks of the Unregulated Market in Human Breast Milk. *BMJ* 350: h1485.

Street, 1615 L., NW, Suite 700 Washington, and DC 20036 202 419 4300 | Main 202 419 4349 | Fax 202 419 4372 | Media Inquiries. Internet Now Main Source of News for Young Adults. *Pew Research Center*. http://www.pewresearch.org/daily-number/internet-now-main-source-of-news-for-young-adults/. Accessed 29 July 2015.

Street, 1615 L., NW, Suite 700 Washington, and DC 20036 202 419 4300 | Main 202 419 4349 | Fax 202 419 4372 | Media Inquiries. Social Networking Fact Sheet. *Pew Research Center: Internet, Science & Tech*. http://www.pewinternet.org/fact-sheets/social-networking-fact-sheet/. Accessed 29 July 2015.

Stuebe, Alison. 2009. The Risks of Not Breastfeeding for Mothers and Infants. *Reviews in Obstetrics and Gynecology* 2 (4): 222–231.

Stuebe, Alison. 2014. Enabling Women to Achieve Their Breastfeeding Goals : Obstetrics & Gynecology. *Obstetrics & Gynecology* 123 (3): 643–652.

Stuebe, Alison M., and Karen Bonuck. 2011. What Predicts Intent to Breastfeed Exclusively? Breastfeeding Knowledge, Attitudes, and Beliefs in a Diverse Urban Population. *Breastfeeding Medicine* 6 (6): 413–420. doi:10.1089/bfm.2010.0088.

Stuebe, Alison M., Karleen D. Gribble, and Aunchalee E.L. Palmquist. 2014. Differences between Online Milk Sales and Peer-to-Peer Milk sharing. (E-Letter Reply to Keim et al., Microbial Contamination of Human Milk Purchased via the Internet). http://scholar.google.com/scholar?cluster=8618325848371141596&hl=en&oi=scholarr.

Sullivan, Sandra, Richard J. Schanler, Jae H. Kim, Aloka L. Patel, Rudolf Trawöger, Ursula Kiechl-Kohlendorfer, Gary M. Chan, et al. 2010. An Exclusively Human Milk-Based Diet Is Associated with a Lower Rate of Necrotizing Enterocolitis than a Diet of Human Milk and Bovine Milk-Based Products. *The Journal of Pediatrics* 156 (4): 562–567.e1. doi:10.1016/j.jpeds.2009.10.040.

Taveras, Elsie M., Ruowei Li, Laurence Grummer-Strawn, Marcie Richardson, Richard Marshall, Virginia H. Rêgo, Irina Miroshnik, and Tracy A. Lieu. 2004. Opinions and Practices of Clinicians Associated With Continuation of Exclusive Breastfeeding. *Pediatrics* 113 (4): e283–290.

Taylor, Erin N., and Lora Ebert Wallace. 2012. Feminist Breastfeeding Promotion and the Problem of Guilt. In *Beyond Health, Beyond Choice:*

Breastfeeding Constraints and Realities, ed. Paige Hall Smith, Bernice L. Hausman, and Miriam Labbok, 193–202. New Brunswick, NJ: Rutgers University Press.

Tesh, Sylvia Noble. 1988. *Hidden Arguments: Political Ideology and Disease Prevention Policy*. New Brunswick, NJ: Rutgers University Press.

The Baby-Friendly Hospital Initiative. *UNICEF*, n.d. http://www.unicef.org/programme/breastfeeding/baby.htm#10.

The Best Nurser. *The Ladies' Home Journal*, 1891.

The Eleventh and Twelfth Months. *The Ladies' Home Journal*, 1903.

The Hays Code Brings Censorship To Motion Pictures. http://www.hollywoodmoviememories.com/articles/hollywood-history/hays-code-brings-censorship-motion.php. Accessed 31 July 2015.

The Ladies' Home Journal and Practical Housekeeper. 1997. *Encyclopedia.com*. http://www.encyclopedia.com/doc/1G2-2536601587.html.

The Mother 'Hood Official Video, n.d.

The Mother of Five. 1885. The Mother of Five. *The Ladies' Home Journal and Practical Housekeeper*, November.

The Motion Picture Production Code of 1930 (Hays Code). http://www.artsreformation.com/a001/hays-code.html. Accessed 31 July 2015.

The Museum of Broadcast Communications - Encyclopedia of Television - Censorship. http://www.museum.tv/eotv/censorship.htm. Accessed 31 July 2015.

The Social-Ecological Model: A Framework for Prevention. Centers for Disease Control and Prevention, March 25, 2015. http://www.cdc.gov/ViolencePrevention/overview/social-ecologicalmodel.html.

The Surgeon General's Call to Action to Support Breastfeeding - Calltoactiontosupportbreastfeeding.pdf. http://www.surgeongeneral.gov/library/calls/breastfeeding/calltoactiontosupportbreastfeeding.pdf. Accessed 28 July 2015.

The Ten Steps to Successful Breastfeeding. *Baby-Friendly USA*, 2012. http://www.babyfriendlyusa.org/about-us/baby-friendly-hospital-initiative/the-ten-steps.

Thulier, Diane, and Judith Mercer. 2009. Variables Associated With Breastfeeding Duration. *Journal of Obstetric, Gynecologic, & Neonatal Nursing* 38 (3): 259–268. doi:10.1111/j.1552-6909.2009.01021.x.

Toby, N.M. 1906. A Mother to Five Hundred Babies: A New York Woman's Beautiful Work. *The Ladies' Home Journal*.

Tomkins, C., and F.D. Slater. 1954. Five Important Rules for Feeding Baby. *Parents*, 1954.

Too Old for Breastfeeding? *Parents*, 1989.

Updegrove, Kimberly. 2013. Nonprofit Human Milk Banking in the United States. *Journal of Midwifery & Women's Health* 58 (5): 502–508. doi:10.1111/j.1542-2011.2012.00267.x.

Urban, Annie. 2012. UPDATE: A Response from Sesame Street on Breastfeeding | Care2 Causes. January 14, 2012. http://www.care2.com/causes/update-a-response-from-sesame-street-on-breastfeeding.html.

Van Esterik, Penny. 1989. *Beyond the Breast-Bottle Controversy*. New Brunswick, NJ: Rutgers University Press.

Vandewark, Aurora C. 2014. Breastfeeding Attitudes and Knowledge in Bachelor of Science in Nursing Candidates. http://www.ingentaconnect.com/content/springer/jpe/2014/00000023/00000003/art00004.

Vari, Patty, Nancy Vogeltanz-Holm, Glenn Olsen, Cindy Anderson, Jeffrey Holm, Heidi Peterson, and Susan Henly. 2013. Community Breastfeeding Attitudes and Beliefs. *Health Care for Women International*, June 6, 2013. http://www.tandfonline.com/doi/abs/10.1080/07399332.2012.655391.

Velez, Mandy. 2014. Here's What Happened When A Mom Posted A Photo Of Herself Breastfeeding At Graduation. *Huffington Post*, June 9, 2014. http://www.huffingtonpost.com/2014/06/09/mom-shamed-by-internet-for-breastfeeding-at-graduation_n_5474420.html.

Verhasselt, Valérie. 2010. Neonatal Tolerance under Breastfeeding Influence: The Presence of Allergen and Transforming Growth Factor-β in Breast Milk Protects the Progeny from Allergic Asthma. *The Journal of Pediatrics* 156 (2): S16–20. doi:10.1016/j.jpeds.2009.11.015.

Villegas, R., Y.-T. Gao, G. Yang, H. L. Li, T. Elasy, W. Zheng, and X.-O. Shu. 2007. Duration of Breast-Feeding and the Incidence of Type 2 Diabetes Mellitus in the Shanghai Women's Health Study. *Diabetologia* 51 (2): 258–266. doi:10.1007/s00125-007-0885-8.

Vogel, Lauren. 2011. Milk Sharing: Boon or Biohazard? *Canadian Medical Association Journal* 183 (3): E155–E156. doi:10.1503/cmaj.109-3767.

Vohr, Betty R., Brenda B. Poindexter, Anna M. Dusick, Leslie T. McKinley, Linda L. Wright, John C. Langer, and W. Kenneth Poole. 2006. Beneficial Effects of Breast Milk in the Neonatal Intensive Care Unit on the Developmental Outcome of Extremely Low Birth Weight Infants at 18 Months of Age. *Pediatrics* 118 (1): e115–e123. doi:10.1542/peds.2005-2382.

Waldburger, Jennifer, and Jill Spivack. 2007. *The Sleepeasy Solution: The Exhausted Parent's Guide to Getting Your Child to Sleep from Birth to Age 5*. Deerfield Beach, FL: HCI.

Wang, Grace. 2010. A Shot at Half-Exposure: Asian Americans in Reality TV Shows. *Television & New Media* 11 (5): 404–427. doi:10.1177/1527476410363482.

Ward, L.Monique, Ann Merriwether, and Allison Caruthers. 2006. Breasts Are for Men: Media, Masculinity Ideologies, and Men's Beliefs About Women's Bodies. *Sex Roles* 55 (9–10): 703–714. doi:10.1007/s11199-006-9125-9.

Watson, Anna. 1888. About the Baby. *The Ladies' Home Journal and Practical Housekeeper*, July 1888.

Watson, E.W. 1887a. Talks with Mothers, By Eminent Physicians: Babies' Summer Hygiene. *The Ladies' Home Journal and Practical Housekeeper*, August 1887.

Watson, E.W. 1887b. Talks with Mothers, By Eminent Physicians: The Care of Babies in Summer-Time. *The Ladies' Home Journal and Practical Housekeeper*, July 1887.

Waxman, Olivia B. 2015. This Ad Perfectly Parodies the 'Mommy Wars.' *Time*, January 30, 2015. http://time.com/3689420/similac-ad-mommy-wars-parody/.

Wessel, M. 1979. Ask Dr. Wessel: Why Give Vitamin Supplements? *Parents*, 1979.

What to Do for a Baby Month by Month. *The Ladies' Home Journal*, 1903.

What to Do When the Baby Has the Rickets. *The Ladies' Home Journal*, 1903.

What to Do When the Baby Is Sick. *The Ladies' Home Journal*, 1903.

What to Expect When You're Expecting, 4th Edition (Description). *Amazon.com*, 2015. http://www.amazon.com/What-Expect-Youre-Expecting-Edition/dp/0761148574/ref=zg_bs_books_67).

Whitacre, Paula Tarnapol, and Sheila Moats. 2011. Updating the USDA National Breastfeeding Campaign - Workshop Summary. http://iom.nationalacademies.org/Reports/2011/Updating-the-USDA-National-Breastfeeding-Campaign-Workshop-Summary.aspx.

WHO | Breastfeeding. *WHO*. http://www.who.int/topics/breastfeeding/en/. Accessed 26 Aug 2014.

Wilder, Laura Ingalls. 2014. *Pioneer Girl*. ed. Hill, Pamela Smith. Pierre: South Dakota Historical Society Press.

Williams, Kaylene, Alfred Petrosky, Edward Hernandez, and Robert Page, Jr. n.d. Product Placement Effectiveness: Revisited and Renewed. *Journal of Management and Marketing Research* 7 (1): 1–24.

Winsten, Jay A. 1993. Promoting Designated Drivers: The Harvard Alcohol Project. *American Journal of Preventive Medicine* 10 (3): 11–14.

Wojcicki, Janet M. 2011. Maternal Prepregnancy Body Mass Index and Initiation and Duration of Breastfeeding: A Review of the Literature. *Journal of Women's Health* 20 (3): 341–347. doi:10.1089/jwh.2010.2248.

Wolf, Jacqueline H. 2001. *Don't Kill Your Baby: Public Health and the Decline of Breastfeeding in the 19th and 20th Centuries*. Columbus: The Ohio State University Press. https://books.google.com/books?hl=en&lr=&id=hHbTD

VfWNU4C&oi=fnd&pg=PR9&dq=don%27t+kill+your+baby&ots=Cb4kjWfqjl&sig=Mg1bK7aR5eKU6iZGi2F1iM0q5pg#v=onepage&q=don%27t%20kill%20your%20baby&f=false.

Wolf, Jacqueline H. 2006. What Feminists Can Do for Breastfeeding and What Breastfeeding Can Do for Feminists. *Signs* 31 (2): 397–424. doi: 10.1086/497279.

Wolf, Jacqueline H. 2012. *Deliver Me from Pain: Anesthesia and Birth in America*. Reprint edition. Baltimore, Md.: Johns Hopkins University Press.

Wolf, Joan B. 2007. Is Breast Really Best? Risk and Total Motherhood in the National Breastfeeding Awareness Campaign. *Journal of Health Politics, Policy and Law* 32 (4): 595–636. doi:10.1215/03616878-2007-018.

Wolf, Joan B. 2010. *Is Breast Best?: Taking on the Breastfeeding Experts and the New High Stakes of Motherhood*. New York: NYU Press.

Wolfberg, Adam J., Karin B. Michels, Wendy Shields, Patricia O'Campo, Yvonne Bronner, and Jessica Bienstock. 2004. Dads as Breastfeeding Advocates: Results from a Randomized Controlled Trial of an Educational Intervention. *American Journal of Obstetrics and Gynecology* 191 (3): 708–712. doi:10.1016/j.ajog.2004.05.019.

Woman Is Publicly Shamed For Breastfeeding In Public. Then She Posts This On Facebook. http://www.tickld.com/x/woman-is-publicly-shamed-for-breast-feeding-in-public. Accessed 29 July 2015.

Women's Bureau (WB) - Quick Facts on Women in the Labor Force in 2010. http://www.dol.gov/wb/factsheets/Qf-laborforce-10.htm. Accessed 30 July 2015.

Wood, James Playsted. 1949. *Magazines in the United States*, 2nd ed. New York: Ronald Press Co.

Woody, R. 1934. Feeding the New Baby. *Parents*, September: 20.

Wright, Anne L., Mark Bauer, Audrey Naylor, Emily Sutcliffe, and Larry Clark. 1998. Increasing Breastfeeding Rates to Reduce Infant Illness at the Community Level. *Pediatrics* 101 (5): 837–844. doi:10.1542/peds.101.5.837.

Wright, Anne L., and Richard J. Schanler. 2001. The Resurgence of Breastfeeding at the End of the Second Millennium. *The Journal of Nutrition* 131 (2): 421S–425S.

Christopher, Walter Shield. 1892. *Summer Complaint and Infant Feeding*. Chicago: Blakely & Rogers, Printers.

Yeaton-Massey, Amanda. 2011. Exclusive Breastfeeding Promotes Postpartum Weight Loss. *American Journal of Obstetrics and Gynecology* 204 (1): 217–218.

Young, Kathryn T. 1990. American Conceptions of Infant Development from 1955 to 1984: What the Experts Are Telling Parents. *Child Development* 61 (1): 17–28. doi:10.1111/j.1467-8624.1990.tb02757.x.

Zanardo, Vincenzo, Giorgia Svegliado, Francesco Cavallin, Arturo Giustardi, Erich Cosmi, Pietro Litta, and Daniele Trevisanuto. 2010. Elective Cesarean Delivery: Does It Have a Negative Effect on Breastfeeding? *Birth* 37 (4): 275–279. doi:10.1111/j.1523-536X.2010.00421.x.

Zhang, Yuanting, Ewa Carlton, and Sara B. Fein. 2013. The Association of Prenatal Media Marketing Exposure Recall with Breastfeeding Intentions, Initiation, and Duration. *Journal of Human Lactation*, May 17. doi:10.1177/0890334413487256.

Zuckerman, Mary Ellen. 1998. *A History of Popular Women's Magazines in the United States, 1792–1995*. Westport, CT: Greenwood Press.

Index

K.A. Foss, *Breastfeeding and Media*,
DOI 10.1007/978-3-319-56442-5

The manufacturer's authorised representative in the EU is Springer Nature Customer Service Centre GmbH, Europaplatz 3, 69115 Heidelberg, Germany. If you have any concerns regarding our products, please contact ProductSafety@springernature.com

Printed and bound by CPI Group (UK) Ltd, Croydon, CR0 4YY
22/09/2026
02221067-0010